FRANCE	Pergamon Press France S.A. 24, rue des Ecoles, 75240 Paris Cedex 05
U.K.	Pergamon Press Ltd, Headington Hill Hall, Oxford OX3 0BW
U.S.A.	Pergamon Press Inc., Maxwell House, Fairview Park, Elmsford, New York 10523
CANADA	Pergamon Press Canada Ltd, Suite 104, 150 Consumers Road, Willowdale, Ontario M2J 1P9
AUSTRALIE	Pergamon Press (Aust.) Pty Ltd, P.O. Box 544, Potts Point, N.S.W. 2011
R.F.A.	Pergamon Press GmbH, 6242 Kronberg- Taunus, Hammerweg 6

ISBN 0.08.027.074.3 (F)
0.08.027.073.5 (H)

Composé par AMP, Paris
Imprimé par SCRIPTA, Avignon

DRUG SAFETY
SÉCURITÉ ET MÉDICAMENT

DRUG SAFETY

PROGRESS AND CONTROVERSIES

SÉCURITÉ ET MÉDICAMENT

PROGRÈS ET CONTROVERSES

Proceedings of the IVth International Congress
of Pharmaceutical Physicians
Comptes rendus du IVe congrès international
des médecins de l'industrie pharmaceutique

Paris, 27/30 April 1981

Editors
Michel Auriche
John Burke
Jacques Duchier

PERGAMON PRESS
Paris Oxford New York Toronto Sydney Frankfurt

LE IVe CONGRES DES MEDECINS DE L'INDUSTRIE PHARMACEUTIQUE
THE 4th INTERNATIONAL MEETING OF PHARMACEUTICAL PHYSICIANS

placé sous le haut Patronage de:
under the patronage of:

Monsieur le Ministre de la Santé et de la Sécurité Sociale

et de | *and of*

Monsieur le Président du Syndicat National de l'Industrie Pharmaceutique (S.N.I.P.)

est organisé par | *has been organised by*

l'Association des Médecins de l'Industrie Pharmaceutique (A.M.I.P)

sous l'égide de | *under the auspices of*

l'International Federation of Associations of Pharmaceutical Physicians (IFAPP)

PARIS, April 27/30 1981

PRESIDENT

Dr M. AURICHE
Président de l'A.M.I.P.

COMITÉS DU CONGRÈS — *CONGRESS COMMITTEES*

COMITÉ D'ORGANISATION — *ORGANIZING COMMITTEE*

Président — Dr R. GARRAUD — *Chairman*

Dr L. CHEYNIER
Dr C. GIGAUT
Dr J.F. HENRY
Dr M. ROBIN

COMITÉ SCIENTIFIQUE — *SCIENTIFIC COMMITTEE*

Président — Dr J.T. BURKE — *Chairman*

Dr AURICHE
Dr P. CARPENTIER
Dr Y. CHAMPEY
Dr J. DUCHIER
Dr J.H. GRIMBERT
Dr J.F. SCHLUMBERGER
Dr C. SPRIET-POURRA

COMITÉ FINANCIER — *FINANCE COMMITTEE*

Président — Dr A. LUMBROSO — *Chairman*

Dr F. TEXIER
Dr M. LOUVET

COMITÉ DES EXPOSITIONS — *EXHIBITION COMMITTEE*

Président — Dr J.F. HENRY — *Chairman*

Dr A. KHER

COMITÉ SOCIAL — *SOCIAL COMMITTEE*

Président — Dr M. LOUVET — *Chairman*

Dr L. CHEYNIER
Dr M. ROBIN

COMITÉ DE RÉDACTION — *PUBLICATIONS COMMITTEE*

Président — Dr J. DUCHIER — *Chairman*

Dr J.F. HENRY

TABLE DES MATIERES

PREFACE

In 1972, the first International Meeting of Pharmaceutical Physicians took place in London. The subject, "International Aspects of Drug Evaluation and Usage" attracted delegates from over thirty nations worldwide and the resulting publication became a standard reference text.

Encouraged by the success of this meeting, the various national Associations of Pharmaceutical Physicians resolved to create an International Federation which would be responsible for organising further meetings and also for arranging a regular exchange of professional and scientific information between the member Associations.

This International Federation of Associations of Pharmaceutical Physicians (I.F.A.P.P.) was officially formed during the second international meeting held in Florence in 1975. On this occasion the topic chosen was "The Rationality of Drug Development" and the organisers enlarged on the theme of the first meeting, examining in some detail the status of international co-operation in the testing of drugs from both the governmental and pharmaceutical industry standpoints. At the end of this meeting the sessional chairmen produced a position paper summarising the situation and making a number of specific recommendations concerning the generation and utilisation of drug evaluation data internationally. This played an important part in the moves that took place then, and later, towards a more rational approach to the international data needs of Health Authorities in many countries, and to some lessening of the data reduplication problems noted by a number of speakers during the meeting.

The third international meeting, now under the sponsorship of I.F.A.P.P., was held in Brussels in 1978. Compared with the two previous gatherings, it focussed less on the scientific and technical aspects of the work of pharmaceutical physicians, and dealt more with their present and future role, as seen both by themselves and by those with whom they interact in the course of their work.

The meeting highlighted a growing awareness of the importance of their function not only as scientist but also as a pivotal link between the various disciplines engaged in developing and utilizing new therapeutic modalities.

This aspect was reflected in the published proceedings, one section of which entitled — "The challenging Role of the Pharmaceutical Physician" — was subsequently extracted and published as a separate booklet for general use.

The present volume contains the proceedings of the fourth international meeting which took place in Paris in April, 1981. The organisers on this occasion have directed attention to general subject of drug safety and to the part that pharmaceutical physicians can and should play in ensuring that the drugs produced by the pharmaceutical industry are not only efficacious but also, as far as is humanly possibly, safe.

This meeting has served to emphasise, yet again, the invaluable role that I.F.A.P.P. now plays in providing an established form for the exchange of practical up-to-date information between pharmaceutical physicians worldwide on all relevant aspects of drug development and usage.

R.K. Rondel
Chairman IFAPP

There are no really
"safe" biologically active drugs.
There are only "safe" physicians.

Harlod A. KAMINETZKY

ALLOCUTION DE BIENVENUE

Il m'est agréable, en ouvrant cette séance inaugurale, de souhaiter la bienvenue à vous tous qui êtes venus, nombreux, assister à ce congrès.

Je tiens à remercier d'emblée ceux qui ont eu l'amabilité de nous accorder leur patronage : je veux nommer M. le Ministre de la Santé et de la Sécurité Sociale, représenté ici, ce matin, par M. Jean Weber, Directeur de la Pharmacie et du Médicament, ainsi que M. Pierre Joly, Président du Syndicat National de l'Industrie Pharmaceutique.

Ce double patronage nous touche et nous honore.

Il y a, bien sûr, parmi vous, une majorité de médecins de l'Industrie Pharmaceutique, puisque nous ouvrons là leur 4e Congrès International. Mais il faut noter qu'ils sont venus non seulement d'Europe, mais de toutes les parties du monde, marquant par là l'intérêt qu'ils portent au sujet que nous avons choisi, Sécurité et Médicament, progrès et controverses.

La sécurité la plus grande, ou mieux encore le meilleur rapport bénéfice/risque, dans l'emploi des médicaments que nous contribuons à mettre à la disposition des médecins et des malades, est en effet pour nous une occupation et une préoccupation majeure et constante.

Je souhaite aussi la bienvenue à ceux qui, bien que n'étant pas médecins de l'Industrie Pharmaceutique, participent pleinement à notre congrès, qu'ils soient concernés plutôt par la toxicologie animale, par la pharmaco-vigilance ou par les problèmes de l'information et de la communication au sujet du médicament.

Je remercie notamment tous ceux qui, souvent venus de très loin, ont accepté avec enthousiasme d'apporter leur participation active à notre congrès, soit par leurs exposés dans des domaines où ils sont particulièrement compétents, soit par leur participation à des Tables Rondes.

Mes remerciements très chaleureux vont aussi à ceux qui, bien que n'assistant pas à la totalité du congrès, ont accepté notre invitation à participer à la séance inaugurale de ce matin. Car ils ont voulu, par là, nous apporter leur encouragement et leur soutien dans nos efforts.

Le sujet que nous avons choisi concerne non seulement très directement et professionnellement toute l'Industrie Pharmaceutique et ses médecins en particulier, les toxicologues, les hospitalo-universitaires, les pouvoirs publics, les médecins prescripteurs et les pharmaciens d'officine ; c'est-à-dire toute la chaîne des responsables de la conception, du développement, de l'autorisation et de la distribution du médicament ; mais il concerne aussi très directement la totalité de la population. Je n'irai pas jusqu'à dire, comme mon distingué confrère le Dr. Knock, que tout homme bien portant est un malade qui s'ignore. Mais je dirai que, par la force des choses, nous sommes tous des consommateurs passés, actuels ou potentiels de médicaments, parfois des consommateurs permanents, à l'exception de ceux qui, dans certains pays n'ont pas la chance d'y avoir accès pour des raisons économiques et financières.

Nous avons, en organisant ce congrès, délibérément choisi de traiter de façon assez approfondie un nombre limité de sujets à l'intérieur du cadre général, et des sujets soit évolutifs, soit controversés. Il nous a donc fallu faire un choix. Et je voudrais, avant de passer la parole, demander votre indulgence si certains acteurs importants sont absents de la scène. Ce n'est pas que nous les ayons méconnus ou ignorés.

Michel AURICHE
Président du Congrès
Président de l'A.M.I.P.

Sécurité et médicaments (1982), pp. 1-5

Introduction

M. AURICHE

Président du Congrès, Rhône-Poulenc Santé, 22 cours Albert 1er, 75008 Paris, France

Sécurité et Médicament, Progrès et Controverses. Pourquoi ce sujet ? Parce que c'est un sujet important et d'actualité.

C'est un sujet important. Le médicament est destiné à prévenir, à guérir et à soulager. Il apparaît choquant qu'il apporte lui-même des maux à l'humanité. Cela est très mal ressenti non seulement par les malades qui les supportent, mais par les médecins qui en sont les auteurs involontaires, par les industriels qui ont donné naissance au coupable, et par les pouvoirs publics qui l'ont autorisé.

Aussi est-il important de mettre en œuvre tout ce qu'il est raisonnable de faire pour obtenir finalement un rapport bénéfice/risque aussi favorable que possible.

C'est un sujet d'actualité. Comparé aux risques de l'alcool, du tabac, de la route, de certains sports et de certaines professions, il est indéniable que le risque médicamenteux est un des plus mal acceptés par la société actuelle dans les pays développés.

On peut même dire que, dans une frange importante de la population et malgré les services rendus, le médicament a mauvaise réputation, ou tout au moins qu'il engendre une anxiété diffuse quant à ses conséquences immédiates et lointaines chez bon nombre de consommateurs.

Comment en est-on arrivé là ? Car il n'en a pas toujours été ainsi. Qu'il était bon le médicament des années 1950 !

C'était, depuis la fin de la guerre, une succession de victoires thérapeutiques. Ceux de ma génération ne l'ont certainement pas oublié. Je voudrais simplement rappeler que, pendant mes études médicales (et je n'ai pas le sentiment d'être tellement vieux), la méningite tuberculeuse, la maladie d'Hodgkin, les leucémies, l'endocardite d'Osler étaient mortelles à 100 % . Le rhumatisme articulaire aigu et la poliomyélite sévissaient largement et faisaient leurs ravages cardiaques et neurologiques. Les fièvres typhoïdes, quand elles ne succombaient pas, quittaient l'hôpital après 2 mois de bains tièdes et de régime lacté, en état de faiblesse et de carence alimentaire. Il y avait de très beaux cas de syphilis nerveuse et viscérale. La thérapeutique psychiatrique était à peu près limitée à l'électrochoc, au gardénal, à l'inoculation du paludisme et à la contention.

L'hypertension artérielle n'avait pas de traitement actif. On traitait son amibiase toute sa vie.

La réanimation était balbutiante, l'immunologie dans l'enfance ; dans les services de chirurgie, les externes pleins de bonne volonté mais peu expérimentés donnaient les anesthésies au masque d'Ombrédanne.

Je me souviens encore avoir fait toutes les trois heures des injections d'une pénicilline récupérée dans l'urine des soldats américains hospitalisés à l'hôpital de La Pitié et des septicémies à staphylocoques miraculeusement guéries avec 100 000 unités par jour.

Que de progrès accomplis depuis !

Il y avait bien eu, aux Etats-Unis, l'affaire de l'élixir de sulfamide qui avait entraîné des obligations légales de vérification d'innocuité. Mais ce n'était pas le médicament lui-même qui était en cause.

On mettait alors sur le marché des médicaments prodigieux, inaugurant de nouvelles classes thérapeutiques, avec des dossiers expérimentaux qui feraient aujourd'hui sourire ou frémir par leur légèreté. C'était l'âge d'or.

Puis les choses se sont gâtées. Il y a eu en France le Stalinon, et le choc que cela a entraîné. Il a fallu peu à peu se rendre à l'évidence : les sulfamides provoquaient des accidents sanguins ou cutanés ; la streptomycine rendait sourd ; la phénylbutazone et le chloramphénicol pouvaient tuer ; la merveilleuse et polyvalente cortisone donnait des effets indésirables graves.

L'aspirine faisait saigner l'estomac, et même la toute bonne pénicilline, si atoxique, pouvait tuer en quelques minutes à doses minimes.

Un des coups les plus graves fut celui de la thalidomide. Le médicament ne s'en est jamais bien remis. Il faut dire qu'on a même vu de vieux amis de l'homme, comme le clioquinol et les sels insolubles de bismuth, devenir soudain méchants sans qu'on ait jamais très bien compris les raisons de ce changement de caractère.

D'accident en tragédie, les législations nationales ont évolué, généralement dans l'ambiance de l'émotion provoquée par une récente affaire, et dans le sens de la prévention d'événements semblables.

Et l'on est arrivé peu à peu à la situation actuelle, où l'on constate non seulement l'existence de réglementations contraignantes, ce qui est compréhensible, mais celle de discordances importantes, en gros et en détail, entre législations de pays de même niveau scientifique, culturel et social, rendant extrêmement complexe, coûteux et prolongé, le développement international de produits pharmaceutiques.

Ne serait-il pas possible de parvenir au plan international à un consensus scientifiquement et matériellement acceptable pour tous ?

Situation actuelle où le développement des épreuves toxicologiques animales imposées est tel que, compte-tenu de l'extrapolabilité inconstante des résultats obtenus de l'animal à l'homme, on peut se demander si le but de sécurité n'a pas été parfois dépassé, si le bilan global des règlementations actuelles est positif ou non pour la santé et le bien-être humain.

Ce sont là les sujets qui vont donner lieu aujourd'hui à des exposés et à des débats.

On peut dire très schématiquement qu'à l'heure actuelle les diverses études pharmacotoxicologiques animales ne laissent subsister que dix molécules sur 10 000 nouvelles candidates. Toujours très schématiquement, de ces 10 molécules une seule sera commercialisée. Les 9 autres auront été éliminées plus ou moins rapidement au cours des essais cliniques et essentiellement pour manque d'efficacité, ou pour intolérance ou toxicité inadmissible. La porte est donc très étroite et le coût global de la recherche très élevé.

Que sait-on du produit qui vient d'être mis sur le marché du point de vue de ses effets indésirables ? En fait, ce que les essais cliniques ayant précédé le visa ont permis de reconnaître, c'est-à-dire les effets indésirables les plus fréquents, dont la fréquence est disons supérieure ou égale à 1 % des malades traités, et dont l'apparition n'est pas trop retardée.

C'est un peu comme un nouveau-né, qui ne présente aucune malformation évidente, mais dont on ne sait s'il deviendra ange ou démon.

Un problème actuellement très à l'ordre du jour est celui de l'identification précise des effets indésirables rares, retardés, ou les 2 à la fois, ou demandant des examens spéciaux pour être reconnus. Cette identification est difficile, laborieuse, reposant parfois sur la chance.

Le monde médical, notamment britannique, a été très ému par les accidents survenus avec le practolol, dont le développement avait pourtant été exemplaire, et la surveillance effective.

Ils montraient en effet que malgré toutes les précautions prises, et l'usage important que font les médecins britanniques de la carte jaune de signalement, le lien entre les accidents, oculaires et autres, et la prise de practolol avait été méconnu pendant assez longtemps.

D'où une impulsion nouvelle donnée à l'utilisation de techniques déjà connues et à la recherche de techniques nouvelles, tendant à identifier qualitativement et si possible quantitativement, les effets indésirables jusque là inconnus des nouveaux produits.

C'est là le sujet central des exposés et des discussions de demain.

Avant de poursuivre, je voudrais vous faire part d'une réflexion. Les législations sur le médicament ont tendance à mettre en situation de symétrie les deux notions et les deux termes d'*Efficacité* et d'*Innocuité*, demandant par exemple que les industriels démontrent l'efficacité et l'innocuité de leurs produits.

Il y a dans ce parallèle quelque chose d'erroné, d'abusif, qui ne peut qu'être source de malentendus :

L'efficacité, c'est quelque chose de positif qui peut se prouver, se mesurer.

L'innocuité est une notion négative, qui n'a qu'une existence virtuelle. L'innocuité ne peut matériellement se prouver ; on ne peut que lui assigner une limite. Ce que l'on peut apprécier, mesurer, c'est la nocivité, l'intolérance, la toxicité. L'innocuité n'en est que le complément, le moule en creux.

Sans doute vaudrait-il mieux parler de niveaux d'intolérance et de toxicité acceptables en fonction de l'efficacité.

Avant de quitter la pharmacovigilance, je voudrais dire maintenant, car on n'aura plus l'occasion d'en parler puisqu'il ne s'agit pas de sécurité, je voudrais dire qu'il me semble que l'on devrait dépenser plus d'énergie et d'imagination à utiliser les techniques de la pharmacovigilance pour découvrir des effets thérapeutiques inattendus. Je ne connais pas d'exemple de recherche systématique dans ce domaine. Pourtant, des ß-bloquants dans l'hypertension artérielle au probénécide et à la benziodarone dans la goutte, des antipaludéens de synthèse, de la pénicillamine et du lévamisole dans l'arthrite rhumatoïde au métronidazole dans les infections anaérobies en passant par l'imipramine dans les dépressions et la carbamazépine dans la névralgie du trijumeau, les exemples sont nombreux de découvertes parfois importantes, imprévues et imprévisibles, faites en clinique.

Peut-être serait-ce un moyen de combler certains vides thérapeutiques, notamment pour des maladies qui n'ont pas de modèle expérimental satisfaisant.

Il n'y a pas, ou très peu, de médicaments dotés seulement de vertus bénéfiques et totalement dépourvus d'inconvénients. Il faut que le public le comprenne et accepte un certain risque médicamenteux comme il accepte les risques de la route ou du sport. Les pouvoirs publics, les caisses de Sécurité Sociale, les media d'information ont un rôle important à jouer dans ce sens.

Il faudrait réussir à dédramatiser les effets indésirables aux yeux des médecins et du public.

Les médecins, les malades, le public en général, ne devraient plus les considérer à priori comme les marques d'une négligence scandaleuse de la part de l'Industrie pharmaceutique. Et celle-ci ne devrait pas les regarder comme une maladie honteuse : ils sont la rançon du progrès thérapeutique et de la difficulté de leur détection.

Dans ce domaine, comme dans bien d'autres, une certaine injustice règne ; c'est-à-dire qu'exposés aux mêmes médicaments, même à doses correctes, les uns auront des effets indésirables et les autres n'en auront pas et nous ne savons pas prévoir, en règle générale, lesquels seront atteints.

Mais, de même que pour la route ou pour le sport l'observance stricte de certaines règles réduit les risques d'accident à leur minimum incompressible, de même les risques d'effets indésirables sont ramenés à leur minimum inévitable par un bon usage des produits et le respect de certaines précautions : il est bien connu qu'un grand nombre d'effets indésirables sérieux sont dus à des posologies inadéquates, à des indications erronées, à des contre-indications non respectées, à des associations connues pour être dangereuses.

Ce respect des bonnes règles et des précautions élémentaires suppose une bonne formation et une bonne information du médecin et du pharmacien, une bonne information et une bonne éducation du public.

C'est à certains de ces aspects que nous consacrerons notre 3e journée, celle du jeudi.

Ce congrès est donc consacré essentiellement aux problèmes concernant la prévention, la limitation et l'identification du risque médicamenteux.

Celui-ci n'étant pas totalement réductible, il faut encore le gérer : une communication du jeudi 30 est consacrée à l'évolution actuelle concernant la responsabilité de l'Industrie pharmaceutique vis-à-vis de ses produits.

Concernant la gestion du risque, je voudrais vous rapporter des extraits d'un éditorial paru en janvier 1979 dans Science, sous la plume du Professeur Cyril L. Comar de la Cornell University et de l'Electric Power Research Institute, Palo Alto, California. Il me paraît marqué au coin de l'intelligence et du bon sens.

Il donne les directives suivantes pour la gestion du risque, en fonction notamment de son importance numérique :

1. Eliminer tout risque qui ne comporte aucun bénéfice ou est facile à éliminer.
2. Eliminer tout risque important (l'auteur donne comme exemple un risque mor-

tel supérieur à 1/10 000 par an) qui n'est pas largement compensé par des bénéfices évidents.

3. Ignorer pour l'instant tout risque minime (l'auteur cite un risque mortel inférieur à 1/100 000 par an) qui n'entre pas dans la première catégorie.

4. Concentrer ses efforts sur les risques compris entre ces limites, sans perdre de vue que le risque que comporte la prise de quelque mesure que ce soit doit être comparé au risque de ne pas la prendre.

L'auteur ajoute : «Concentrer son attention sur des actions réellement susceptibles d'améliorer la santé et le bien-être, tout en évitant de gaspiller des ressources à tenter de réduire des risques faibles tandis que de plus importants ne sont pas pris en considération.

Eviter de répondre par l'anxiété, l'apathie ou la dérision à la prise de conscience du fait que nous vivons apparemment dans un océan de substances carcinogènes (le risque d'aujourd'hui).»

Nous avons essayé de réaliser un congrès qui ne soit ni contemplatif, ni polémique, mais qui incite toutes les parties prenantes à réfléchir et à discuter sur les meilleures façons d'utiliser, au mieux des intérêts des malades, des moyens et des ressources qui ne sont pas illimités.

Nous souhaitons que la salle se manifeste de façon très active pendant ces 3 jours, et que de vos discussions sortent quelques propositions concrètes et quelques idées nouvelles.

Le moraliste français Joseph Joubert disait : «Il vaut mieux débattre d'une question sans la régler que de la régler sans la débattre».

Puissent vos débats contribuer à faire évoluer un certain nombre d'entre elles.

I

DRUG SAFETY: A MULTIFACETED PROBLEM

DIVERSITE DES PROBLEMES POSES PAR L'EVALUATION DE LA SECURITE EN MATIERE DE MEDICAMENTS

Sécurité et médicaments (1981), pp. 9-18

The Scientific Basis of Drug Safety Regulations

F. H. Gross

Pharmakologisches Institut der Universitat. Im Neuenheimer Feld 366, D. 6900 Heidelberg, West Germany

"Efficacy and safety of drugs" is a widely used slogan, which, however, should never be applied without adding the adjective "relative". In the WHO Technical Report N°. 563, "Guidelines for Evaluation of Drugs for Use in man", issued in 1975[1], there is the statement : "Current procedures for the evaluation of the safety and efficacy of drugs, although greatly improved during the past decade, still leave much to be desired. Therefore, no matter how well performed, it is necessary to emphasize that there can be no guarantee of absolute safety". The assessment of the relative safety of a drug is based on both toxicity studies in animals and drug monitoring in man, the first being regulated in most countries, the second generally left to the keen observation and detecting ability of doctors. Attempts to conduct monitoring after marketing of a drug are made in the form of postmarketing surveillance, but the complex and costly operations involved have limited the number of drugs for which this form of monitoring has been and will be practised. In addition, a new problem has arisen for such studies, since recently the Central Ethical Committee of the British Medical Association has asked that patients treated with monitored drugs should consent to this procedure[2].

In dealing further with the topic, let us ask and answer several questions :

HOW CAN DRUG SAFETY BE REGULATED ?

Preclinical toxicity studies in animals still form the basis for a drug to be accepted by regulatory agencies. However, it also holds true that, as was stated by a WHO Scientific Group 15 years ago[3], "... many toxic effects may (also) be predicted from observations made in animals, but, in the present state of knowledge, there are some important toxic effects that are not predictable from animal studies, and this is their main limitation... Every effort should be made to build up knowledge of species differences and similarities in toxicological responses". This is a typical WHO statement, a clear analysis of the present situation and a well-meant recommendation for the future, to which, however, WHO will not and cannot contribute in any way and which is little more than wishful thinking. Of course, some progress has been made in recent years, but there are still severe adverse reactions in man, for which no equivalent changes are seen in animals. On the other hand, there are various toxic reactions in the animal species mostly used for chronic toxicity studies, for which no corresponding damage is found in man.

The drug regulatory agency does not take into consideration all these discrepancies, but tries to simplify according to what may be called the "least minimal risk". This procedure does not necessarily increase drug safety, since it will not make unpredictable responses more predictable, but it may prolong preclinical toxicity studies, especially when testing for carcinogenicity is requested. In a recent paper on "Scientific and regulatory tendencies in drug toxicology," Zbinden[4] stressed the dilemma of drug toxicology, which finds itself encompassed by scientific conviction on the one hand and regulatory responsibility on the other. In his opinion, the so far dominant role that regulation plays in drug toxicology will be replaced more and more by scientific considerations, with the effect that regulatory requirements will be reduced. However, where and how to diminish what has been requested so far will be the matter of long debate and will not be generally accepted at all by the various regulatory agencies. As long as major toxic responses remain unpredictable on the basis of toxicity studies in animals, every reduction in such studies will be illusionary, since regulatory agencies may not dare to alleviate the rules as long as they have to face the blame of having neglected the necessary care[5].

Much will be gained, if, in future, drug regulators will be cautious in asking for the introduction of additional methods by which drug safety should be increased. Tests for mutagenicity are one recent example ; they are not yet compulsory in all countries, but are requested in some, although it is not at all clear what the results obtained in in-vitro studies with bacteria (Ames test) or mammalian cells mean for drug safety in man[4, 6]. On the other hand, a positive result in these tests may suffice to induce a manufacturer not to follow up the drug any further, because he is afraid of either facing problems with the acceptance of the drug or being forced to undertake costly postmarketing surveillance. Hydralazine and dihydralazine, marketed nearly 30 years ago and being most useful therapeutics in the treatment of high blood pressure, have recently been found to be mutagenic in the Ames test[7]. If such an observation were made today, the drug would be dropped, since it would be regarded as a potential human carcinogen.

Progress in toxicology will help to strengthen the scientific basis of drug safety, and it is to be hoped that the regulatory agencies will be open-minded and listen to the advice of the toxicologists with respect to establishing a minimum requirement list of methods and studies serving to ensure drug safety. A symposium organised recently by the Drug Regulatory Agency of the Federal Republic of Germany, the Bundesgesundheitsamt, dealt with the problems of chronic toxicity studies, their aim, their conduct, and their evaluation[8]. This is a good example of cooperation between experts and drug regulators and should be followed by others.

DO DRUG SAFETY REQUIREMENTS IMPEDE DRUG INNOVATION ?

A recent editorial[14] claimed that "unscientific and irrational bureaucracy is strangling innovation in the British drug industry..." and the unduly long periods were criticized that elapse until permission to start clinical trials or, even more so, to market a new drug is granted by the Committee on Safety of Medicines. In the meantime, the situation with respect to the first application of a new drug in man has been revised, and the new U.

K. Clinical Trial Exemption Scheme, based on a summary of preclinical data, will definitely speed up the onset of clinical trials and facilitate their early phases. However, the delay in approving drugs for either clinical trials or marketing has never been the crucial point by which drug regulation affected drug innovation. It is the number of studies, mainly on the toxicity of a new drug, and the amount of work, which is a heavy charge on a research department and does not leave the necessary capacity for untargeted research, a prerequisite for developing new drugs that are original and not mere copies.

As a consequence of regulatory requirements for drug safety, the percentage of expenditure for basic research in the American drug industry fell from 15.4 % to 11.4 % in the ten years between 1968 and 1978[9]. Both figures are insufficient to support the activities necessary today to be successful in drug innovation and not only in drug imitation. It is the easy way of reasoning to make influences from outside responsible for the declining number of new drugs instead of looking for possible causes within the industrial enterprises. A few months ago, it was reported that one of the leading Dutch drug companies "had been forced by rising costs and increasing regulatory pressure" to give up traditional drug research which was "simply not big enough to generate results ; no new product had emerged for the last ten years". It was stated, however, that developmental activities to improve existing drugs will go on. On the other hand, the company plans to concentrate research on the new field of genetic engineering, an area where at least initial progress is fast, but of which the definite position in drug research has yet to be found[10].

It is not only the work load which requirements of drug safety have imposed on drug companies, but also the scarcity of true inventorship and creativity in drug research, which is responsible for the deplorable reduction in drugs which may be considered novel. Industrial research is hampered today by a rapidly growing bureaucracy, which develops inversely to success and will curb individual research activities instead of stimulating them. Drug regulations in general, including those for drug safety, have definitely improved practices and standards of the drug industry. The often repeated complaint that this has been achieved only at the cost of drug innovation is not justified ; it is up to industry to change their research policy and to invest more in basic research, instead of just trying to achieve rapid and easy success. Research asks for endeavour and courage and of course for new ideas and imagination, none of which is restrained by drug regulations[11].

WHAT IS THE SIGNIFICANCE OF THE BENEFIT-TO-RISK RATIO ?

Since drug safety is relative, it cannot be assessed as such, but only in relation to the possible benefit to be expected from the drug. However, benefit, too, is not at all certain and has to be rated with reserve. The balance between benefit and risk implies that the therapeutic aims of the drug be considered in relation to the possible risks demonstrated by the early studies. To estimate the danger or to quantify the risk is as difficult as to value the benefit that a drug may have, and for this reason drug regulatory agencies should welcome the advice of experts, helping them to reach a decision. The question what risk might be acceptable in treating a certain disease cannot be formally answered, but only on the basis of professional experience and expert knowledge, of which the drug regulators should make ample use.

Both, benefit and risk, can only be assessed after a drug has been marketed, because efficacy has to be demonstrated in a much larger group of patients than the relatively small number who received the drug during the clinical trials period. The same is the case for detecting severe adverse reactions, which are the real risk of a drug. It has been argued that drugs for indications which may be considered trivial, such as sleeplessness, anxiety, or mild to moderate pain, and for which there is no urgent need should undergo more extensive toxicity studies to minimize their possible risk.

However, such a procedure is no justified, since prolongation or extension of preclinical toxicological studies does not reduce the risk of unpredictable adverse reactions. The statement made by the former FDA Commissioner Donald Kennedy [12] that "the FDA's decision to require long-term carcinogenic-effect testing before clinical use has spared patients in the United States a potentially dangerous kind of exposure" is not correct, since it refers to practolol, the adverse reactions of which cannot at all be related to a carcinogenic potential. Furthermore, no data are available which demonstrate that the risk of new drugs has really been diminished by carcinogenicity tests.

The matter of benefit-to-risk ratio cannot be settled on the preclinical basis, but only by careful monitoring after marketing, not necessarily in the form of a strict post-marketing surveillance study, but also by means of traditional methods, including information about drug consumption. In case suspicion arises that a drug may be responsible for an adverse reaction, a retrospective case-control study should be undertaken, which may be helpful in either strengthening or alleviating the guess, but cannot give a definite proof. The cost of such a study has not inevitably to be borne by the drug manufacturer, but the drug regulatory agency may also contribute to it.

There is a special need for estimating the risk of drugs which have to be given over prolonged periods, such as antihypertensives, oral antidiabetics, hypolipidaemic drugs, and others. The recent experience made with the five years' administration of clofibrate is an example[13] of what the risks of long-term administration may be and of how drug regulators may react to the results of such a study. In most countries, the regulatory agencies responded to the small reduction in serum cholesterol levels, the somewhat lower incidence of myocardial infarction, and the higher incidence of gall-stone formation with subsequent cholecystitis, which occured in the clofibrate group, by stricter labelling of the drug. Clofibrate was no longer considered a safe drug for community-wide primary prevention of ischaemic heart disease, but its use should be limited to patients with definite hypercholesterolaemia[14]. In the Federal Republic of Germany, however, the drug had to be taken off the market, mainly because of the somewhat higher death rate in the treatment group, obviously unrelated to the hypolipidaemic activity of the drug. The fact that clofibrate may favour the formation of gall stones and cholecystitis had been known before, and the higher incidence of tumor formation in the treatment group was not clearly related to the administration of the drug[15].

It is evident that not only scientific considerations were the basis of the various decisions made after the publication of the clofibrate study, but that some agencies were influenced by bias and emotion rather than by sober arguments. It would be difficult, if not impossible, to estimate approximately only whether the risk attributable to the administration of clofibrate has outweighed the relative risk caused by the withdrawal of the drug in a country where clofibrate had been banned completely compared to countries where a more restricted use only had been recommended. Better and more reliable assessment of risk will contribute to improved drug safety, but to obtain the information necessary for the estimation of risk may be extremely difficult. Drug regulatory agencies should actively support studies which will help to improve the valuation of the benefit-to-risk ratio.

WHERE ARE THE LIMITS OF SAFETY REGULATIONS ?

The significance attributed to experimental toxicological studies for the assessment of drug safety may induce regulatory agencies to apply the same measures also to other chemicals. The Delaney Clause in the legislation of the United States, which orders withdrawal of every food ingredient for which a positive carcinogenicity test has been obtained in animals, was responsible for the disappearance of the artificial sweetener cyclamate from the American market about 12 years ago. In other countries, cyclamate is still available, obviously without having any damaging effect on the large number of people who regularly take it. However, in the United States, the situation became critical, when the only remaining sugar substitute, saccharine, also seemed to cause malignant tumors in animals, although the experiments were anything but clear. The Food and Drug Administration recommended the removal of saccharine, but for once political intervention from Congress prevented the ban[16]. Scientific advice had apparently been too weak to convince the regulatory bureaucrats of the fact that the experimental studies were not a sufficiently sound basis to deprive of their sugar substitute the American people as well as those of other countries where drug regulatory agencies usually follow the recommendations of the FDA blindly. Meanwhile, the turmoil has calmed down, and for the time being nobody in the United States seems concerned at the possibility that artificial sweetness might pose a safety problem. However, in Italy, according to recent legislation, saccharine and other sweeteners are only available in pharmacies and on prescription[10]. Let us hope that people there will find a way "all'Italiana" to get what they need.

Today, if it is not sweeteners, it is coffee which causes apprehension in the United States. The FDA undertook a study to examine the safety of caffeine, which, when fed by gavage in doses of 40, 80, and 125 mg/kg to rats during the first 19 days of gestation, caused birth defects. This observation resulted in a warning to pregnant women "to eliminate or limit their consumption of caffeine-containing products"[17]. Considering that 40 mg/kg of caffeine, given in a single dose, would correspond to 2 g for a woman with a weight of 50 kg, or to 40 cups of coffee, once more makes obvious the problem of drawing parallels between toxicity studies in animals and possible drug safety. Nevertheless, the results of the study made the FDA propose that caffeine be removed from the list of substances classified as "Generally Recognized As Safe (GRAS)". It will be up to the manufacturers of beverages to initiate further studies to determine the real risk.

Furthermore, caffeine has been incriminated of being carcinogenic, since, in a case-control study of patients suffering from cancer of the pancreas, the relative risk associated with the daily intake of two cups of coffee was 1.8, and that with three or more cups per days was 2.7[18]. The authors conclude that "if the association between coffee consumption and pancreatic cancer is confirmed and found to be causal, the relation will have some importance in quantitative terms. ..., we estimate the proportion of pancreatic cancer that is potentially attributable to coffee consumption to be slightly more than 50 per cent". How safe is it then to drink coffee, and what steps have to be taken to warn consumers ?

Another safety problem related to a drug has been the possible formation of nitrosamine in the stomach after intake of amino-phenazone together with food containing nitrates for preservation[19]. The demonstration that nitrosamines may be found in the rat stomach was enough to induce some regulatory agencies to require the replacement of aminophenazone by propyphenazone in numerous analgesic mixtures still on the market in European countries. This is an example of the often inconsistent handling of safety matters by drug regulation. While agranulocytosis, a proven severe adverse reaction caused by aminophenazone, was not considered sufficiently serious — although it had been responsible for quite a few fatal complications — experimental evidence of nitrosamine formation was reason enough to ask drug manufacturers to quickly and quietly substitute the well-known drug by a hardly used pyrazolone derivative. No long-term toxicity studies have ever been performed for propyphenazone, not to speak of carcinogenicity or teratogenicity tests.

Such a procedure of replacing one drug by another without adequate data being available is a serious precedent. In addition, it not only violates drug safety regulations in various respects, but also deceives the consumer, who — unexpectedly — under the same brandname receives a drug which differs in its composition from that he has used before. If, in order to avoid a possible adverse reaction, the method of replacing a drug by a chemically related one were generally applied, one might ask for exemption from long-term toxicity studies on the basis of chemical similarity. However, marked and in various respects unpredictable differences may exist between drugs which are chemically closely related to one another. Such differences are observed not only with respect to toxicity, but also regarding the pharmacodynamic profile and pharmacokinetics. Practolol is a recent example of how little one may conclude from chemical and pharmacological similarities with respect to the occurrence of severe adverse reactions, and glutethimide and thalidomide are older examples, the former being free of teratogenicity, despite its close chemical relation to thalidomide.

It has been suggested that a newly developed active drug may have better chances of being exempted from some long-term toxicity studies, if it is related to a drug already on the market. This "me too" philosophy[20] may be applicable with respect to efficacy, but is certainly not valid to satisfy safety requirements. Regulation of drug safety has to regard also a closely related substance as a new chemical entity, which is diversely handled by the organism and may have a toxicological profile which markedly differs from that of the drug already in use. Hence, on scientific grounds, it cannot be recommended to reduce toxicology requirements for a new substance, even if it is chemically closely related to a known one. We have as little information of structure-activity as of structure-toxicity relationships.

CAN CLINICAL TRIALS BE EXPEDITED WITHOUT NEGLECTING DRUG SAFETY ?

In various European countries, e. g. the Federal Republic of Germany, France, Switzerland, and Austria, clinical trials of a new chemical entity may be started without waiting for the permission from the drug regulatory agency. It suffices to deposit with the regulatory office all the experimental data which have to be obtained according to the standards of pharmacodynamic, pharmacokinetic, and toxicity studies. In other countries, a clinical trials certificate is still requested, e. g. in Italy, whereas in Britain the clinical trials exemption scheme has been accepted quite recently, and it is expected that exemptions will be the rule in the future[21]. The experience made in countries without a regulatory control of clinical trials has shown that renouncing a clinical trials certificate does not weaken drug safety. Practice has rather confirmed the old observation that the time of investigation of a drug before it is marketed is the safest period in its whole life-span. The facilitation of clinical trials in man and consequently the possibility of initiating human studies earlier will probably not reduce, but rather increase drug safety. Since it will be possible to submit a large number of new chemical entities to at least a preliminary clinical testing, the chance of discovering favourable quantitative and qualitative differences is definitely better than on the basis of animal experiments exclusively.

This first step which makes easier the administration of new drugs to man should be followed by further efforts to reduce the safety requirements for the early phases of clinical trials. The standard procedures and guidelines which are issued by national regulatory agencies as well as by international bodies correspond only in part to scientific knowledge and experience and do not take into account sufficiently the individual situation for a given drug. It is not justified to apply to such an experimental phase, as are early studies in man, the same strict rules as to a drug that is going to be marketed and will thus be generally available to the medical profession. The individualization of toxicity studies according to the nature of the substance, the selection of appropriate procedures and the assessment of their reliability for establishing safety is a scientific challenge for toxicologists and clinical investigators experienced in early studies of new drugs in man.

It may be argued that it is not ethical to expose patients and healthy volunteers to a large number of chemical substances which later on will not be marketed as drugs and to enhance the number of experiments in human beings unnecessarily. However, it has to be realized that progress in drug research depends on effective clinical trials. It is essential that ethics of clinical trials are strictly observed, and this includes the best possible guarantee for safety aspects to have been duly considered.

HOW CAN THE SCIENTIFIC BASIS OF DRUG SAFETY BE IMPROVED ?

Drug safety cannot be enhanced by regulation, but only by scientific progress. Consequently, the contribution of drug regulation to drug safety can only consist of transferring results of toxicological research to the regulatory procedures. Today, one of the most important aims of toxicology is to develop methods permitting to predict adverse reactions which may occur in man and to obtain this information within a relatively short period, i. e. not on the basis of life-span studies. However, toxicological studies alone cannot give the desired information, but should be considered together with pharmacokinetics, which give insight into drug metabolism. The rate of metabolisation, the type of metabolites, which may be species-dependent, the trapping in deep compartments, the excretion, and other pharmacokinetic characteristics affect the toxicity of a drug in animals as well as in man. Genetic differences may be of significance and may make certain groups of people more susceptible than others to adverse drug responses.

Attempts to discover, in animal experiments, damages which may allow at least some conclusions as to what may have to be expected when a substance is given to man over a prolonged period have already resulted in some progress. The development of toxicological models which are based on the known relationship between the intake of certain drugs and the occurrence of delayed toxic reactions has been proposed by Zbinden[22] as a suitable means to discover a distinct type of damage. By fine-needle liver biopsies in rats which had received a liver carcinogen it was possible to demonstrate already after a few weeks, the occurrence of premalignant cells. Similarly, carcinogens for the urinary bladder affected the synthesis of nucleic acids in the epithelial cells of the rat's bladder after a short period of treatment[23, 24]. Other examples of such an early manifestation of precancerous changes and of other characteristic lesions have been given, which, although not frequent so far, furnish more rapid information than life-span carcinogenicity studies in rats and may be as reliable.

Chronic toxicological studies, required for new chemical entities in the frame of new drug applications, may also indicate possible cancerogenic activities[25]. These preneoplastic changes may be useful in deciding whether proper carcinogenicity studies have to be undertaken or whether the drug may be exempted from them. In animals, clinical observations, results of laboratory tests, as well as morphological studies may all give hints as to the direction in which a search for possible damage should be started. On the other hand, if a new chemical entity is clean with respect to these various directions of investigation, it does not make sense to ask for special carcinogenicity or mutagenicity studies.

It is the aim of toxicological studies to enlarge the basis for the regulation of drug safety, to increase the number of studies which are directed towards discovering damages or changes in certain organs and tissues, instead of exploring the whole organism of the laboratory animal for alterations caused by the drug[22]. Of course, the latter method will remain useful, even indispensable, in case no directed studies can be undertaken. It has to be stressed again that safety cannot be achieved by simply prolonging studies. If, today, in most European countries a toxicological study of six months' duration is considered satisfactory, the 12 or even 18 months requested by the American FDA or the Canadian Drug Directorate do not at all warrant a greater degree of safety.

Much is said today about the harmonisation of regulations and guidelines, and many meetings and symposia have been held and discussions taken place between the various parties concerned, but little has been achieved[26, 10]. Dr. Richard Crout, the former director of the Bureau of Drugs of the American FDA, a few years ago expressed the opinion that international agreement on data for the acceptance of new drugs is not a scientific problem, but "a matter of reconciling legal standards and decision-making processes among the nations with strong drug regulatory agencies"[27]. Since it happens that the nations with strong drug regulatory agencies also contribute most substantially to drug research and to biomedical progress, including pharmacology and toxicology, it should not be too difficult on a national basis to lay the foundations for an international cooperation. It does not contribute to drug safety, if repetition of toxicology studies is requested in cases where they have already been performed outside the country according to present standards. In December last year, the FDA Commissioner Jere E. Goyan stated : "When it is well established in the scientific literature that a drug is safe and effective for a particular use, there is no valid scientific reason for requiring more tests in animals and humans. Duplicate testing is a needless waste of already scarce scientific talent and facilities"[28]. It is to be hoped that Dr. Goyan's successor will adopt this statement and continue this line of open-mindedness.

In Europe, within the EEC, steps have been taken to adapt to one another the drug regulations of the various countries. So far, expert advice and new scientific developments have not had much impact on the text of the document which has been prepared by the Commission for the Council of the European Economic Community. However, it is to be hoped that the scientific influence will increase, and that experts will be invited, not only to express their opinion, but to give continuous advice according to the progress that is made. The example given by the British regulatory authorities in asking a competent clinical pharmacologist, such as is Dr. Grahame Smith, to prepare a report on the safety requirements for the administration of a drug to man should be accepted also by other countries as well as by the EEC. If scientific considerations prevail legal aspects and get better access to regulatory agencies, drug safety will not be reduced, but enhanced.

REFERENCES

1. Report of a WHO Scientific Group, Guidelines for Evaluation of Drugs for Use in Man, World Health Organization Technical Report Series N° 563, Geneva, 1975.
2. Gist-Brocades ready for R & D shift, *Scrip* **564**, February 11, 1981, (p. 6).
3. Report of a WHO Scientific Group, Principles for Pre-Clinical Testing of Drug Safety, World Health Organization Technical Report Series N° 341, Geneva, 1966.
4. Zbinden G., "Wissenschaftliche und regulatorische Tendenzen in der Arzneimittel-toxikologie", *in : Sicherheit versus Innovation in der Arzneimittelforschung. Symposium mit Paneldiskussion. 18. GDCH-Hauptversammlung, Berlin, 19. September 1979*, Ed. MPS Medizinisch Pharmazeutische Studiengesellschaft e. V., Mainz, 1980, p. 30-42.
5. Smith T., Are the drug-regulatory agencies paper villains ?, *Brit. Med. J.* **281** (1980), 1333-35.
6. Draper M.F. and J.P. Griffin, *Draft CPMP guidelines on mutagenicity testing*, Arch. Toxicol., in press
7. Williams G.M., G. Mazue, C.A. McQueen and T. Shimada, Genotoxicity of the antihypertensive drugs hydralazine and dihydralazine, *Science* **210** (1980), 329-30.
8. AMI-Berichte, *Zur Problematik von chronischen Toxizitätsprünfungen. Ziel, Durchführung und Bewertung. Wissenschaftliches Symposium des Instituts für Arzneimittel des Bundesgesundheitsamtes, Berlin, 26.-28. Februar 1979*, B. Schnieders und P. Grosdanoff eds, Berlin, Dietrich Reimer Verlag, 1980.

9. Steward F. and G. Wibberley, Drug innovation — what's slowing it down ?, *Nature* **284** (1980), 118-20.

10. Dukes M.N.G., Harmonisation of pharmaceutical regulation : a personal view, *Scrip* **561**, February 2nd, 1981 (pp. 5-7).

11. Gibson W.C., The cost of not doing medical research, *J. Am. Med. Assoc.* **244** (1980), 1817-19.

12. Kennedy D., A calm look at "drug lag", *J. Am. Med. Assoc.* **239** (1978), 423-26.

13. Report from the Committee of Principal Investigators, A co-operative trial in the primary prevention of ischaemic heart disease using clofibrate, *Brit. Heart J.* **40** (1978), 1069-18.

14. Editorial, Drug innovation bureaucracy, *Brit. Med. J.* **280** (1980), 1484-85.

15. Report of the Committee of Principal Investigators, WHO cooperative trial on primary prevention of ischaemic heart disease using clofibrate to lower serum cholesterol : mortality follow-up, *Lancet* **1980**, II, 379-85.

16. Lasagna L., Toxicological barriers to providing better drugs, *Arch. Toxicol.* **43** (1979), 27-33.

17. Caffeine and pregnancy, *FDA Drug Bulletin* **10**, 3 (1980), 19-20.

18. MacMahon B., S. Yen, D. Trichopoulos, K. Warren and G. Nardi, Coffee and cancer of the pancreas, *New Engl. J. Med.* **304** (1981), 630-33.

19. Eisenbrand G., B. Spiegelhalder, J. Kann, R. Klein and R. Preussmann, Carcinogenic N-nitrosodimethylamine as a contamination in drugs containing 4-dimethylamino-2,3-dimethyl-1-phenyl-3-pyrazolin-5-one (Amidopyrine, Aminophenazone), *Arzneim.-Forsch*, (Drug Res.) **29** (1979), 867-69.

20. Joyce C.R.B., "Me-toos", "me-agains" and the risk of drugs, *Brit. Med. J.* **281** (1980), 286-87.

21. Medicines Act 1968, Addendum of 1981 : Data requirements for clinical trial certificates — MLX 130, January 1981. Department of Health and Social Security, London.

22. Zbinden G., "Toxikologische Modellversuche in der Prognose von Langzeitschäden", *in : Zur Problematik von chronischen Toxizitätsprüfungen. Ziel, Durchführung und Bewertung (AMI-Berichte 1/1980)*, B. Schnieders und P. Grosdanoff eds, Berlin, Dietrich Reimer Verlag, 1980, p. 87-89.

23. Lawson T.A., "Replication and permeability in the animal model", *in : Health and Sugar Substitutes, Proc. ERGOB Conference*, G. Guggenheim ed., Basel, Karger, 1978, pp. 48-53.

24. Boelsterli U., and G. Zbinden, *Application of fine-needle aspiration biopsy for the diagnosis of dysplastic and neoplastic liver cell changes induced by N-nitrosomorpholine in rats*, to be published.

25. Frohberg H., "Zur Korrelation chronischer Effekte mit kanzerogenen, mutagenen und embryotoxischen Wirkungen im Tierversuch", *in : Zur Problematik von chronischen Toxizitätsprüfungen. Ziel, Durchführung und Bewertung* (AMI-Berichte 1/1980), B. Schnieders und P. Grosdanoff eds, Berlin, Dietrich Reimer Verlag, 1980, pp. 94-100.

26. WHO-FDA meeting produces directory, but little else : harmonisation fails, *Scrip* **539**, November 10, 1980 (p. 9).

27. Crout J.R., "Influence of statutory requirements. Viewpoint of the regulatory agencies", *in : Trends and Prospects in Drug Research and Development*, XIth CIOMS Round Table Conference, Geneva, 8-9 December 1977, Z. Bankowski and J.F. Dunne eds, published by *Scrip* for the Council for International Organisations of Medical Sciences, 1977, p. 87-88.

28. Goyan J.E., *in : HHS News* (US Department of Health and Human Services), Food and Drug Administration, December 8, 1980.

29. Editorial, Clofibrate and the primary prevention of ischaemic heart disease, *Brit. Med. J.* **1978**, 4, 1585-86.

30. Saccharin goes on prescription-only in Italy, *Scrip* **522**, September 10, 1980 (p. 3).

31. Southampton PMS unit concern over BMA caveats, *Scrip* **578**, April 1, 1981 (p. 3).

Sécurité et médicaments (1982), pp. 19-31

The Effects of Drug Regulation on Iatrogenic Disease

M. N. G. DUKES* and I. LUNDE**

* Netherlands Committee for the Evaluation of Medicines, Rijswijk, Netherland
** Norwegian Center for Medicinal Products Control, Oslo 9, Norway

Abstract — Within the framework of the "European Studies of Drug Regulation" sponsored by the World Health Organization a number of investigations are being performed to determine the extent to which drug regulatory activity succeeds in reducing the incidence or severity of drug induced injury. A number of techniques have been developed for this purpose and comparative studies in several countries are under way. The present paper will describe the methods of investigation and present preliminary results from Europe and elsewhere.

On the north side of the Strand in London there stands a remarkable but not undignified building known as the Royal Courts of Justice. The Law Courts, as they are known, were opened in 1882 by Queen Victoria. There is a story about their opening. It seems that, shortly beforehand, the Lord Chancellor called a meeting of the judges, at which the draft of an address to the Queen was considered. It contained the phrase : "Your Majesty's Judges are 'deeply sensible of their own many shortcomings..." whereat a learned judge named Jessel strongly objected, saying "I am not conscious of "many shortcomings", and if I were I should not be fit to sit upon the bench." After some wrangling as to the terms of the address, Lord Justice Bowen suggested a compromise. As he put it : "Instead of saying that we are 'deeply sensible of our own many shortcomings' why not say that we are 'deeply sensible of the many shortcomings of each other' ?"[1].

Drug Regulators, when one stops to think about it, have something in common with judges. There is no opportunity to examine the parallel at this point, but there is very little doubt that when a drug regulator sets out to study critically the way in which his profession serves the community he is likely to find it easier to examine the performance of his brethren than his own. That is just one of the tenets of the European Studies of Drug Regulation which we together established a little over two years ago and which we are now continuing under the auspices of the World Health Organization. Gradually the realization has grown that it is time to look at drug regulation critically but constructively so as to plan for the future. That involves a very careful analysis of the repercussions which various forms of drug regulation have had for the community. Those repercussions may be of many types ; drug control can have effects upon medical treatment, upon drug safety, upon creative research and upon the economy. One by one these must be examined on the basis of hard facts and international comparisons. Several of these matters we have examined in published or ongoing studies in this series. In this present paper, and in view of the theme of this meeting, we shall limit ourselves to one aspect only, namely the effect of drug regulatory systems on the incidence and severity of drug induced disease. One of the original purposes of instituting drug control was, after all, to reduce the risk of new drug tragedies and of adverse reactions in general. If that purpose has to any extent been accomplished, the effects should in course of time become demonstrable, and perhaps even quantifiable.

In one of our earliest papers in this series[2] we pointed to the pitfalls which one can encounter in studying this matter. Even if one can show that the rise of drug control has co-incided with a decline in some types of drug-induced disease, this does not prove cause-and-effect ; the two phenomena may have been contemporaneous by mere chance, or because they have some common cause. On the other hand, any positive effect which drug control has had may be entirely masked or overshadowed by other influences ; coarse parameters such as gross morbidity or mortality are for this reason unlikely to be of any great value.

Nevertheless we have developed a number of techniques to study this topic ; some of these, and a number of preliminary results, will be presented in this paper.

A FOLLOW-UP STUDY OF REJECTIONS

To get our bearings, we began with a relatively simple method and we tested it in one of our own countries, namely Norway. When a regulatory agency believes that it has identified a safety problem, the bluntest weapon which it can use to tackle that problem is to reject the drug completely. Now in one of our first studies[3] we analyzed a hundred consecutive rejections in Norway (Table 1).

As one can see, of the 100 drug rejections, 30 were based largely or entirely on safety considerations. In 25 of these cases the human safety data were considered to be

Table 1. Drugs rejected in Norway 1974-1977

Total rejections :	100
30 rejections for safety reasons :	
a. Animal data :	3
Human data :	25
Animal & Human data :	2
	30
b. Data inadequate :	18
Risk suspected :	12
	30

insufficient, in 3 the animal data, in 2 both types of safety data. This is a start, but we have to go much further. In 18 of the 30 instances, the Specialty Board rejected the drug simply because the safety data were not up to its prescribed standards. In the other 12, however, it was considered that a specific safety problem appeared to arise, and it is on these twelve that we would like to concentrate our attention. Of these 12 cases (Table 2) 4 were instances in which the suspicion was based on animal data ; in the other eight the evidence that the drug was harmful came from the human investigational material.

Table 2. Norwegian rejections for suspected risk

Animal evidence :	4
Human evidence :	8
	12

With this type of data to hand, the question which obviously arises is whether the Norwegian Specialty Board was right or not. One can tackle this question, in the light of the knowledge now available, but first we must formulate it very carefully. In these twelve cases, the Norwegian Regulatory Agency did two things :
firstly, it identified what it regarded as a safety problem ;
then, it took that problem as a ground (or one of the grounds) for rejecting the drug.

In the interests of objective analysis we have to confine our attention to the first point, i. e. whether the problem was correctly identified ; that is the essence of the matter, after all, and by looking carefully at the literature which has appeared since that time we can decide reasonably objectively whether the problem really existed or not. Whether that problem justified a rejection, or whether it would have been sufficient to require further studies or to issue appropriate warnings is a matter we shall set aside, because these things depend very much upon the national situation and it is impossible to be objective about them when one makes international comparisons.

Especially interesting are the first four cases, in all of which the evidence of a safety problem came from animal studies (Table 3). The first two relate to drugs in which some hepatotoxicity was found. Up to 1981 this has not proved to be a clinical problem, though liver enzymes have occasionally been elevated. The third case, also con-

Table 3. Norwegian rejections on animal evidence 1974-1977

Drug type	Suspicion	Literature 1981
NSAI	Hepatic & renal toxicity	Very rare
Antibiotic	Hepatotoxicity	Slight, rare
Relaxant	Tumour induction	probably not

Table 4. Norwegian rejections on human evidence 1974-1977

Drug type	Suspicion	Literature 1981
1. Antiarrytmic	Multitoxic	Correct
2. Ca-antagonist	Interaction	Can be severe
3. Anorexic	Metabolic effects	Unimportant
4. Anorexic	CNS effects	Can be common
5. Eyedrop (comb.)	React. Hyperaemia	Can occur
6. Dietary aid	Inappropriate	Theoretically so
7. Skin steroid	Cushing	Risk
8. IUD	Perforation	Theoretically so

cerning hepatoxicity, involved a prediction which one can reasonably consider correct, though jaundice only has occured with high doses. The fourth drug appeared induce tumours. Anno 1981, the possibility that such an effect might occur in man is still disputed. In these 4 cases, therefore, the animal studies to predict safety were not entirely valueless, but they tended to produce somewhat misleading or uncertain trails.

We can now look at the eight instances in which a problem was considered to have been identified on the basis of the clinical data in the registration file (Table 4) or in three instances on what one might call theoretical clinical grounds, in other words, matters of clinical principle. As you can see, correct predictions of problems were made in five of the eight cases, and marginally correct predictions of limited importance in the other three. The record of the clinical material thus seems to be considerably better than that of the animal data.

Having gained these impressions, we then decided to develop the method much further and to apply it more broadly, taking now as our basic material the practice of the Australian Drug Evaluation Committee.

A RETROSPECTIVE STUDY OF RESTRICTIVE DECISIONS

As we have already said, rejection is a blunt weapon, and often it is not an appropriate one. Quite apart from amending data sheets and labelling, which happens all the time

Table 5. Australia : applications leading to restrictive decisions (1976-1978)

New drugs	33
New dosages or forms	8
New ındications	6
Clinical trials	2
New safety claims	1
	50

Table 6. Australia : 50 restrictive decisions (1976-1978)

	Rejected	Deferred	Limited	TOTAL
Licences	12	16	5	33
Forms/Schedules	6	1	1	8
Indications	5	1	0	6
Trials	1	0	1	2
Safety claims	0	1	0	1
TOTAL	24	19	7	50

in the interest of safety, an agency can, when it is faced with a safety problem on a new drug, do three things. It can reject the drug outright, or it can defer its decision so that further evidence can be obtained, or else it can impose certain limitations so as to minimalise the risk. These are the three matters we looked at when we turned to Australia.

Our Australian material related to 50 consecutive restrictive decisions of one or the other of these three types ; they were taken over a total period of 27 months, running from March 1976 to June 1978 (Table 5). The table shows what the topics were ; 33 involved applications for a new drug licence, 8 applications for a new pharmaceutical form or a new dosage schedule, 6 applications for a new indication. Table 6 shows the type of restrictive decision which emerged ; in 24 cases the request or application was refused, in 19 the matter was deferred for further evidence, in 7 a limitation was imposed.

As in Norway, we then set out, using a number of standard reference works such as Meyler's Side Effects, Iatrogenic Diseases, and Adverse Reactions Titles, to discover whether in the light of present day knowledge the problems which the Australian Drug Evaluation Committee considered it has identified really have been found to exist in practice. At this point we have to make once more the distinction between the action taken and the problem identified, particularly because in this case ten of the drugs con-

Table 7. Australia : reliability of predictions

	N	%
Correct	32	53
Marginally correct	6	10
Incorrect	5	8
Not known	17	29
	60	100

Table 8. Australia : primary evidence of risk

Clinical only	26
Clinical + theoretical	8
Clinical + animal	5
Animal only	16
Animal theoretical	1
Theoretical only	4
TOTAL	60

cerned actually raised two distinct safety problems — in other words, in the fifty cases we examined there were not fifty but 60 underlying problems.

Our analysis is given in Table 7. Still being as objective as we can, we conclude that in 32 cases, or 53 % of instances, the Australian Committee had indeed identified and taken action on what subsequently proved to be a significant and genuine clinical problem. In a further 10 % of cases the prediction was marginally correct ; in 8 % it was apparently incorrect, and in 29 % of cases we still do not know, 3-5 years later, whether the problem exists in the clinic or not.

With these figures in mind, we can then go ahead as we did in Norway and look at the evidence on the basis of which the problems were identified (Table 8). In 39 instances the problem was predicted entirely or largely on the basis of human data, in 17 cases entirely or largely on the basis of animal data, in 4 cases only on theoretical considerations.

We can now try to correlate the nature of the evidence of safety problem and the reliability of the prediction. Our analysis is outlined in Table 9. If we group together the first three lines, in other words all the cases in which there was clinical reason to anticipate a safety problem at the time when the Committee had to take its decision, we see that in 31 of 39 cases the prediction proved to have been reliable — a very high scoring rate indeed.

Table 9. Australia : reliability of evidence

Primary evidence	Correct	Marginally correct	Incorrect	Not Known	TOTAL
Clinical only	20	1	1	4	26
Clinical + theoretical	7	0	0	1	8
Clinical + animal	4	0	1	0	5
Animal only	0	5	1	10	16
Animal + theoretical	0	0	0	1	1
Theoretical only	1	0	2	1	4
TOTAL	32	6	5	17	60

By contrast, where the primary evidence of a safety problem was derived from animal studies, as in the fourth and fifth lines of the table, there were no instances in which we can be really sure that a truly correct prediction was made. Naturally this reflects to a large extent the fact that much of the animal evidence relating to safety problems concerns possible long-term effects such as carcinogenicity or mutagenicity ; it may be many years before clinical experience and investigations can confirm or exclude such an effect in man, if indeed this ever happens at all ; eleven of these 17 cases fall into this category.

One can do a lot more with this material. Very recently we have been looking at the five instances in which animal studies suggested and acute safety problem, and where the prediction was marginally correct. Rather like the Norwegian cases of marginally correct predictions from animal studies they tend to involve problems which do in fact exist in the clinical literature but which are quantitatively not important. One of the cases related, for example, to an animal prediction that a vasodilator drug was cardiotoxic ; this is true, but in fact many cardiovascular drugs are to a degree cardiotoxic. Animal studies like this do not indicate whether there is a degree of cardiotoxicity disproportionate to the clinical effect. This question inevitably has to be studied in man, and it is the human evidence which will weigh almost exclusively when a decision on the drug is taken.

MAJOR IATROGENIC ACCIDENTS IN RETROSPECT

There are of course quite different ways of studying the predictability of iatrogenic problems and the extent to which these actually have been or could have been predicted. One is to look retrospectively at some of the recognized iatrogenic accidents of our time and then to attempt to determine in retrospect whether they were or could have been foreseen by even the most competent agency. Table 10 comprises a list of the most important iatrogenic drug reactions since thalidomide and it was compiled by Dr. Geoffrey Venning of Britain's Department of Health (Venning, personal communication) after he had obtained evidence from quite a number of physicians and regulatory agencies. What one would like to know is to what extent drug regulatory agencies anticipated these problems or might have been able to do so using currently available methods. What is immediately evident is that most of these problems would not have been predicted by animals studies — pharmacological or toxicological — as they are presently performed. Nor would most of them have been predicted in preregistration studies of the type currently required ; the incidence of most of these reactions is too low for that, or the time of their occurrence to late in treatment. Some of these drug accidents have been the subject of detailed histories — for examole that by Dr Nicholls of ICI on practolol[4] or that compiled by the Tokyo District Court on clioquinol and SMON[5]. When one goes through the list it is clear that most of these problems could have been (and in a few cases were) picked up on the basis of post-marketing surveillance in one form or another. The list is also instructive in that it reminds us of various regional variations in adverse effects ; most of these problems have in fact been much more prominent In one country than another. Finally the list underlines a point

Table 10. Major drug problems since thalidomide (G.R. Venning)

PRACTOLOL	Practolol sydrome
ORAL CONTRACEPTIVES	Tromboembolism
ANALGESICS	Nephropathy
PHENFORMIN	Lactic acidosis
SYMP. AEROSOLS	Asthma deaths
CLIOQUINOL	S.M.O.N.
STILBOESTROL	Vaginal Cancer
CHLORAMPHENICOL	Aplastic anemia
HALOTHANE	Jaundice
METHYSERGIDE	Fibrosis
CLINDA/LINCOMYCIN	Colitis
PHENBUTAZONE	Aplastic anaemia
PHENOTHIAZINES	Dyskinesias

we made earlier, namely that prohibition of a drug is a blunt and sometimes inappropriate weapon ; only three of the drugs on this list have been widely removed from the market — namely phenacetin, phenformin and clioquinol. In most other cases regulatory agencies have taken less extreme action so as to minimise the harm done whilst retaining the product for the good which it does. In the case of practolol, for example, the oral form was removed but the injectable form retained in many countries ; in many other instances — halothane, the sympathicomimetic aerosols and the phenothiazines, for example, physician eduction by the authorities has been the most dominant measure.

EFFICIENCY OF REGULATORY ACTIVITY ON SAFETY MATTERS

Let us now turn to quite a different approach ; this one involves looking at the degree of efficiency — or inefficiency — with which regulatory agencies have in the course of the years dealt with existing safety problems. Let us take the case of clioquinol, which was listed in Dr. Venning's table. The time-course of the clioquinol/SMON story is a very strange one indeed. The first human reports in the literature dated from 1935. Animal data pointing to a degree of neurotoxicity was obtained in 1939 and elsewhere in 1965. The astonishing SMON epidemic in Japan occurred in the period 1967-1970. Clioquinol was found in the urine of SMON patients in June of that year, and sales were suspended in Japan three months later. Regulatory restrictions elsewhere were introduced from 1972 onwards and in many countries no action has been taken. Now one could argue that this shows regulation at its worst, but in some respects it shows regulation at its best. Firstly, because in Japan it took only 12 weeks to remove clioquinol from the market when it had been biologically identified as the cause — or one of the causes — of SMON. Secondly, because regulatory agencies have taken their own national decisions based on the national situation ; there has been no wild rush to emulate the example of Japan, where special factors may have been involved. By and large, agencies have restricted or banned clioquinol only where they have found evidence of a national problem, as for example in Sweden or the Netherlands[5, 6].

A very recent study of this type, which has just been incorporated in the European Series, is that by John Griffin and Philip D'Arcy published in the 1981 Side Effects of Drugs Annual[7].

Briefly, Griffin and d'Arcy set out to determine how a large number of drug safety problems had been discovered, and when and how regulatory agencies had done something about them. Their findings are not particularly complementary to the control authorities. Typical is their analysis of the history of phenformin-induced lactic acidosis, the first reports of which dated from 1968. By 1972 there were 41 papers in print, making it quite clear that the complication was a serious one. Yet various major agencies did nothing about it, even to the extent of issuing warnings, until around 1975-1977. This type of time-course suggests that agencies sometimes neglect a problem for a long time, and then suddenly catalyze one another into action, and perhaps even into over-reaction, at a fairly late stage. Lactic acidosis was never a frequent complication, but it was a serious, and agencies could probably do better in the future at monitoring and providing information on problems of this type.

OTHER TECHNIQUES

There are of course other ways of studying the influence of drug regulation in iatrogenic disease ; we still have a lot to do. One very promising approach involves our collaborative studies with individual drug firms, reconstructing the registration history of some individual drugs. These investigations, which are now under way, are promising to throw a lot of light on the merits and shortcomings of the regulatory process, including its ability to cope with safety problems in an appropriate manner.

AN INVALID TECHNIQUE

It has been evident from the start of our series of investigations of drug control that we had to be extraordinarily careful to avoid bias, since we would be dealing all the time with material which can all too easily be distorted in order to prove what one wants to prove. We may present here one example of that, bearing on the safety field. One could argue that it should be possible to show there are greater problems with iatrogenic disease in countries without a strict regulatory system than in those where a critical drug control system has existed for a long time. We therefore approached W.H.O.'s International Drug Monitoring Centre in Uppsala with a list of 18 drugs commonly regarded as problematical (Table 11). Most of the drugs on this list are widely considered to pose a delicate problem as regards their efficacy/safety balance, and some of them have disappeared for this reason. We asked the W.H.O. to compile for us the total number of reports received on these drugs over the last 12 years, broken down by country. We then looked at the record of each participating country. What we very well

Table 11. Problematical and disputed drugs

Tilidine	dihydrostreptomycin
aprindine	oxyphenisatin
perhexiline	glafenine
metamizole	clozapine
phenacetin	oral. preg. test
clioquinol	amiodarone
esculin etc.	glutamate HBr
aminorex	mefenamic acid
crotoniazide	fenclofenac

knew was that this would be difficult data to analyze, data which could all too easily be distorted to serve a purpose. To give you an example of what we mean, we compiled Fig. 1 This was drawn to prove the unlikely hypothesis that the more stringent drug control is in a particular country, the greater the risk that problems will arise. If this diagram is to be believed, one can say that the fewest problems with the drugs in question arose in Italy and Indonesia, which were no more at risk than Norway, with its stringent control system. Similarly, the Netherlands and Australia come out at the same risk level as western Germany, which for much of that period had no adequate control system.

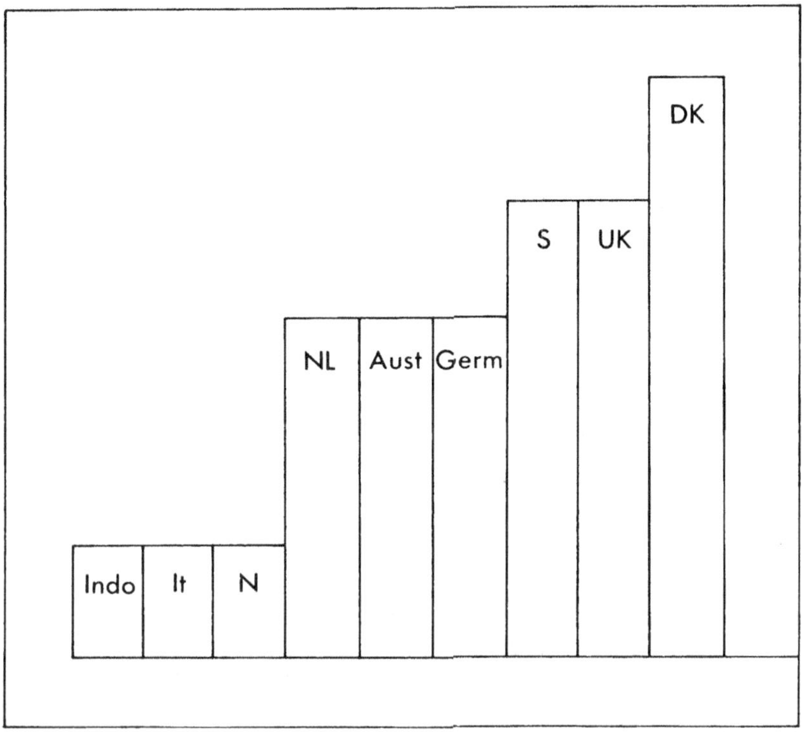

Fig. 1. Numbers of "problem drugs" involved in iatrogenic disease (distorted analysis)

Table 12. W.H.O. monitoring centre

"Cut-off" effect around 1975
Dihydrostreptomycin
Venopyrone
Phenacetin
Aminorex
Clioquinol
Geographical shift around 1975
Metamizol
Glafenine
Tilidine
Mefenamic Acid

The dangerous places to live appear to be Sweden, the U. K., and Denmark. This is we must stress, nonsense ; we produced this diagram by selecting our drugs carefully, ignoring the time curve of these events, and conveniently forgetting the fact that a country with a well-run control system is also likely to monitor adverse reactions more efficiently. Contrasting with this dangerous example, Table 13 suggests what one can indeed do with this type of information. The W. H. O. material points in a very interesting fashion to the marked change in reporting patterns around the mid seventies. Around that time, existing problems with quite a number of drugs, such as aminorex and venopyrone, were largely eliminated by appropriate regulatory measures. On the other hand, one encounters several drugs where there was simply a geographical shift in the problem. As the problems with metamizol, glafenine, tilidine and mefenamic acid were solved in some countries (either by restrictive activity or by giving the doctor appropriate information) so they raised their head in others, particularly countries with incomplete or relatively immature regulatory systems. The W.H.O. material does also indicate to some extent the greater risk of iatrogenic problems encountered in a country such as Germany during the early seventies when the number of drugs marketed was very large, consumption apparently high, and control still minimal. However one cannot determine which of these three factors, if any, was responsible for the problem, and analysis is further complicated by the fact that some countries have contributed very irregularly to the central file, and others (despite their participation in the system) not at all.

CONCLUSIONS

So much for the W.H.O. material, which we are continuing to study. In closing this paper, we would like to present at least some preliminary conclusions from the various types of work we have done.

Firstly, we see that well-organized drug regulatory agencies are, all the time, identifying safety problems and acting on them. In retrospect, they have a fairly high scoring rate in identifying problems correctly, which is the best proof that they succeed in representing the public interest. To that extent, one can conclude that it is a good thing that the pharmaceutical industry is required to submit its data to an impartial arbiter.

Secondly, agencies succeed in identifying problems primarily on the basis of the preliminary clinical material. Short-term animal studies unconfirmed in the clinic are often of very little use clinically and may even be misleading. We do not, as yet, know how valid longer-term animal data are. Such studies leave one with an uneasy feeling that something disagreeable may turn up in the clinic without any indication as to how reliable this indicator is. There is quite a lot of literature which we can commend to the reader on the prediction of adverse reactions from animal studies[8, 9] : most of it is not encouraging ; we probably need better techniques in this field than we have at the moment.

Thirdly, the role of post-marketing surveillance conducted simultaneously in several countries needs to be stressed again. Many of the major drug problems of the last two decades could not have been predicted on the basis of the pre-registration material currently required.

Fourthly, and finally, the Griffin and d'Arcy study suggests very strongly that regulatory agencies are not particularly good at keeping the physician abreast of the serious drug problems which he should know about.
These studies are very far from being completed. What we hope, however, is that as we proceed with them, so other people will do the same. The future of drug control is too important a matter to be settled by mere argument and political debate. What we have to demonstrate is what measure of drug control — and what type of drug control — the community needs, in its own interests, and then to create it.

REFERENCES

1. Megarry R. A., *Miscellany-at-Law*, London, 1955.
2. Dukes M.N.G. and I. Lunde, Measuring the repercussions of Drug Control : An Emerging Challenge, *Pharm. J.* **223** (1979), 511-13.
3. Lunde I. and M.N.G. Dukes, Les Répercussions du contrôle administratif des médicaments, *Ind. Santé* **49** (1980), 37-57.
4. Nicholls J.T., The Practolol Syndrome : A Retrospective Analysis, London, Medico-Pharmaceutical Forum, 1978.
5. Decision of the Tokyo District Court, August 3rd 1978, Kicadis, Tokyo, 1979.

6. Soda T. ed., *Drug-Induced Sufferings : Medical, Pharmaceutical and Legal Aspects*, Amsterdam-Oxford-Princeton, Excerpta Medica, 1980.

7. Griffin J. and P. d'Arcy, "Adverse Reactions to Drugs : the Information Lag", *in* : *Side Effects of Drugs Annual*, M.N.G. Dukes ed., 5, Amsterdam-Oxford-Princeton, Excerpta Medica, 1981.

8. Hill R., "Toxicological Testing : Predictive Value for Clinical Experience", *in* : *International Aspects of Drug Evaluation and Usage*, A.J. Jouhar and M.F. Grayson eds, London, Churchill Livingstone, 1973.

9. Baker S.B. de C. ed., *The Correlation of Adverse Effects in Man with Observations in Animals*, Amsterdam, Excerpta Medica, 1971.

Sécurité et médicaments (1982), pp. 33-40
© Pergamon Press France

Deregulation of Drug Development: If Effective, Can it be Safe ?

W. M. WARDELL

Center for the Study of Drug Development, Department of Pharmacology, University of Rochester Medical Center, Rochester, New York 14642

Abstract — Preliminary results from the update of our survey of new drug development in nearly all (38) U.S. — owned, research-based pharmaceutical firms showed that the decline in the number of new chemical entities (NCEs) under clinical investigation which occurred in the mid-1970s, was maintained through 1979. The mean number of NCEs first taken into man in 1977-1979 was 29 per year, about half the number investigated annually in the previous decade. This decline was reflected in a reduced number of Investigational New Drug Exemption (IND) filings. In addition, the proportion of INDs filed on drugs which are self-originated (i.e., not licensed or otherwise acquired) fell to 59 % in 1979 and averaged 68 % in 1976-1979, a decline from a mean of 82 % self-originated in the previous 13 years. The trend toward initial clinical testing of drugs outside the U.S.A. appears to have diminished. The percentage of self-originated NCEs first given to man abroad, which rose in the early 1970s to approach 40 % in 1976, declined to less than 20 % in 1977-1979. The time involved in clinical investigation of new drugs remains at the mid-1970s level of eight years. Self-originated NCEs approved for marketing in 1977-1979 spent six years in the IND filing phase and two years in the New Drug Application (NDA) review phase. The success rate in U.S. drug development was approximately the same in 1977-1979 as in the mid-1970s. Eleven percent of INDs filed on self-originated NCEs prior to 1972 had reached NDA approval by the end of 1979.

Now that it has been officially recognized that the process of developing and approving new drugs has become excessively long and expensive over the past decade[1-5], attempts are underway to encourage innovation by making the process simpler and more efficient. In the United States, these efforts are part of the general government move towards "deregulation"*.

Judging from the large, rapid swing of the regulatory pendulum from leniency to stringency over the past two decades, we should not be surprised by similar swings

* Although the movement to reduce government regulation actually had its genesis in the Ford and Carter administrations, the Reagan administration's pursuit of "deregulation" has been considerably more intense. For example, the President's Executive Order of 17 February 1981 requires not only that executive agencies formally scrutinize the potential costs of all new "major" regulations (already a Carter rule), but also that the agency choose "the alternative involving the least net cost to society." The Order establishes the Presidential Task Force on Regulatory Relief, now headed by Vice President George Bush, to oversee the process. (See U.S., President, Executive Order 12291, "Federal Regulation," *Federal Register* **46**, 13193 (1981). The mood unquestionably extends to Congress where the provisions of the first House bill of the new (97 th) session – H.R. 1 – require agencies to be more careful about the costs of regulation and allow courts to overturn more easily regulations already in force. (*New York Times*, 19 February 1981)

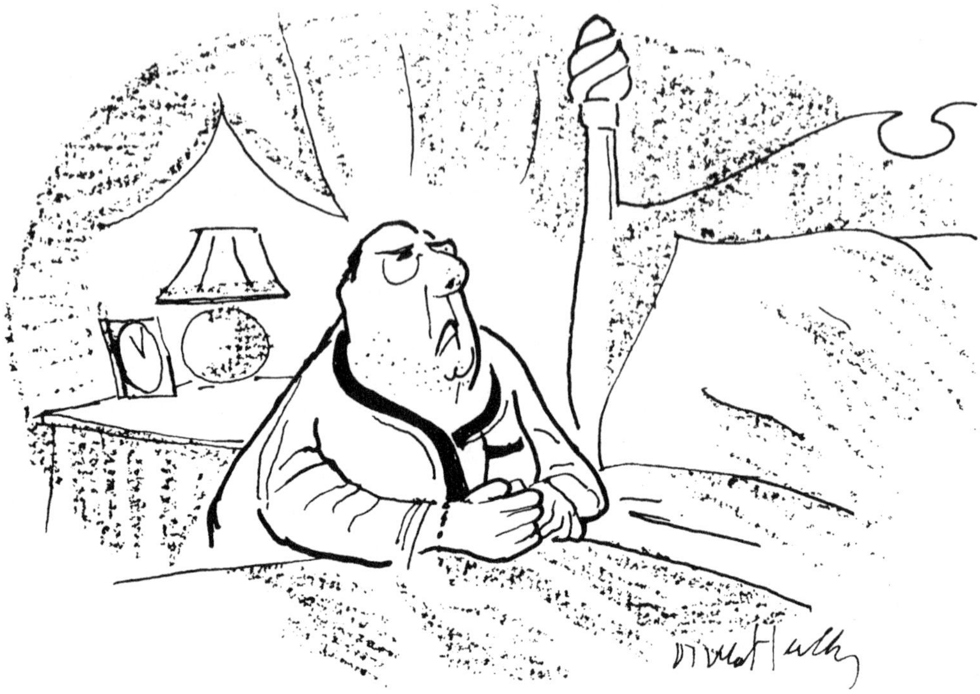

"...and please grant me and the rest of the board the grace not to abuse deregulation."

Fig. 1. March 16th issue of the *New Yorker*, drawing by Donald Reilly.

— in either direction — in the future. Thus, we should now be examining the possible consequences of deregulation to detect any backlash, particularly that based on real or imagined threats to public safety. Indeed, consumer organizations have already expressed concern that the efficacy requirement, in particular, will be scrapped or made meaningless[6].

The deregulation movement has become orthodox enough to be the subject of a charicature and the theme of the *New Yorker* cartoon reproduced here (Fig. 1). Whether the pharmaceutical industry in particular will be able to avoid what could *appear* to be abuse is a valid concern. The history of drug regulation and legislation, at least in the U.S., shows that most increases in regulation have ben based on disasters — whether real (as with the 1938 and 1962 drug laws), contrived (as with the clinical portions of the Bioresearch Monitoring Program), or imagined (as with the 1976 Medical Device Amendments). Almost any irregularity, regardless of its real importance, can provide the stimulus for stricter legislation and regulation.

Because absolute safety cannot be guaranteed by the present state of the art, we can be fairly certain that new episodes of drug toxicity will arise in the future. These should continue to diminish in scale as our mechanisms for preventing, detecting, and stopping them steadily improve. Nevertheless, even modest or minor incidents of toxicity might be portrayed as disasters and blamed on deficiencies in the regulatory process. Deregulation programs are natural scapegoats for such blame. Should this occur, the entire deregulation effort might be discredited, halted or even reversed — whether or not it was in any way a contributing factor*.

Now, at the beginning of the deregulation era, is the time to identify and deal with potential problems by evaluating current deregulation proposals in terms of *their* safety and efficacy — much as one might review a new drug application. Making deregulation as safe and effective as possible is in the interest of everyone : government, industry, academe, practicing physicians and, most of all, the patient.

Politically, overall safety will probably be the most important determinant of the survival of deregulation programs (although safety is not always the most crucial need of individual patients). The effectiveness (in terms of reducing the regulatory burden) of each element of deregulation should be critically examined, too : it would be unwise to include anything in the deregulation program that would not achieve its intended goals or that could be interpreted (now or later) as a reduction in safety.

When one examines the major U.S. proposals to deregulate the process of drug development and approval, it becomes apparent that a large proportion have virtually no conceivable effect on safety. Thus, if they are effective, these proposals can be supported without reservation.

Certain other deregulation proposals do have potential effects on safety — or could be portrayed as having such. It is essential that these safety issues be fully identified now and carefully analyzed and solved at the time of implementation in order to counter any future charges that safety was inadequately considered.

Table 1 shows some specific U.S. deregulation proposals that will be analyzed in this paper in terms of safety and efficacy. Although they obviously vary in the extent of probable impact, all have been specifically mentioned in the deregulation proposals of the Reagan administration.

THE EARLY STAGES : LESS-STRINGENT CONTROL

The attitude of the present U.S. administration toward the early stages of drug research follows several years of debate that included numerous hearings on the various drug reform bills proposed since 1976. The intent is to lessen FDA involvement by increasing the review and approval responsibilities of the local IRB for the first human studies**. Although this change would certainly achieve deregulation, it is not at all clear that it would actually work, at least with existing IRBs. For example, the IRB on which I

* Two examples of this have occurred already in the U.S., both involving drugs that were withdrawn from the market. In the case of azaribine (Triazure), the alleged use of postmarketing studies instead of further Phase III work was challenged at a hearing held by the House Subcommittee on Intergovernmental Relations and Human Resources on 27 October 1976. (For a thorough discussion, see Seymour Shubin, "Triazure and Public Drug Policies", *Perspectives in Biology and Medecine*, Winter 1979, 185-204)

** Some have even proposed that Phase I and early Phase II studies not be regulated at all by FDA and that simple reporting be the requirement. (See Gilbert F. McMahon, Talk presented at the legislative debate regarding S.2755, 95th Congress, Washington, D.C., 8 May 1978, p. 4 and Scheweiker, "Remarks", 28 May 1980, p. 7.)

Table 1. Current "deregulation" proposals in the U.S.

Preclinical Review
- Devolve responsibility to local IRBs, less for the FDA

Clinical Research
- Phase I: extent of FDA monitoring decreased; increases in responsability of local IRBs and researcher
- Review by stages: (the "developing NDA")

Review/Approval Process
- Minimize paperwork
- Greater reliance on summaries
- More efficient organisation (including "fast track")
- Submission of evidence by stages and by discipline
- Revision of efficacy standards:
  - "significant" rather than "substantial" evidence
  - special consideration for "breakthrough" drugs and "treatment INDs"
- Greater importance assigned to data from foreign studies
- Improved procedures for dispute resolution
- Reviewers' performance more closely monitored (for deadlines, etc.)

Postmarketing Issues
- PMS as remplacement for some Phase III studies
- Restoration of effective patent life

serve at the University of Rochester not only lacks the specialized manpower to make IND-type decisions quicker than the FDA, but would also be confronted by numerous other obstacles such as legal liability and insurance coverage for its members.

The effectiveness of local IRBs for this purpose might be improved if they received more funding and were more appropriately or specifically structured to make drug-study decisions. Special funding for local or regional IRBs might facilitate more rapid reviews, but perhaps at the risk of creating a number of FDA-like bureaucracies with widely varying, idiosyncratic requirements and different degrees of competence. One obvious effect of this could be to make multi-center studies impossible.

The efficacy or overall gain from deregulating Phase I depends on how badly regulations slow Phase I studies at present. In the U.K., concern that the requirements for the CTC (Clinical Trial Certificate) were responsible for forcing clinical studies abroad resulted in the 1981 Medicines Order which essentially replaces the CTC procedure with a clinical trial exemption (CTE) scheme[5, 7, 8]. In the U.S., our own informal enquiries of a few U.S. firms suggest that the degree of delay at the IND stage varies significantly: some firms reported that INDs were usually approved within the 30-day period; others experienced numerous delays and rejections not only during the first 30 days but also when the protocols were expanded subsequently. Although the potential for improving Phase I regulation is obviously there, assessments of the magnitude of possible relief are approximate at best.

Given the excellent acute safety record of Phase I studies, relaxing regulation there poses little or no hazard provided the current high standards of preclinical testing are maintained. The only real safety issue involved is the question of what to do if concurrent long-term animal tests show toxicity — a problem that exists with or without deregulation. Clearly, heavy chronic exposure of man to new chemicals should be avoided until the results of appropriate chronic animal toxicity tests are available. Pharmaceutical firms will need to be especially careful to maintain their standards on this in an era of deregulation.

SEQUENTIAL SUBMISSION AND REVIEW

There have been several proposals to restructure the submission and review of data, as alternatives to the present single, massive submission at the time of the NDA. One of these, the FDA's "developing NDA" concept, seems a good idea, but was deemed inefficient in practice because the final reviewer was required to repeat all the work of the earlier reviewers. Current proposals (in the IND/NDA revision program, for example[9]) entail earlier submission of the pharmaceutical and chemical data : most of the deficiencies are currently found in this area but at the same time these data could be reviewed long before submission of the NDA.

There is already ample evidence that greater efficiency can be achieved by reorganizing the sequence of review (e.g., in the "fast-track" priority-review procedure[10, 11]). To the extent that these can be achieved without compromising the quality of the review, they merit unreserved support and the appropriation of all resources necessary to implement such changes. These improvements carry no risk at all.

Likewise, measures to facilitate the mechanics of the review procedure could greatly speed the process with no risk. The staggering volume and notorious slowness of the requisite paperwork could be reduced by greater reliance on summaries and by efforts to speed the flow of paperwork both within the agency and between it and the companies. A significant amount of cooperative work will be needed from industry if the agency is to achieve greater efficiency through such measures.

REALISTIC STANDARDS OF EVIDENCE FOR EFFICACY

I doubt that there is a serious move in the U.S. to abolish the efficacy standard — that would be a retrograde step scientifically, medically, and politically. Current legal and regulatory requirements are satisfactory as *written* ; nevertheless, there is much in the FDA's actual requirements for proof of efficacy that so exceeds the legal definitions as to be unrealistic. Much unnecessary work could be eliminated by simply making the FDA adhere strictly to the 1962 legal definition of "substantial evidence" and to the agency's own 1970 regulations that define the "well-controlled clinical investigations" needed to supply such evidence[12, 13]. This involves no sacrifice of either safety or efficacy and can be supported without reservation.

ACCEPTANCE OF FOREIGN AND IRREGULAR DATA

In the past, there has been a real problem in assessing the validity of some studies done by unknown persons, in unfamiliar places, documented inadequately (or not at all), and analyzed in idiosyncratic ways. I believe that this problem is rapidly disappearing as efforts to raise standards of study design and reporting bear fruit. Such activities, undertaken by regulatory agencies at the national and international levels, by pharmaceutical companies and by academic and professional societies are reducing international differences through a general rise in scientific standards.

While some judgment will continue to be necessary to determine how much weight should be given to any particular study (including foreign studies), it is my impression that well-done studies are increasingly being evaluated according to their intrinsic merit regardless of source. If this trend does not proceed spontaneously, then specific regulatory attention should be given it.

The potential gain in regulatory efficiency from this development is considerable provided both the company and the agency structure their development and review plans to take maximum advantage of the opportunities. Similarly, the effect on safety can me made negligible by appropriate planning for the timely completion of any necessary supplemental studies.

IMPROVED ADMINISTRATIVE AND MANAGEMENT TECHNIQUES

HHS Secretary Schweiker has poposed a new procedure intended to facilitate the resolution of disputes and to make reviewers more accountable for correspondence with the company and for meeting deadlines[2]. These reasonable approaches offer some potential for improvment but only if sufficient personnel and other resources are available to the agency. There is no safety risk from implementation of this program.

POSTMARKETING ISSUES

Patent restoration

Products subject to premarket clearance requirements have experienced much erosion of their effective patent life ; in the case of new drugs marketed in the U.S. in 1979, the mean effective patent life had fallen to 9.5 years compared with the 17-year patent protection envisaged in the patent law[10]. Restoring patent life is an important incentive to innovation that carries no health risks for the consumer and should be pursued vigorously. The issue has been receiving considerable attention in Congress : a study has been requested from the Office of Technology Assessment and hearings have been held in both houses. A favorable report to the full Senate is likely from the Judiciary Committee where fifteen of the eighteen members have joined Senator Mathias in sponsoring S. 255, the Patent Term Restoration Act of 1981.

Postmarketing surveillance (PMS)

Dependable and effective PMS is the single most important requirement both for existing systems of drug development-and-approval and for many of the deregulation proposals considered above. Even those deregulation actions that are intrinsically safe could conceivably add some overall risk simply by causing earlier marketing of a new compound. A truly effective PMS system can forestall this and minimize existing and future problems of drug toxicity. The better the system, the more confident we can be that any undesirable incidents will be few and quickly handled.

But implementation of an effective PMS system faces a major obstacle at present : although PMS was officially envisaged as a substitute for excessive premarketing testing[14], no substitution has yet been achieved. The present PMS system is in real danger of becoming a burdensome add-on to the existing premarket requirements. The original objective can still be achieved if the trade-off is made explicit by specifying exactly what portions of the premarketing investigation process (e.g. all of Phase III) can be wholly or partially replaced by an adequate PMS system. To ensure that the PMS plan is adequate, it may be necessary to institute other safeguards such as voluntary marketing restraints designed in accordance with the particular PMS system chosen.

It would be beneficial to the overall drug development and approval process if new and workable approaches to PMS were devised and implemented by the companies themselves rather than by the regulatory agencies. Such efforts would not only be in the spirit of deregulation but could also help improve the unproductive, adversarial relationship that sometimes exists between regulatory agencies and industry. In the U.S., precedents for restrained promotion coupled with PMS include the initial marketing of L-Dopa, most anticancer drugs, azaribine, and certain prostaglandins.

CONCLUSIONS

As we have shown, some of the deregulation proposals are entirely risk-free ; patent restoration is the best example. The bulk of the proposals entail no *intrinsic* risk to the public and would result in earlier marketing by increasing the efficiency of the development and approval process. Any conceivable increase in risk that might arise from such earlier introduction can be minimized by adequate postmarketing surveillance.

Special, intensive PMS — perhaps combined with initial marketing restraints — may be necessary in some instances. This would be true particularly if several of the deregulation proposals were applied simultaneously to the same drug, yielding much earlier marketing approval.

Under the existing system, there is every reason for responsible companies to organize these safeguards themselves since the legal and financial penalties for failure are deservedly high. In the new era of deregulation (assuming it eventuates), companies must strive — with a firm sense of history and an awareness of past mistakes and their consequences — to avoid any suggestion of compromise with safety. In particular, they must act resolutely to apply and maintain the very highest standards of intensive

PMS — especially for new products in early marketing — and demonstrate that they can restrain marketing when public safety warrants. Deregulation is potentially one of the most important facilitators of drug development to appear in the last 20 years, but if mishandled it could set the pendulum swinging in the wrong direction for the rest of this century.

REFERENCES

1. Halperin J.A., "Pharmaceutical regulation in the 1980's — Predictions", speech presented at the 50th BPA Conference and Annual Meeting, New York, 26 February 1981.

2. Schweiker R.S., "Remarks", speech presented to the Pharmaceutical Manufacturers' Association, Boca Raton, Florida, 6 April 1981.

3. U.S. Congress, House, Subcommittee on Science, Research and Technology, *The Food and Drug Administration's Process for Approving New Drugs*, Report, 97th Congress, November 1980.

4. U.S. General Accounting Office, *FDA Drug Approval : A Lengthy Process that Delays the Availability of Important New Drugs*, Report to the Subcommittee on Science, Research and Technology, 28 May 1980.

5. Proposed scheme for exemption for certification of clinical trials. Letter to interested organizations from J.R. Long, Medicines Division, Department of Health and Social Services, United Kingdom, 17 April 1980 (MLX 125).

6. Wolfe S. and B. Gordon, Comments on the Drug Lag, Report submitted to Congressman H. Waxman about drug reform bills, 13 May 1980.

7. U.K. CTC exemption procedure now offical, *Scrip* **568**, 25 February 1981 (p. 3).

8. New U.K. exemption procedure means virtual end of CTS, *Scrip* **569**, 2 March 1981 (p. 5).

9. U.S., Department of Health, Education and Welfare, Food and Drug Administration, "Investigational and New Drug Regulations — Revisions — Concept Document", October 1979.

10. Eisman M.M. and W.M. Wardell, Incremental time study : an analysis of time spent in the development and approval of drugs for the U.S. market, *Economic Costs of FDA Regulations : A Set of Studies of Some Economic Effects of Food and Drug Administration Regulation of Human Pharmaceuticals*, Washington, D.C., Pharmaceutical Manufacturers' Association, March 1981, pp. 53-81.

11. U.S., Department of Health and Human Services, Food and Drug Administration, Bureau of Drugs, "New Drug Evaluation Project Briefing Book", March 1981.

12. Department of Health, Education and Welfare, Food and Drug Administration, "New Drug Regulations Under the Federal Food Drug, and Cosmetic Act", *Federal Register* **35**, 7250-53, 8 May 1970.

13. *United States Statutes at Large*, Vol. 76, In One Part, Washington, D.C., U.S. Government Printing Office, 1963, p. 781.

14. To be supplied.

Sécurité et médicaments (1982), pp. 41-50

Les grands médicaments d'hier auraient-ils franchi avec succès le barrage de la réglementation préclinique actuelle ?

P. DUCHENE-MARULLAZ

Pharmacologie Médicale, Faculté de Médecine, 28, place Henri Dunant,
63001 Clermont-Ferrand Cedex, France

Résumé — La réglementation pré-clinique telle qu'elle existe dans la plupart des pays crée un double et regrettable obstacle à l'innovation thérapeutique, l'un provenant des firmes pharmaceutiques, l'autre dépendant directement des autorités officielles.

Tout d'abord, étant donné le coût des essais exigés (de l'ordre de 6 à 10 millions de francs), on hésitera de plus en plus à pousser les molécules jusqu'au stade des essais cliniques. C'est ainsi que, dans les réunions successives qui précèdent de tels essais, il est beaucoup plus facile de jouer le rôle du cadre responsable et prudent qui met en garde contre certains inconvénients potentiels de la molécule, plutôt que celui de l'audacieux qui engagera la société à poursuivre les essais. Ce deuxième personnage a plus de chance que l'autre d'être démenti par les faits puisque seulement 17 p. 100 des molécules ayant fait l'objet d'essais cliniques parviendront à la commercialisation, c'est-à-dire jusqu'à la rentabilité financière.

Mais pour des raisons peut-être pas tellement différentes, crainte aussi d'être démenties par les faits, les autorités adoptent des attitudes de prudence de plus en plus marquées. Elles ne sauraient, sous peine d'être accusées de négligence, ignorer les progrès de la biologie, tout en étant le plus souvent dans l'incapacité de connaître la valeur prévisionnelle pour l'espèce humaine d'essais réalisés chez l'animal, voire sur la cellule ou un fragment de cellule. Si bien que, du fait des exigences actuelles, bien des grands médicaments d'hier — plusieurs exemples sont donnés — n'auraient pu franchir le double obstacle des réglementations elles-mêmes et de l'attitude de prudence qu'elles ont fait naître dans l'industrie pharmaceutique.

Dans la sélection des médicaments essentiels, établie par un comité d'experts de l'O.M.S.[1], on rencontre un certain nombre de produits très anciens. Ne figure-t-il pas, notamment, dans cette liste l'éphédrine, utilisée depuis plus de 5 000 ans en Chine avant que d'être introduite en 1924 dans la pharmacopée occidentale ? Mais on peut se demander si l'aspirine, la colchicine, la morphine, l'atropine, la chloroquine, la digitoxine etc., tous médicaments retenus par les experts sauraient satisfaire, en 1981, les exigences légales ? Toutefois, il importe de se poser une autre interrogation : est-ce que les laboratoires pharmaceutiques pousseraient ces produits jusqu'au stade où ils auraient à être examinés par les autorités ?

LES COMMISSIONS D'AGREMENT

Il n'est pas besoin de souligner combien les autorités responsables de la mise sur le marché des médicaments ont, depuis plusieurs années, accru leurs exigences.

Certes, une telle attitude est en partie la conséquence de connaissances scientifiques de plus en plus vastes. Mais elle découle surtout peut-être de l'importance des sentiments de responsabilité qu'éprouvent les membres des commissions vis-à-vis de leur propre conscience comme au regard de l'opinion publique.

Or, il est curieux de constater le manque d'indulgence et de compréhension de l'opinion publique en ce qui concerne le médicament ou, plus exactement, l'industrie pharmaceutique. On admet, tout en le déplorant, que l'automobile soit responsable de tant de drames. Or il n'y a pas de commission examinant si tel ou tel matériau, telles ou telles modifications techniques n'auraient pas été préférables pour la sécurité dans un nouveau modèle avant sa fabrication en grande série. On connaît désormais les dangers du tabac, dont pourtant l'industrie est, en France, un privilège d'Etat. L'alcoolisme représente, pour la santé publique, un gouffre budgétaire dont la profondeur plusieurs fois explorée n'a suscité aucune réaction des mass media. Le chirurgien bénéficie d'un privilège et d'un capital de confiance, refusé au médicament. C'est ainsi que les pontages coronariens se compliquent d'une mortalité qui est encore de l'ordre de 3 p. 100, pour un bénéfice que l'on a mis longtemps à mesurer. Mais un médicament, qui serait capable de guérir de façon totale et définitive la maladie coronarienne, ce à quoi la chirurgie ne prétend pas, en entraînant la mort d'une personne sur cent traitées, verrait-il le jour ? La réponse est forcément négative. Mais n'est-ce pas là une hypothèse à méditer par tous ?

L'esprit humain n'a-t-il pas une très grande tolérance et un certain fatalisme au regard des dangers bien connus et une méfiance systématique vis-à-vis des nouveautés ? Des incidents dans une centrale atomique seront relatés à la première page de tous les quotidiens du monde. Des morts dues à une explosion de gaz ou à une électrocution n'occuperont que quelques lignes du seul journal local et ne susciteront une émotion que dans l'entourage des victimes.

Dans un essai de carcinogenèse, le saccharose[2] a été pris comme référence pour l'étude d'un autre glucide. Or le nombre de cancers, développés au niveau des foies de souris traitées, a été significativement plus élevé que chez les témoins. Le fait a été signalé, oublié. En aurait-il été de même s'il s'était agi d'un médicament, voire d'un édulcorant ?

Alimenter des souris ou des rats avec des sardines grillées c'est accroître, là encore, de façon considérable le pourcentage de tumeurs[3]. Va-t-on pour cela cesser de pêcher les sardines, ou désormais les manger bouillies ?

Ainsi soumises à de telles pressions conscientes et inconscientes, les autorités gouvernementales redoublent de prudence ou s'entourent du maximum d'alibi et alors multiplient les exigences.

Toutefois, on est en droit de se demander si l'accroissement des précautions prises est totalement au bénéfice de la Santé Publique. Si l'on excepte la médecine vétérinaire, le médicament est fait pour l'homme malade. Or est-il raisonable de se baser systématiquement sur les seules réactions du rat ou du chien pour juger de l'opportunité d'essais chez l'homme ? Doit-on attendre que le produit soit inoffensif pour tout le règne animal, y compris le rhinocéros blanc de Ceylan, avant de l'essayer chez l'homme ? Faut-il envisager toutes les souches dans toutes les espèces ? Et quelle réponse choisir ? En théorie, les choses sont claires : celle de l'espèce dont la pharmacocinétique et les métabolites du produit considéré seront identiques à ce qui est observé chez l'homme. Mais pour combien de molécules la chose est-elle possible ? Intervient d'ailleurs le problème de la souche. Le N-méthyl N'-nitro N-nitrosoguanidine, produit des cancers d'estomac chez tous les rats de la souche ACI, mais aucun chez ceux de la souche Buffalo[3]. Encore faut-il que les réactions, la susceptibilité, la pathologie spontanée des espèces animales et des souches soient bien connues. C'est avec un tel argument que l'on continue à utiliser le chien Beagle. Or la valeur prévisionnelle pour l'espèce humaine des résultats obtenus est très souvent discutable ou indiscutablement mauvaise. De plus, il importe de faire attention au type d'aliments dont la composition, mais aussi la quantité, intervient de façon étonnante dans les variations de pourcentage de cancers[4].

N'existe-t-il pas de nombreux produits mieux tolérés par l'espèce humaine que par les espèces animales, habituellement utilisées dans les essais de toxicologie ? Cette possibilité est reconnue pour les médicaments du passé, est-elle vraiment offerte pour les nouveaux produits ? La phénylbutazone a d'abord été utilisée comme solvant de l'amidopyrine. Mais qui aurait osé l'employer chez l'homme, si les essais de toxicologie actuellement obligatoires avaient été préalablement exigés ? La meilleure tolérance de la phénylbutazone chez l'homme et constatée plus tard chez l'animal n'a-t-elle pas été un exemple sur lequel on s'est appuyé pour se permettre d'essayer d'autres antiinflammatoires ? Certes commercialiser un produit dangereux s'expose à des conséquences évidentes, préjudiciables pour le malade et qu'il est possible d'estimer en terme de dommages et intérêts. Mais comment apprécier le préjudice causé par l'abandon prématuré d'un produit mal supporté par telle ou telle souche de rat et qui aurait sauvé des vies humaines ? Il serait plus facile, certes, de mesurer les conséquences d'un retard à une commercialisation d'un produit ! Cependant qui tenterait de le faire en reprochant aux pouvoirs publics un excès de prudence ? Le fonctionnaire tatillon, qui aurait retardé le visa du thalidomide sous prétexte qu'à son avis les dossiers étaient trop pauvres en enregistrements électro-encéphalographiques, n'aurait-il pas quand même protégé la santé de son pays et mérité la reconnaissance de tous ?

LE PRIX ET LA DURÉE DES ESSAIS PRÉCLINIQUES

Les exigences, pour ne pas parler de surenchères, des commissions d'agrément entraînent des dépenses considérables d'argent et de temps. Il n'est d'ailleurs pas évident que tous les membres des dites commissions soient pleinement conscients de ce fait.

Ces dépenses d'argent éloignent peu à peu de la compétition les petites firmes dont pourtant les possibilités d'innovation sont loin d'être négligeables. Il est prévisible que, devant l'accroissement des sommes à dépenser, seules quelques firmes mondiales pourront subsister dans le futur. Certains esprits chagrins pensent d'ailleurs qu'il existe un semblant de complicité entre certaines administrations et quelques grands laboratoires pharmaceutiques mondiaux pour, en élevant le niveau de ces exigences, hâter cette évolution.

Aux U.S.A.[5], une étude préclinique chez l'animal revenait, en 1967, à 97 000 dollars et à 177 000 dollars en 1976. Or sur 100 produits faisant l'objet d'une étude de toxicité, 29 seulement permettent la poursuite des essais. D'ailleurs, sur 100 produits introduits en phase I, 50 atteignent la phase II et 19 la phase III. Toujours aux U.S.A.[5], qui bien souvent servent de référence en matière de médications, on estime qu'en moyenne la phase I ne dure que 9,1 mois mais que la phase II s'étend à 23,2 mois et que la phase III se prolonge 33,6 mois. La toxicologie seule pour le développement international d'un produit revient, en 1981, à plus de 9 millions de francs. Si l'on ajoute, à cela les délais des études pharmacologiques, les inévitables délais administratifs, le fait que l'indispensable protection par un brevet doit être assurée avant toute étude approfondie, on mesure la durée de l'aventure et la foi indispensable qu'il faut avoir dans le projet pour le mener à bien. Cela fait que le temps de protection de l'invention aura singulièrement raccourci et les réalisations faites pourront bientôt être partagées par les laboratoires qui exploiteront le produit comme générique.

LES LABORATOIRES DE RECHERCHE PHARMACEUTIQUE

L'ensemble de ces faits bien connus des responsables des laboratoires de recherche pharmaceutique est certainement un facteur de démobilisation des esprits. La prudence étouffe l'enthousiasme et inhibe les initiatives. Tout projet est soumis à l'examen de commissions successives, tout d'abord au sein même du centre de recherches. Quelle va être l'attitude d'un chercheur qui, après avoir vivement recommandé la poursuite des essais de différentes molécules, aura été successivement contrarié par les résultats de la toxicologie, de la tératologie ou des essais de reproduction chez l'animal ? Il est certain qu'une attitude de prudence dubitative expose à beaucoup moins de déboires. Proposer l'abandon d'un projet est bien loin d'engager autant la responsabilité que de pousser à sa poursuite malgré les aléas. Si un brevet a été pris ou une publication réalisée sur les premiers résultats, il est fort improbable qu'une autre firme s'empare de l'idée pour la pousser plus loin. Un démenti est donc pratiquement impossible. Il ne sera jamais donné et l'homme prudent ne sera jamais désavoué. Il sera considéré et promu à des postes de plus en plus grande responsabilité. Ainsi tout projet poussé trop loin et abandonné par la suite est une source de dépenses telles qu'il importe de savoir s'arrêter à temps. Cela explique les chemins de facilité parcourus par beaucoup, ceux sur lesquels on sait qu'il n'y a que peu de pièges et qui, en fait, amènent au unième dérivé propionique, au unième bêta-bloquant adrénergique et qui multiplient les "me too". Il est donc facile d'imaginer l'existence, dans les poubelles des centres de recherches ou parmi les brevets pris et jamais exploités, de molécules susceptibles de soulager certaines affections. Les motifs d'abandon auront été parfois une susceptibilité particulière de telle ou telle souche de rats, mais aussi le veto d'un département de marketing qui aura estimé les possibilités du marché insuffisantes pour couvrir la somme considérable de frais engagés ou à engager.

Tout cela est-il bien raisonnable ? Un des moyens de le savoir est de choisir certains grands produits du passé, toujours largement utilisés, et de les considérer à la lumière des exigences actuelles.

QUELQUES DOSSIERS DE GRANDS MÉDICAMENTS ANCIENS

L'aspirine

On connaît le succès commercial de l'aspirine, dont la vente dans le monde a atteint 33 250 tonnes en 1977. L'acide acétyl salicylique est apparu en 1899, l'acide salicylique avait été extrait en 1844 et préparé par synthèse en 1860. Toutefois, les salycilates que l'on trouve en abondance dans l'écorce, les feuilles et les fruits de beaucoup d'arbres et de plantes étaient utilisés en thérapeutique depuis la plus haute antiquité. C'est ainsi que les Phéniciens employaient couramment l'écorce de saule pour combattre la fièvre. On en trouve mention dans les aphorismes d'Hippocrate rédigés il y a quelques 2 400 ans comme dans les écrits de Galien datant du IIe siècle de notre ère.

On connaît les effets secondaires provoqués par l'aspirine : irritation de la muqueuse gastrique, à l'origine de saignements le plus souvent occultes, beaucoup plus rarement syndrome d'hypersensibilité pouvant entraîner la mort par œdème laryngé ou collapsus cardiovasculaire. Toutefois, les conclusions formulées par un groupe de travail en 1977[6], après avoir examiné toutes les publications parues et avoir mis en balance les avantages et les inconvénients de cette thérapeutique, ont été que «Aspirin is a safe and effective popular antalgic when given at the recommended doses of 325 to 650 mg every 4 hours». Toutefois, de telles conclusions n'ont pu être réalisées qu'après 90 ans d'utilisation clinique intensive.

Il importe donc d'imaginer le chemin qu'aurait à parcourir l'acide acétyl salicylique si on proposait cette molécule successivement au pharmacologue, au toxicologue avant de la présenter aux autorités d'enregistrement.

Au cours d'un screening pharmacologique, le produit serait soumis notamment à des tests permettant de retenir les produits analgésiques et anti-inflammatoires. Comme méthode d'étude des analgésiques, les techniques de la plaque chauffante ou celle des torsions induites par injection intrapéritonéale de phénylbenzoquinone, chez la souris, sont très généralement utilisées. Dans la première, la dose efficace 50 (DE_{50} de l'aspirine, donnée per os, est de 800 mg/kg contre 75 pour l'aminopyrine, 30 pour la codéïne, 5 pour le dextromoramide. Dans la seconde, la DE_{50} de l'aspirine est de 100 mg/kg contre 13 pour la glaphénine, 12 pour la codéïne, 9 pour l'aminopyrine. Quand on sait que la DL_{50} de l'aspirine est de 1 100 mg/kg, il est vraisemblable que le produit ne serait pas retenu comme analgésique par le pharmacologue.

Pour reconnaître les anti-inflammatoires, différentes méthodes sont classiquement utilisées par tous. Dans l'oédème induit par la carragénine sur la patte du rat, la DE_{50} de l'aspirine est de 200 mg/kg contre 25 pour la phénylbutazone, 5 pour le kétoprofen et 3,5 pour l'indométacine. L'aspirine est inactive dans le granulome provoqué par un pellet de coton introduit sous la peau du rat, alors que les DE_{50} sont de 5 mg/kg pour le kétoprofen et de 0,1 mg/kg pour l'indométacine. Dans le modèle de polyarthrite créé par injection d'adjuvant de Freund, les traitements étant réalisés pendant plusieurs cemaines, la DE_{50} est de 200 mg/kg pour l'aspirine contre 25 mg/kg pour la phénylbutazone, 2,5 mg/kg pour le kétoprofen, 0,5 mg/kg pour l'indométacine. Ainsi, dans l'état actuel de nos méthodes, il est plus que vraisemblable que le pharmacologue ne recommanderait pas la poursuite des essais concernant cette molécule considérée comme peu active.

En admettant qu'il en soit allé de façon différente, le toxicologue aurait souligné combien le chien supportait mal ce produit. En tératologie, il aurait été montré que 250 mg/kg donnés à des rats du 7e au 10e jours de la gestation, entraînaient 23,8 p. 100 de malformations chez des sujets nourris à satiété mais 95,8 p. 100 lorsqu'une restriction alimentaire était associée[8]. De plus, 200 mg/kg administrés durant les six derniers jours de la gestation provoquent un retard à la mise bas et des dystocies pouvant créer des morts in utero[9]. Il est vrai que l'on sait qu'il en va ainsi avec tous les inhibiteurs de la prostaglandine synthétase.

Donc l'acide acétyl salicylique se présente comme une molécule faiblement active, dont la DE_{50} est, dans quelques tests, très proche de la dose léthale, mal supportée par certaines espèces animales et susceptible d'entraîner des malformations chez le rongeur nouveau-né. Ainsi il semble bien, qu'en 1981, l'aspirine n'aurait pas obtenu d'autorisation de mise sur le marché, non pas parce qu'elle aurait été rejetée par les autorités compétentes mais parce que les promesses d'efficacité apparaîtraient trop faibles devant l'investissement financier à réaliser et les effets secondaires à redouter.

Les psychotropes

L'histoire de la découverte de la chlorpromazine est, désormais, bien connue grâce, notamment, au livre de Judith P. Swazey, fruit d'une enquête mondiale sérieuse et bien documentée[10].

Le pouvoir anthelminthique de la phénothiazine, décrit par Harwood en 1938 a été largement utilisé en médecine vétérinaire. Il était donc normal de travailler autour de cette structure. Deux équipes, l'une américaine, l'autre française, se fixent indépendamment l'une de l'autre le but de préparer de nouveaux antiparasitaires. L'échec et l'abandon de cette voie de recherche par les américains, en 1944, restent ignorés de l'équipe française qui dévia de l'objectif initial pour s'orienter vers la préparation d'antihistaminiques. La découverte de la prométhazine vint couronner cet effort. Mais, lors de l'utilisation clinique, les effets sédatifs et hypnogènes de cette nouvelle médication, plus importants que ceux présents par les précédents antihistaminiques, devaient être soulignés. Cette constatation devait orienter les recherches vers la préparation de dérivés de la phénothiazine possédant, en dehors de toute activité antihistaminique, une forte activité centrale. Ce programme devait aboutir à la découverte de la chlorpromazine, synthétisée en décembre 1950. Il faut noter que les premières études pharmacologiques se sont poursuivies de décembre 1950 à avril 1951, que les premières études cliniques se sont situées entre avril et septembre 1951 et que le largactil a été mis à la disposition du corps médical en France en décembre 1952 dans de vastes indications puisque comprenant la psychiatrie, l'anesthésiologie, les vomissements. Entre temps,

Laborit et Huguenard soulignaient, le 13 février 1952, l'intérêt du produit en anesthésiologie réanimation ; Delay, Deniker et Harl, le 26 mai 1952, les perspectives ouvertes en psychiatrie. Les laboratoires S.K.F. devaient introduire la chlorpromazine sur le marché américain en mai 1954 sous le nom de Thorazine. Il s'est donc écoulé deux ans entre la synthèse du produit et sa commercialisation, deux ans seulement, le temps désormais demandé pour une seule toxicité chronique, quatre ans si l'on considère le marché américain. Les études de toxicité, réalisées par la suite chez le rat et le chien pendant des durées relativement courtes, ne devaient pas faire apparaître d'anomalies susceptibles, si elles avaient été réalisées plus tôt, d'empêcher les essais cliniques. La chlorpromazine ne devait pas, non plus, se révéler tératogène chez l'animal bien que certains auteurs aient signalé la persistance de fentes palatines chez la souris.

L'histoire de la chlorpromazine est donc tout à fait "convenable". Il s'agit d'un produit qui serait encore retenu par les comités scientifiques, les centres de recherches pharmaceutiques, accepté par les toxicologues, reconnu par les cliniciens selon le même enchaînement de circonstances que celui vécu, et pour lequel une autorisation de mise sur le marché serait certainement accordée. Mais ce n'est là qu'une probabilité statistique et non pas une certitude absolue. En effet, car deux firmes américaines, contactées avant que S.K.F. ne le soit, avaient rejeté le produit. Dans l'une d'elles, la raison invoquée avait été «because the management didn't want to gamble on a new drug that had no clear-cut marketing areas with large sales potential». C'est souligner, si besoin en était, la toute-puissance du management.

Sans le succès de la chlorpromazine, aurions-nous eu des antidépresseurs ? La pharmacologie-fiction est un art difficile, mais la réponse semble bien devoir être négative. C'est l'étroite parenté chimique entre l'imipramine et la chlorpromazine qui a fait essayer en clinique, là encore sans précaution toxicologique exagérée, un produit dont le profil pharmacodynamique n'était guère enthousiasmant : un peu antihistaminique, un peu sédatif à fortes doses. Seul le génie intuitif de Kuhn, constatant l'aggravation de l'état des psychotiques l'a fait utiliser dans les dépressions nerveuses et surtout peut-être avoir la patience d'attendre les 2 à 3 semaines nécessaires pour que l'efficacité se manifeste. Que se serait-il passé, si l'on avait suivi la filière aujourd'hui obligatoire ? Un toxicologue prudent n'aurait-il pas arrêté tout projet parce que le produit à la dose de 20 mg/kg i.v., c'est-à-dire à cinq fois seulement la dose thérapeutique, entraîne des convulsions graves chez le chien ?

Divers produits[11]

L'atropine est le seul antispasmodique sélectionné parmi les médicaments essentiels. Les doses thérapeutiques sont de l'ordre de 0,5 à 1 mg. Or ce n'est pas pour rien que Linné dénomma la belladone, dont l'atropine est un des alcaloïdes, "Atropa belladonna" du nom d'Atropos, la plus âgée des trois Parques, celle chargée de couper le fil de vie. Dès la dose de 2 mg, des effets secondaires gênants apparaissent. Des hallucinations, des délires, un coma s'installent pour une posologie égale ou à peine supérieure à 10 mg. Qui voudrait désormais d'un produit dont la dose léthale est à peu près dix fois la dose thérapeutique ?

Qui, selon les normes actuelles, oserait proposer d'essayer *la colchicine* dans le traitement de la goutte, ainsi que le fit Von Störck en 1763 ? Voici un produit qui n'a aucun effet analgésique, qui n'influence pas l'excrétion de l'acide urique et qui ne fait qu'inhiber la migration des polynucléaires dans un foyer inflammatoire. Les comprimés sont à 1 mg. On conseille trois comprimés le premier jour, soit 3 mg, alors qu'à la dose de 7 mg, on a pu observer des accidents mortels. La F.D.A. aurait-elle permis à Benjamin Franklin d'introduire ce produit aux U.S.A. ?

La chloroquine est le résultat d'un effort poursuivi lors du dernier conflit mondial. Il s'agissait donc de trouver des médicaments efficaces contre le paludisme. Elle fait partie d'une large série de 4-aminoquinolines. Dix d'entre elles, après des essais sommaires de pharmacologie chez l'oiseau infecté et de toxicologie chez le rat, ont fait l'objet d'épreuves de pharmacologie clinique que le climat de guerre autorisait. Des volontaires avaient accepté d'être inoculés avec du plasmodium falciparum. La chloroquine, retenue à l'issue de cette épreuve, a largement été utilisée depuis. On devait découvrir qu'en fait la molécule avait déjà été synthétisée et étudiée dès 1934 par les allemands sous le nom de Résochin. Mais on devait s'apercevoir aussi que la valeur de la DL_{50} de la chloroquine, chez le chien, était sensiblement la même que celle de la dose thérapeutique : 20 mg/kg. Et si l'on avait suivi les recommandations actuellement imposées ? Il faut, en effet, rappeler qu'une administration a longtemps retardé et freiné encore l'usage dans son pays d'un antagoniste des mouvements du calcium parce qu'il entraîne des cataractes chez le chien Beagle. Or, ce produit est sur le marché thérapeutique depuis plus de dix ans, dans la vieille Europe, sans qu'aucun accident oculaire n'ait été signalé.

L'acétaminophène ou *paracétamol* est utilisé en thérapeutique depuis 1893. Mais sa vogue comme antalgique a sourtout commencé en 1949, quand il a été reconnu comme étant le principal métabolite à la fois de l'acétanilide et de la phénacétine. Produit souvent considéré sans danger, en vente libre dans bien des pays, il provoque à doses toxiques des nécroses hépatiques, des nécroses tubulaires, des comas hypoglycémiques. Une consommation trop importante en quantité ou en durée peut entraîner chez l'homme une anémie hémolytique. La dose thérapeutique est d'environ 60 mg/kg/jour. Or, à 200 mg/kg/j, le paracétamol tue tous les chiens d'anémie hémolytique[12]. Qui accepterait désormais de poursuivre des essais avec un produit, dont l'activité pharmacologique comme le coefficient de sécurité chez le chien sont si faibles ?

La phénylbutazone et autres anti-inflammatoires. On sait que la phénylbutazone a été tout d'abord utilisée comme solvant de l'aminopyrine. Mais il est très vraisemblable que, dans le contexte actuel, le produit ne serait pas poussé très loin lors des essais précliniques. On peut d'ailleurs se demander si un autre anti-inflammatoire, très utilisé dans le monde entier, serait proposé à l'enregistrement. Il s'agit d'une molécule dont la DL_{50} est, chez le rat, 3 fois supérieure à la dose thérapeutique, dont la dose maximale tolérée en administration chronique, chez le chien, est 1,9 fois cette dose ; un effet embryotoxique apparaît à 2,6 fois la posologie utilisée chez l'homme. Il semble que, devant l'efficacité clinique et la relativement bonne tolérance dans l'espèce humaine, le produit obtiendrait les autorisations nécessaires pour une commercialisation. Mais il a été dit que les responsables actuels de la firme concernée ne prendraient plus le risque d'essais chez l'homme.

Toutefois, on sait désormais combien les anti-inflammatoires sont, de façon générale, beaucoup mieux tolérés par l'homme que par l'animal. Mais comment le sait-on ? Tout simplement parce que les essais thérapeutiques ont été réalisés avant que la lourdeur administrative ait été mise en place, avant que l'on soit devenu trop savant.

CONCLUSIONS

Ainsi, il apparaît que bien des médicaments du passé, dont l'efficacité reste tout à fait actuelle, ne seraient plus maintenant à la disposition des malades. L'obstacle serait vraisemblablement beaucoup plus venu des firmes pharmaceutiques elles-mêmes que des commissions d'enregistrement. L'homme est un animal unique. L'efficacité et la tolérance d'un médicament destiné à notre espèce ne peuvent, en réalité, être connues qu'après utilisation chez l'homme. Les responsables, qu'ils travaillent dans l'industrie ou au sein des commissions officielles, doivent se garder de deux dangers opposés : le premier serait de permettre l'utilisation de produits sans grande efficacité, ou plus encore de produits dangereux pour le malade ; le second serait de freiner l'initiative, d'empêcher les progrès thérapeutiques alors que trop de maladies encore demeurent invaincues, d'oublier que les modèles animaux n'ont qu'une valeur prévisionnelle limitée et que, finalement, beaucoup de progrès thérapeutiques n'ont été que le fait de chance, de hasard ou d'intuition, quand cela n'a pas été de fausses prévisions. Mais, généralement, ils ont été issus d'essais faits chez l'homme.

Ainsi, être médecin de l'industrie pharmaceutique est un métier difficile. Mais qui, à part lui-même, pourrait le savoir ?

Remerciements — Nous tenons à remercier vivement le Docteur Vétérinaire JULOU de l'aide cordiale qu'il a bien voulu apporter à la préparation de ce texte.

REFERENCES

1. *La sélection des médicaments essentiels*, second rapport du comité d'experts de l' O.M.S., série de rapports techniques 641, Genève, O.M.S., 1980.

2. Edited transcripted of Dr Arje Scheihin's speech to the C.D.A. convention in Quebec city on September 12, 1979.

3. Sugimura T., The Rationalization of the Interpretation of Animal Carcinogenesis Experiments, rapport présenté au Eight International Congress of Pharmacology, Tokyo, 19-24 July 1981.

4. Roe F.J. and J.J. Tucker, "Recent developments in the design of carcinogenicity . Tests on laboratory animals", proceedings of the European Society for the Study of Drug Toxicity, *Excerpta Med.* **15** (1974), 171-77.

5. Hansen R.W., "The pharmaceutical development process : estimates of development costs and time and the effects of proposed regulatory changes", *in : Issues in pharmaceutical economics*, R.I. Chien ed., Lexington Books, D.C. Heath & Company, 1979.

6. Analgesics, *Federal Register* **42**, 131 (1977), 35 381-412.

7. Tous les résultats pharmacodynamiques sont issus du CERM (Riom — France) et du laboratoire de Pharmacologie médicale (Faculté de médecine, 63001 Clermont-Ferrand Cedex).

8. Beall J.R. and M.F. Klein, Enhancement of Aspirin-Induced Teratogenicity by Food Restriction in Rats, cité dans *Federal Register*.

9. Tuchmann-Duplessis H., D. Hiss, G. Mottot and I. Rosner, Effects of prenatal administration of acetyl salicylic acid in rats, *Toxicology* **3** (1975), 207-11.

10. Swazey, Chlorpromazine in Psychiatry : A Study of Therapeutic Innovation, Cambridge, Mass. & London, MIT Press, 1974.

11. Goodmann and Gilman's, "The pharmacological basis of therapeutics" *in* : A. Goodmann-Gilman, L.S. Goodmann and A. Gilman eds, New York, McMillan, 1980.

12. Conquet P., communication personnelle.

Sécurité et médicaments (1982), pp. 51-53

The International Transfer of Information Regarding Drug Safety : Benefits, Difficulties and Solutions*

J. F. DUNNE

Senior Medical Officer Pharmaceuticals, W.H.O., 1211 Geneve 27, Switzerland

Abstract — For many years, the research-based pharmaceutical industry has been organized on an international basis, whereas drug regulation remains firmly entrenched in the national domain. Public health considerations demand that adequate information on the benefits and risks of pharmaceutical products in international circulation should be accessible wherever they are available. On the other hand, national drug regulatory authorities, in their capacity as trustees of privileged information, have a clear obligation to ensure confidentiality operates to protect legitimate commercial interests.

In many countries resources do not exist to enable the State to commission an independent review of all products marketed under their aegis. Dependable information from external sources then becomes essential to the development of any meaningful system of drug control.

Over the years, a series of resolutions has been passed by the governing bodies of WHO and by the UN General Assembly itself that aims to promote freer exchange of information concerning the safety and efficacy of pharmaceutical products moving in international commerce. Recent developments relevant to these resolutions will be reviewed.

Within a healthy, vigorous and socially conscious society, drug safety can readily be portrayed as an emotive issue, but the sick are likely to take a more indulgent view. There can be no serious doubt that, within the developed world, medicine has been remarkably well served by pharmaceutical innovation over the past fifty years, and it is mandatory to make that point whenever attention is centred upon drug-induced injury. This is said, of course, not to underplay the impact of the emotive drug-induced tragedies that have forcefully sensitised public opinion over the general question of drug safety, nor unreservedly to endorse contemporary trends in new drug development, but rather to establish the fact that modern synthetic drugs are characteristically potent biologically-active compounds that have an inherent potential to produce unwanted as well as beneficial effects. Society is bound to accept a measure of risk as the price for therapeutic progress, but it has a right to assume that professional skills will be dutifully applied to minimize the hazards.

Given this situation it is axiomatic that risks identified in the use of drugs should be

* Opinions expressed in this article are personal and do not necessarily represent offical policy of the World Health Organization

appreciated at the earliest possible juncture everywhere that they are used. The need for unconstrained flow of information on the safety and efficacy of drugs is accepted without reservation at national level, and it is self-evident that an identical need exists internationally. The same basic range of products is used worldwide, although only the more affluent of the developed nations command the resources to undertake an entirely independent assessment of their benefits and risks. Indeed, virtually every country is in some measure dependent upon external sources of information in implementing drug control policies.

The importance of effective intergovernmental exchange of relevant information has been recognized from the time the W.H.O. constitution was adopted in 1946, but the frequency with which Member States have subsequently adopted resolutions calling for implementation of these provisions suggests that their fulfilment is not readily realised. W.H.O. is notified of the circumstances in which drugs are withdrawn from national markets in only a proportion of cases, even when safety is at issue. In part, this reflects the fact that no formal regulatory action is taken in many instances. The preference of manufacturers to assume the initiative in withdrawing products voluntarily in the face of administrative pressure is understandable, but public health considerations are not advanced when this compromises international channels of communication.

Understandings on confidentiality of information also have relevance. Regulatory authorities operate within a framework of national law. Their international obligations are rarely defined by statute, and they are further constrained in inter-communication because they operate as privileged trustees of commercial information. Without a clear exposition of their discretionary powers, agencies are bound to adopt a cautious stance over disclosure of information.

Whereas protection of property rights demands respect for confidentiality within governmental agencies that have privileged access to restricted information, an untenable conflict of interest arises when this impedes communication between countries on substantive public health issues. Fortunately, however, implementation of the 1976 Freedom of Information Act in the United States of America has shown that the situation is amenable to effective compromise. Private property rights are still rigorously observed in the USA and confidentiality of information of commercial value remains protected. Nonetheless, substantial information on the safety and efficacy of drugs registered by the Food and Drug administration is now in the public domain without any apparent untoward erosion of commercial interests.

These legal provisions are singled out because they have exerted influence internationally, and particularly because they constitute an important precedent that several other countries now seem set to follow. In the meantime, however, W.H.O. needs to respond without delay to the demands of drug-importing countries for adequate information on the quality, safety and efficacy of all drugs in international commerce. Resolutions persuing this aim have been adopted not only by the Organization's own governing bodies, but most recently within the United Nations General Assembly itself. One possibility is to canvas countries to accept an extension of the provisions of the existing W.H.O. Drug Certification Scheme in which 71 nations, including virtually all the major manufacturing countries, now participate. At present, the scheme is concerned dominantly with assurance of quality through the provision of a Certificate issued, at the request of the importing country, by the regulatory authority of the exporting country. If these countries were also to provide an officially approved product control document, such as the data sheet or package insert, the importing country would immediately have a tangible basis for checking labelling and advertising claims. No administrative or political difficulties are apparent ; nonetheless, the suggestion is entirely speculative and formal consultation with both Member States and the official representatives of the pharmaceutical industry would be required should the proposal ever be taken further.

Meanwhile, plans are already in hand to create a formal international mechanism by which communication between national drug regulatory authorities may be facilitated. Senior officials from several representative countries have already been engaged in consultations to this end, and a recommendation has emerged for the creation of an Advisory Committee on Drug Information and Regulation. The primary objective of this body would be to promote an echange of information on the efficacy and safety of drugs between regulatory authorities ; it would operate under the aegis of W.H.O., and its members would be drawn from officials responsible for the technical aspects of drug assessment within the regulatory authority of each Member State.

The potential size of the Committee would preclude regular meetings but its promulgation would provide an international panel of officials that could subserve a vital liaison function provided effective administrative procedures can be developed. A cardinal principle accepted by all those involved is that regulatory officials should themselves contribute to the administrative apparatus through a Steering Committee that would encourage all countries actively to participate in the collaborative effort.

The formation of such a body would inevitably lead to a more precise and generally-accepted definition of the national commitment to intercommunication in the drug sector, and it would provide importing countries with a forum from which they could better establish their informational needs. There is every hope that the pharmaceutical industry might come to regard such a development with approbation rather than suspicion particularly if other issues such as the harmonization of regulatory requirements were brought into focus.

Reservations over innovations of this nature are bound to be voiced, despite confidence that the vast majority of drugs widely used in medicine today are established securely enough to withstand any degree of unbiased public scrutiny. The investment that has been directed to drug monitoring at both national and international levels over the past decade offers a reassuring analogy since the results have operated more to allay unfounded concerns than to identify unanticipated hazards. In the absence of these data banks it would be virtually impossible to dispel doubts, for example, that the long-term adverse effects of practolol might be shared by other beta-adrenergic blocking agents. One can only hope that, as memories of thalidomide retreat from consciousness, drug monitoring will not be allowed to regress under the pressure of strained economic circumstances.

There is no difficulty, of course, in taking an assured stand from a position of detachment on the need for increased accessibility to information on the safety of drugs. However, there can surely be little doubt that open and candid handling of these data is of prime importance not only to standards of public health, but also to the public image of the international pharmaceutical industry.

Sécurité et médicaments (1982), pp. 55-62

Ethical Considerations in Drug Safety Evaluation

Michael P. HAMILTON

Canon, Washington Cathedral, Mt St Alban, Washington DC 20016, USA

Abstract — This paper discusses the contemporary social context for ethical choices regarding research and marketing of drugs, and identifies the major conflicting forces involved. The ethical decision points in the conduct of clinical trials are identified, and the role of non-medical members in policy review boards is examined. Some of the difficult moral issues involved in testing and marketing of drugs in non-industrial countries are discussed, and the paper ends with some suggestions for the long-term care and feeding of pharmaceutical doctors.

In our time of rapid technological and cultural change, it is sometimes helpful to listen to a lay person — someone outside your professional community — speak on how the developments within your profession are viewed by the larger world. It is ethical implications of the developments within your work that I shall be discussing today, and I hope you will find the experience worthwhile, not too painful and perhaps even enjoyable at times.

First, permit me to tell a story to show you a simple means by which you can make the crucial distinction between what should be changed within your practice of pharmacy and what will inevitably abide. It is a true story concerning Winston Churchill during World War II :

> One evening at a small dinner party, as was his custom, Churchill drank a considerable amount of wine and liquor. He was preoccupied with this own thoughts when the lady on his right, in disgust at his unsociable behavior, turned to him and said, "Mr. Prime Minister, you are drunk !" Churchill slowly turned around to face her and replied, "I know. However, you are ugly, and tomorrow I will be sober !"

I suggest our society has changed and the former naive trust in the benefits of scientific research has dissipated. It is not necessary for me to describe the environmental dangers which have accompanied industrialization, the perils of atomic war attendant on the discovery of nuclear fission, nor the political and social temptations of manipulating the DNA-RNA genetic mechanisms, for we are all too familiar with both the hopes and anxieties these technologies have produced. If the general public was ignorant of the inevitable, costly implications of technological development, then scientists were unconcerned about the political and social implications of their research. There was a time when scientists said that they felt no responsability for how society might use their discoveries and that they had no obligation to assist in assessing the moral implications of what they were doing. However, those attitudes of mind became untenable after the destruction of Hiroshima.

In this paper I shall be using illustrations primarily drawn from American experience, but the underlying principles, I believe, are recognizable elsewhere. In the United States particular events have contributed to a public skepticism regarding political and scientific leadership. Thus, the significant loss of faith in the wisdom and integrity of leadership came as a result of both the follies of the Vietnam War and the corruption revealed by the Watergate crisis.

Similar skepticism has developed in the field of medical research due to such publicized scandals as the non-treatment of syphilitic research patients at the Tuskegee Institute and cancer-cell injections given to unsuspecting old people by physicians of the Sloan-Kettering Institute. The most serious, the thalidomide tragedy, has frightened and angered us all.

In response the American public, characteristically activist, has produced a "Consumerism Movement" which demands both information about, involvement in, and review of the decision-making processes in much medical research and regulation. Hitherto, these matters were left largely to medical professionals. For us to discuss whether the public should be involved in medical policy in the United States would be futile. Americans insist on being involved. The task is to learn how this public influence can be most creatively exercised without adding unproductive bureaucratic regulations.

I will also be discussing matters which are central to the work of the pharmacists and some matters which arise when they are members of a research team or are a link in the production and marketing process. In both areas, how you use your influence on future policy, be it large or small, is the responsibility I want you to reflect on today.

CONFLICT OF INTEREST IN RESEARCH

Within this context of continuing hope regarding the benefits of modern technology mixed with disillusionment over its disappointments, there arise a number of ethical problems in drug research and marketing. Rather than just list and comment on them, I would like to go to a deeper level and attempt to identify the underlying conflicts of interest from which particular ethical problems arise.

In the field of drug research there is inevitably a conflict of priorities between the investigator (pharmacist, physician, or scientist), the patient or subject, and the source of funding. The institution which funds the research is concerned in finding cheaply, and as soon as possible, a reliable, positive answer to the treatment hypothesis so that it can enhance its reputation and profit from the production and sales of the drug.

The medical investigator as scientist is curious about the validity of the research hypothesis, impatient to enhance his status amongst his peers by publishing his findings, and concerned for the welfare of the individual enrolled in the research. Individual doctors will vary their emphasis among these three goals from one piece of research to another. The temptation for the investigator is to play down the danger of the discomforts visited upon the subjects so that enrollment can be as quick and as easy as possible. Naturally, he does not appreciate having his time consumed by review procedures and regulation requirements.

The patient's concern is to be cured with as little financial cost or personal inconvenience as possible. Thus, if the patient is in a drug trial, he would prefer being the recipient of the new drug being tested rather than receiving the normal treatment or a placebo. The patient is in a highly dependent state. He may be sick and wishes to please, as much as possible, the doctor upon whom he hopes his cure will come. While he may fear experimentation, he probably fears even more the disapproval of his physician. He is not in the best position to assess the scientific soundness of the research, the adequacy of the consent form, or the ethical character of the whole venture.

From this *resume* of the different perspectives, the different elements of self-interest which are present within the parties to medical research, one can easily see the ethical problems which result. In no way am I condemning the investigator, the donor or the patient for having conflicting self-interests. If anything is to be condemned, it is unwillingness to face up to them and modify them when community welfare or individual rights require. Even when the conflicts are apparent, there is no totally satisfactory way of resolving them. For example, we must trust donors of research funds not to corrupt professionals and academic consultants by giving them large honoraria for many contracts so that the independent nature of their judgement is threatened.

In the United States it is legally mandated that for all government-funded research an Institutional Review Committee be established to pass, recommend changes in, or table each protocol. Membership includes not only medical and sometimes statistical personnel, but also at least one representative from the public. The latter is usually a minister, priest, social worker or lawyer. The importance of this non-medical person has been considerable because he or she has none of the inhibiting self-interests, previously outlined, of the other parties to the research. He does not need to be cured, he is not paying any bills and he is not employed full-time by any of the parties. While his competence does not extend to making judgements on the merits of medical and scientific research, he can ensure that the consent form is plainly written and includes all the information regarding risks and dangers which are mentioned in the protocol.

Physicians are usually overworked and undereducated. The world comes to you on your terms because of its medical needs. However, lay representatives come to you on their terms and they have different, if not broader, perspectives than you on the conduct of your research. After the initial period of anger amongst physicians that these outsiders were being forced upon them, recent interdisciplinary evaluations of the lay representatives and the function of the Institutional Review Boards have been favorable[1].

ETHICAL ISSUES IN CLINICAL DRUG TRIALS

Because clinical drug trials play such an important role in pharmaceutical research, I would like to pay special attention to the ethical issues which arise in double-blind, randomized, clinical trials. I am a strong supporter of these trials and believe that good science is good ethics, and that inadequately planned research is necessarily unethical because it can produce misleading results which cause harm in consequent therapy. There is no better substitute for unbiased research than clinical trials for evaluation of both old remedies and new preparations.

Clinical trials, of course, can only take place ethically when there is sufficient uncertainty about the therapeutic value of the new drugs or when doubts arise regarding the efficacy or harm caused by traditional therapy. Once the trial is started, it is essential that recruitment and randomization continue until a statistically reliable result has come to light. If during the course of the trial one form of treatment appears to be more successful than the other, but still has not reached that critical point of reliability, recruitment must continue. Anyone familiar with the progress of clinical trials knows that both positive and negative trends can arise by chance during the course of the trial. It is not only bad science but also unethical to change the procedures (particularly that of randomization) before that degree of reliability, which was the prior goal of the experiment, has been reached. In this connection it is useful to have a separate committee composed of people who are not themselves investigators to monitor the incoming data and to inform the blinded investigators when a reliable conclusion has been reached so that the trial may be halted. This committee, often called a "Data Safety Committee", can also monitor the conduct of the trial to see if serious side-effects are occuring. They have the key to learn who receives the drug and who receives the placebo and therefore, they alone are in the position to know when harm is being done and when the trial should be halted.

Of course, in addition to these special problems, clinical trials raise the familiar ethical issues in research. These include the evaluation of risk versus benefits, the appropriate dosage and its interactions with other medications, the adequacy of the consent form, the need for prior animal tests before the drug is given to humans, and the avoidance of selection of a patient population which is socially discriminatory.

Incidently, the patient can also fall into unethical behavior. For instance, if for financial or therapeutic reasons he wants to be a subject in an investigation or trial, he may withhold information about his health which would inhibit his enrollment. Such a deception resulted in a death during a National Institutes of Health sponsored sleep study in 1980.

THE MARKETING AND USE OF DRUGS

Turning to the marketing and use of drugs, I will identify some major conflicts of interest underlying the ethical issues.

First there is the desire of the drug company to maximize its profits while maintaining its public status of being trustworthy and responsible. There is the concern of most governments to avoid abuses in advertising, the protection of citizens from undue risks in using drugs, and the need to learn side-effects of drugs both during the research and marketing stages. The interest of the patient is to have access to drugs of reliable quality which are truly therapeutic and available at affordable prices. The dispensing pharmacist is concerned for an adequate financial return on his or her labor while ensuring that the patient's health be maintained through proper prescribing. The physician shares most of these concerns, and in addition has his own prescribing "habits" which govern his practice.

There is an occasional and serious conflict of interest arising when practicing physicians have a financial interest or ownership of dispensing pharmacies. I do not believe this practice can be ethical and it should be forbidden by law. The temptations are just too great for such physicians to adjust their prescribing orders to financial profit as opposed to the welfare of their patients. Informing the patients of this conflict of interest is not sufficient protection, for many patients would neither understand the significance of the conflict, nor be sufficiently emotionally independant of their personal physician to question his prescribing judgement.

The role of the pharmaceutical physician with his expert knowledge is crucial in areas of marketing and drug use. As in research procedures (either as an investigator or member of a review board) when advising clinicians, his judgement on dosage, interaction with other drugs and their side-effects are of prime importance in prescribing treatment.

The pharmacist is the resource for information on drugs and the problem, which is so difficult to solve, is how best he can communicate his knowledge to others around him. The family doctor needs up-to-date information on drugs, but as often as not it comes to him more from manufacturers' literature and representatives than from learned journals or a professional pharmacist. Misleading drug advertising is the bane of drug promotion and sours the practice of medicine in the minds of both doctors and patients. While government regulation of advertising is the major means of achieving the necessary degree of honesty, the pharmacist has also much that he or she can do. Pharmacists can organize educational conferences at local hospitals and make as many friendly relationships with prescribing doctors as possible which not only helps promote good business, but also can be the channel by which errors in prescriptions can be pointed out. A pharmaceutical physician who is an employee of an industrial company needs to work hard to uphold non-deceptive standards of advertising of his firm's products. I am aware that this is not an easy responsibility, and I would be interested in learning from you your experiences in this field.

In spite of the apparent clash of self-interest between these parties, there is in fact the common interest shared by the pharmacist, the doctor, the government, the patient and the drug company that they all maintain the long-term welfare of the communities they represent. Because these communities are interdependent, responsible behavior from each of them is continually necessary. To achieve this measure of social viability, each one of the parties must be both truthful and open to new truth, and this principle and those of community welfare and individual civil rights are the best ethical standards by which their actions can be judged.

DRUGS IN THE THIRD WORLD

There are a number of ethical problems peculiar to the Third World in relation to the research and marketing of drugs. By the Third World I mean to include the Fourth

World and all those countries designated "developing" for those who prefer that terminology. I would like to offer seven commandments and two dilemmas :

Commandments

1. Thou shalt not take advantage of the poverty and lack of education of citizens of the Third World.
2. Thou shalt not sell drugs in the Third World which, in the context of their educational standards, sanitation, economic resources and health-care delivery services, do more harm than good.
3. Thou shalt not advertise in the Third World the benefits of new drugs without full mention of the risks and adverse side-effects.
4. Thou shalt not expose citizens of the Third World to research with drugs which will not later be provided to those citizens at a cost they can afford if the drug is found to be beneficial.
5. Thou shalt at least live up to the scientific and ethical standards of each Third World country where one conducts research or markets drugs.
6. Thou shalt live up to thine own national, scientific and ethical standards of medical research and marketing of drugs wherever possible.
7. Thou shalt always live up to the scientific and ethical standards of the Code of Nuremberg and the Declarations of Helsinki and Tokyo.

Dilemma N° 1

How do investigators proceed when no thought has been given by a Third World government to ethical standards of medical research, or when their standards, in effect, disregard the basic civil rights of subjects in research ? These conditions can quite understandably occur when the government of a poor nation has more desperate priorities upon which to exercise its energy and financial resources than the oversight of medical research. Some would argue that, in this situation, for the incoming drug company to live up to its own national standards would be to practice cultural imperialism. Under the guise of the sophistic claim of not wanting to be "imperialistic", the drug company might plan to disregard elements of the informed consent procedure or adequate monitoring of adverse side effects. This is obviously unethical.

However, I personally do not believe that the demanding, safety requirements of countries with a high standard of health need necessarily apply in all Third World nations. For example, if a drug is being tested for later marketing in a poor Third World country to alleviate a serious health or population problem, the risk-/benefit judgement would have to be different from that in a highly developed country. It seems to me to be unrealistic not to take that difference into account when an ethical judgement is to be made on whether or not to proceed with research and marketing. Greater risks can, and sometimes should, be taken when greater benefits are expected to result.

The World Health Organization is currently studying research procedures in the Third World and their conclusions, I understand, should emerge in the Fall of this year. In the meantime, the Code of Nuremberg in 1947, the Declaration of Helsinki of 1964 and the Declaration of Tokyo in 1975 provide minimum standards for self-regulation. However, as anyone who has been involved in the review of protocols and the practice of research knows, each individual piece of projected research also needs to be evaluated by an independent body to judge how well the relevant, scientific and ethical standards have been met. Would it be possible for the World Health Organization to organize regional bodies, composed of both professional and lay people, to make evaluations of projected research in those Third World countries that do not yet have adequate procedures to conduct reviews themselves ?

Dilemma N° 2

How shall research be encouraged and funded whose goal is the relief of diseases in Third World countries ? Poverty in these nations have precluded their own funding of research directed towards indigenous diseases. The drug companies have understandably been limited in their ventures in this field because profits from marketing are not sufficient to reimburse costs of research. However, the plight of unnecessary suffering appalls us all. Perhaps research costs could be financed by a combination of international sources similar to those assembled for famine relief, as well as from donations from the large drug companies in the industrial nations.

Incidently, the actual costs of marketing new drugs in the Third World can be less than expected. This is because there is no competitive treatment alternative and therefore lower promotional costs. The government can buy the drug in great quantities and thus make savings, and the people themselves — if the drug relieves a serious health condition — have an incentive to promote and distribute it.

THE CARE AND FEEDING OF PHARMACEUTICAL PHYSICIANS

In conclusion, I would like to turn to what is needed to keep your profession healthy — how to provide for the care and feeding of pharmaceutical physicians. First you need to remind each other that as physicians you are essentially here to serve the public. You deserve a fair wage but you should not be greedy in making money, and the normal financial rewards should not be so great that young men and women enter your profession more for the love of money than for the love of your art or concern for people's health.

For your own professional welfare you need to make continuous efforts to keep the medical community, the public and the governing authorities, bureaucratic and legislative, informed about the ongoing nature of pharmaceutical research. You should speak and write in such a way that people catch the excitement of your task. To do this you need to be open and honest to individuals whom you treat as patients, research subjects and to the general public. You need to share what you know, what you don't know, and speak of the dangers as well as the benefits of new and old drugs. For a mature, educated public and individually informed patients are the best evidence for the integrity and quality of your work. A knowledgeable public and government is likely to want to help further your work, not hinder it by excessive regulations born of fear and ignorance. Finally, openness and honesty is an essential part of counteracting that anxiety and skepticism towards leaders, which I suggested in my opening remarks, are characteristic of our changing times.

On a more profound level we are confronted with an abiding malaise and only those who have a perspective on it are free from the worst of its implications. There is no totally reliable research conclusion, no one hundred percent safe drug, no faultless pharmacist or priest, and no fully just and equitable system of marketing. It is not true that there always have been profound failures throughout human society and its institutions and a chaotic quality to our natural environment ? Injustices and dislocations in economic and political institutions have arisen in every age, in every nation, and while reforms can improve our corporate life, the causes cannot be eradicated even by systematic change. Rather, these continuing tragedies also reflect psychological and spiritual realities — the love and hate which battle silently deep within ourselves. All wells are poisoned — all souls are selfish. Our existence is contingent upon forces, both natural and human, which we have never been able fully to control. Alexander Pope, the 19th century poet, said, "Everything that is made has a crack in it." The earth — this creation — is crying out, waiting impatiently for its own healing and redemption. This hope is shared, not just by members of the judeo-christian tradition, but by members of all religions and of most secular humanist philosophies.

Whoever, then, would venture to heal by prescribing drugs, to restore normalacy, to make whole, to bring Shalom, embarks on a mysterious and sacred task. The pharmacist, in his or her work, is a vivid symbol of that universal human desire to participate in a new wholeness and a new creation.

So finally, I wish to remind you of how important your work really is. Because it participates in the fulfillment of deep human longings and answers to some degree the hope of overcoming sickness, your work and person is of unusual significance to those with whom you live. When you succeed and establish truly humane and healing relationships, then people's hearts and minds are profoundly affected. On the other hand when you fail, when you either corporately or individually do not live up to the public's estimation of what ethically you can achieve, then condemnation of you is angry and your fall is great. It is both joy and responsability which your vocation provides. You must therefore remind each other of the high standards of your profession and encourage each other to work in that truly humane way which has always been the hallmark of your own best ideals.

REFERENCES

1. Gray Bradford H., An Assessment of Institutional Review Committees in Human Experimentation, *Medical Care* **13**, 4, April 1975.
"The Performance of Institutional Review Boards. A Report to the National Commission for the Protection of Human Subjects of Biomedical and Behavioral Research", Survey Research Center, Institute for Social Research, The University of Michigan, May 28, 1977, appendix to report dated November 1, 1977, DHEW publication N° (OS) 78-00009.

Sécurité et médicaments (1982), pp. 63-66

A Comparison of International Guidelines for the Clinical Evaluation of Psychotropic Drugs The Price of Safety

V. H. VAN LANDEGHEM

L.E.R.S., 58, rue de la Glacière, 75013 Paris, France

Abstract — A comparison of the rules governing the clinical evaluation of new psychotropic drugs in Europe and in the United States shows there are substantial differences between the two. Although in Europe the CPMP is studying a plan for harmonisation on an E.E.C. level, each country at present has its own guidelines and none of these apply to psychotropic drugs as a particular class.

In contrast, the U.S. FDA issues guidelines which are stricter but which, while they do not guarantee the granting of a registration, give reasonable assurance that a dossier observing them will be given a favorable reception.

The guidelines appropriate to CNS drugs are established by the most qualified specialists and incorporate the most recent discoveries and techniques.

However an inevitable consequence of a system with stricter guidelines is a limitation on the number of new drugs available. This may not be in the patients' best interest since a theoretical over-concern for side effects may exclude or delay the introduction of drugs which can in fact provide greater safety for the patient. Several examples exist in the fields of hypnotic, antidepressant and anticonvulsant drugs. The most desirable system therefore is one which strikes a proper balance between rules which are too imprecise to serve as a useful guide for the investigator and those which are too restrictive and prevent the timely marketing of worthwile drugs.

The subject of this talk is "A comparison of international guidelines for the clinical evaluation of psychotropic drugs", and one of the themes will be : the price of safety.

However, the only country with guidelines specific to psychotropic drugs is the U.S.A. In Europe or elsewhere, there are no formal guidelines of the American type and certainly none specifically for psychotropic drugs.

To a large extent, therefore, I find I am addressing myself to the subject of the advisability and nature of detailed guidelines in general and only incidentally as they apply to psychotropic drugs in particular.

The American guidelines issued by the U.S. Department of Health, Education and Welfare are, as we all know, very comprehensive and very detailed. In the CNS field there are separate ones for hypnotics, antianxiety drugs, anticonvulsants, antidepressants and psychoactive drugs in children.

They offer obvious advantages :

— Firstly they incorporate much of the best and latest thinking on the subject by renowned experts ;

— There is also little doubt that the need to follow the guidelines has resulted in an improvement of the overall quality of our clinical investigations ;
— Moreover guidelines give a reasonable assurance that, if they are followed, the dossier submitted will be accepted for review and not refused a priori for, as an example, lack of one specific study ;
— And also, guidelines give in principle the maximum assurance for safety.
However, these guidelines present some problems. For example,
— Although the FDA describes the guidelines as being "recommendations for clinical studies" "recognized as desirable approaches" and "not to be interpreted as mandatory" one is only too conscious that they are to be ignored at one's risk and peril.
Thus it is difficult not to submit to their constraints even when they are not, as they obviously cannot always be, entirely suitable for the particular molecule in question.
— They are also in the opinion of many of us one of the major factors in preventing new molecules to get a registration in the U.S.

A major drug in the prevention of epileptic seizures, sodium valproate, was marketed several years after it was marketed in France, and in the U.K. Thus, as pointed out by the National Commission for the Control of epilepsy and its Consequences, subjecting American patients to approximately 1 million unnecessary seizures a year.
— They are also an obstacle in getting a new indication for a registered drug approved. The classical examples here are propranolol in essential tremor and agitation, clonidine in migraine.
— They can also limit the number of me-too drugs which in the field of psychiatry and major tranquillizers will prevent the physician from tailoring a drug to the individual patient.
— They make the international use of research reports very difficult, thus multiplying the investigations unnecessarily.

And finally there is the problem that, although the intention is to update the guidelines every two years, this is often not happening.

This is particularly important in the relatively young area of clinical psychopharmacology where the state-of-the-art evoluates very quickly and still requires the development of newer and better techniques.

In sum, although guidelines can be a great help and guidelines addressed to an overall therapeutic class such as psychotropic drugs even more so, the detail in which the FDA guidelines enter tends to be a handicap when we are dealing with a specific subclass such antidepressants, anxiolytics or hypnotics, each with their peculiar characteristics.

Isn't it slightly exaggerated to read page 5 of the guidelines for the clinical evaluation of antianxiety drug : numerically balanced or imbalanced parallel group design may be used, for example 20 drugs vs. 20 placebo, 12 drugs vs. 8 placebo, or 30 drugs vs. 10 placebo.

I think that we could have worked this out for ourselves.

Furthermore, I do not believe that such detail makes a contribution to the issue of safety. I'll address this theme in a few minutes.

Now let us look at the situation in Europe. Here, guidelines similar in clarity and specificity to the FDA ones do not exist. There is much more reliance on precedent, consultation and eventual compromise. This leaves the investigator with greater freedom but also with greater uncertainty about the outcome.

While the system has worked in this way in the past, we must recognize that the criteria by which the European regulatory authorities judge a new product dossier are becoming more exigent and more specific.

Thus to continue as now, without authoritative guidelines, will result in a situation where there will be the disadvantages of the American system without its advantages.

There is great awareness of this and already at the level of the E.E.C., efforts are being made to establish a certain number of directives. The only one I am aware of which affects the CNS area deals with anti-epileptic drugs and is being reviewed by Dukes' working group.

On an international level, an ad hoc working group issued in 1977 guidelines for conducting clinical trials of psychotropic drugs. Although the group did this work independently of any regulatory agency or other organisation, it is considered likely that the FDA will make use of these recommendations in revising their guidelines for psychotropic drugs.

And finally in June 1980, W.H.O.'s planning Group on the evaluation of Drugs and Diagnostic substances met in Copenhagen to formulate a general outline of future guidelines for Clinical trials.

One of their propositions was that a working party be established in order to develop guidelines on minor tranquillizers and sedatives.

As far as I am aware, this sums up the situation in Europe.

Let us now try to measure the impact of the ultra-cautious U.S. approach, as expressed in its detailed guidelines and more stringent regulations, in terms of safety. For we have to keep in mind that safety is the main justification for having such strict regulations.

First of all, the price paid to achieve this degree of safety.

A few figures :

We know that from 1976 to 1979 the cost of developing a drug in the U.S.A. increased from 55 to over 70 million dollars, while the cost in Europe has remained much lower.

Based on data assembled from 9 PMA member companies, one study concluded that the U.S. pharmaceutical industry spent $ 300 million in 1978 to satisfy regulatory requirements which were unnecessary.

We can now put the question whether the price paid, directly or indirectly by the delays in registering new molecules really provides an increased degree of safety.

It is obvious that there can be no side-effects or toxicity from a product which is not on the market.

A good example is thalidomide which because of the usual delays was not being marketed in the U.S.A. when problems became apparent in Europe. But, following this reasoning further, the rest of the world becomes America'guinea-pigs, as was pointed out in a recent meeting of the society for Clinical Pharmacology and Therapeutics at New-Orleans.

Keeping certain products from the market can have the opposite result. An example of this is the anti-depressants. The new anti-depressants such as viloxazine, nomifensine, mianserin, maprotilin, may or may not offer an advantage in efficacy over the existing products but they certainly offer one in safety.

Viloxazine is virtually devoid of toxicity in cases of acute over-dosage, an indisputable gain in terms of safety in a disease such as depression.

We can perhaps compare this with the reduction in successful suicide attempts since the benzodiazepines took the place of barbiturates.

Apart from real toxicity, the side-effects of new molecules are often considerably reduced, a factor perhaps of greater importance in depression than in other fields where side-effects can easily be mistaken for symptoms of the disease itself.

We could agree that strict regulations containing every possible precaution will give the greatest certainty of safety. But even then, how can they protect patients against toxic effects that are unforeseeable ?

How many years of experience are necessary to avoid incidents such as the cases of agranulocytosis resulting from the administration of carbamazepine or clozapine or cases of retro-peritoneal fibrosis with methysergide frequently used for migraine. How could one have foreseen the accidents of photosensitization or the cornean deposits of phenothiazines ?
There is almost no end to such a list.

Again, how can all the cases of drug interactions be foreseen before a drug enters into general use ? A single example suffices to illustrate this point : that of the hallucinations, delirium and general agitation observed in non-psychiatric patients treated with idrocilamide, a myorelaxant drug. These side-effects have now been established to be the result of an inter-action with caffeine.

Many more examples could be cited.

What conclusion can be drawn from what I have said ?

The present system is obviously far from perfect on either side of the Atlantic. On one side over-regulation, on the other maybe too little.

The solution lies in the harmonization of the systems in the middle ground. Obviously the subject is too complex and too important for me to enter into it in this presentation. There is an awareness of the problem and considerable efforts are devoted to solving it. For example, a meeting of drug regulatory agencies took place at Annapolis last October under the auspices of the FDA and W.H.O. but the results were inconclusive.

Nevertheless, in a world — and certainly in our industry — where the problems are truly international and drug research must be undertaken on an international basis, harmonization is a necessity.

Sécurité et médicaments (1982), pp. 67-70

USA et FDA Versus CEE et CSP
Une étude comparative ouverte des médicaments anti-angoreux

J. R. ESPIE

Laboratoires MSD-Chibret, 3 avenue Hoche, 75008 Paris, France

Résumé — La FDA et le Comité des Spécialités Pharmaceutiques (CSP) de la C.E.E. ont publié des guides ou directives destinés à orienter les études cliniques des médicaments anti-angoreux. Le médicament ayant actuellement une diffusion mondiale, il est instructif et utile de comparer les exigences de la FDA qui est souvent l'inspiratrice à celles qui sont en cours d'élaboration au niveau du CSP.

En préambule les deux Services d'enregistrement demandent aux utilisateurs de relire les directives générales concernant la méthodologie des essais cliniques. Le seul objectif de la directive traitant des médicaments anti-angoreux est d'aider les demandeurs à interpréter les directives générales compte tenu des problèmes spécifiques liés à ces médicaments.

Les deux agences attachent une grande importance aux méthodes de diagnostic et à la sélection des malades. Les directives de la FDA sont plus précises, plus descriptives, celles du CSP plus qualitatives. La FDA souhaite inclure des sujets normaux au stade I, le CSP les ignore. Le CSP n'envisage pas de fiche d'auto-évaluation remplie par le malade, par contre la FDA attache une grande importance à celle-ci. Les paramètres concernant l'efficacité sont nettement décrits et précisés par la FDA, ils ne sont que qualitatifs pour le CSP. La FDA recommande une durée de traitement contrôlée limitée à trois mois avant la mise sur le marché, puis des études d'innocuité à long terme d'une durée variable selon le cas après la mise sur le marché. Le CSP recommande de poursuivre les études pendant un an sans précision en rapport avec la mise sur le marché.

En conclusion : les directives des deux Services d'enregistrement ne sont pas conflictuelles, celle de la FDA est précise, très contraignante, parfois trop, celle du CSP laisse un grand degré de liberté qui peut embarrasser le fabricant. Une directive trop vague reste-elle une directive ? Ces différences ne seront-elles pas annulées par l'interprétation des textes apparemment plus libéraux du CSP et par une application tout aussi contraignante que ceux de la FDA ?

La réglementation concernant les essais cliniques destinés à l'enregistrement d'un nouveau médicament devient de plus en plus exigeante et précise. Il est intéressant d'analyser l'orientation que les autorités administratives proposent :
— celle de la C.E.E. (CSP) dont nous dépendons et
— celle des U.S.A. (FDA) qui sert souvent de référence.

Les organisateurs m'ont demandé de vous parler de la réglementation des médicaments anti-angoreux à titre d'exemple, mais je pense qu'il serait instructif d'analyser d'autres "directives" comme celle des anti-inflammatoires ou celle des médicaments du système nerveux central.

Dans le domaine des anti-angoreux les deux services d'enregistrement que sont le CSP et la FDA demandent aux utilisateurs de relire les directives générales concernant la méthodologie des essais cliniques détaillés au niveau des "considérations générales" FDA 3040 et des "Normes et protocoles" C.E.E. 75/318.

La FDA et le CSP rappellent que tout essai clinique doit être précédé par des études précliniques in vitro et chez l'animal appropriées au médicament à tester et soumises à une analyse critique sérieuse.

Les "guidelines" FDA séparent nettement les critères de diagnostic de l'angor des critères de sélection des malades, ce qui n'existe pas au niveau de la "directive" CSP.

Les critères de diagnostic de l'angor décrits par le Guideline FDA sont très détaillés et précis.

Les symptômes cliniques rapportés par le malade, caractéristiques de l'affection sont définis avec précision...

— description des symptômes déclenchés par l'effort, calmés par le repos et/ou Trinitrine.

De même que les signes électrocardiographiques...

— anomalies du segment ST sous décalage au repos
sous décalage à l'effort

Et même les anomalies angiographiques pouvant être retrouvées...

— sténose 60 % de la lumière d'une coronaire ou d'une collatérale.

Seuls peuvent être considérés comme répondant au diagnostic d'Angor tel qu'il est défini par la FDA, les malades présentant soit une association des signes cliniques et électrocardiographiques, soit une association de signes cliniques et angiographiques, soit enfin l'association des signes cliniques d'Angor et d'antécédents d'infarctus du myocarde confirmé. Au contraire le CSP recommande simplement que les malades présentent un Angor d'effort et que l'intensité de l'effort provoquant la douleur soit quantifiée. Il appartient apparemment au clinicien de définir les critères permettant de poser ce diagnostic.

La sélection des malades est très bien définie au niveau du guide de la FDA et rappelle que l'Angor doit être conforme aux critères diagnostiques définis précédemment. Le nombre de crises spontanées au cours de la vie courante doit être au minimum de 5 par semaine mais peut être ramené à une crise au cours d'une épreuve d'effort ou à des modifications caractéristiques et reproductibles de l'électrocardiogramme lors d'une épreuve d'effort.

La stabilité de l'Angor doit exister depuis 3 mois au moins ou encore être établie par une fréquence stable des crises au cours d'une semaine et prendre le temps nécessaire pour y parvenir.

L'ECG au repos devra être normal ou ne pas présenter d'anomalies du segment ST susceptible d'interférer avec les modifications de ST liées à la crise d'angine de poitrine.

Les malades atteints d'anémie, porteurs d'une valvulopathie ou traités par la digitaline ne seront pas retenus car les signes ECG de ces maladies sont identiques ou très voisins de ceux de l'Angor.

L'existence d'un infarctus au cours des six derniers mois ne permet pas la sélection du malade. En général les femmes non ménopausées ne sont pas sélectionnées.

Les critères de sélection requis par le CSP sont limités à la présence d'un Angor d'effort stable depuis 3 mois.

Le CSP demande de tenir compte soigneusement des facteurs de risque tels que le fait de fumer, l'hypertension, l'hypercholestérolémie, la prise d'autres médicaments.

La fréquence des crises constitue pour la FDA un facteur important pour apprécier l'efficacité du médicament.

En conséquence, le "Guideline" énumère les facteurs capables de modifier la fréquence des crises et demande qu'il en soit tenu compte pour évaluer l'efficacité du médicament quand ils sont présents. Citons, les causes qui réduisent l'apport d'oxygène au myocarde comme l'anémie ou l'hypotension orthostatique, les causes qui modifient la fréquence cardiaque ou la pression artérielle.

Le CSP dans sa directive précise que l'Angor au repos (Prinzmetal) et l'Angor organique consécutifs à une anémie grave ou à une sténose aortique doivent être exclus de l'étude.

Les méthodes d'étude proposées par chaque organisme pour apprécier la fréquence et/ou la gravité des crises d'angine de poitrine méritent d'être commentées.

La méthode proposée par la FDA préconise que des ECG effectués au repos et à l'effort sur des sujets normaux servent de base de comparaison.

La méthode du "Journal" qui permet au malade de noter le nombre, l'intensité et la circonstance de survenue des crises ainsi que la consommation de Trinitrine paraît souhaitable.

L'analyse de l'ECG après épreuve d'effort standardisée est à retenir. Il convient de quantifier l'importance de l'effort en notant sa durée, la consommation d'oxygène, la pression artérielle, la fréquence cardiaque, la puissance de travail en watts ou l'inclinaison et la vitesse du tapis roulant. Arrêter l'épreuve dès l'apparition de la douleur angineuse.

La mesure des effets hémodynamiques du médicament sous stimulation auriculaire ou lors d'un Angor d'effort en utilisant l'ECG, la pression télédiastolique ventriculaire gauche permet une étude quantifiée de l'Angor. L'étude sera faite en double aveugle et le cross-over préférable à la méthode parallèle. La durée n'est pas précisée.

Une étude à long terme après la mise sur le marché du médicament permettrait d'étudier la tolérance, l'action sur la morbidité et la variation de l'espérance de vie.

La directive du CSP ne mentionne pas le volontaire sain et distingue une phase aiguë et une phase à long terme.

La phase aiguë permet d'étudier l'Angor provoqué par une épreuve d'effort en utilisant des paramètres quantifiés.

La phase long terme est destinée à une étude en double aveugle pendant un an des effets du médicament sur des malades ambulatoires.

L'évaluation des résultats proposée par la FDA porte sur une diminution de 50 % des crises, sur une amélioration des signes cliniques et ECG à l'effort ainsi que de l'indice de consommation d'oxygène.

L'évaluation statistique des résultats sera faite sur la réponse moyenne du groupe et sur la réponse de chaque malade.

Le CSP propose une évaluation des résultats basée sur le nombre de crises, la consommation de Trinitrine et l'amélioration du test de tolérance à l'effort. Cet organisme préconise de soigneusement étudier et enregistrer le nombre d'abandons de traitement (infarctus, effets secondaires).

L'arrêt brutal du traitement peut entraîner une aggravation des symptômes. Il est souhaitable d'étudier soigneusement ce phénomène.

Cette analyse comparative des textes de la FDA et du CSP met en évidence des différences. Il apparaît nettement que le "Guideline" de la FDA est plus précis, plus quantitatif que celui du CSP qui est plus qualitatif et plus vague.

Peut-on avancer que cette différence est liée au fait que la FDA est impliquée tout au long du processus d'enrgistrement et que le CSP n'est pour l'instant qu'un organisme conseil ?

Si la FDA décide et juge, le CSP oriente et conseille.

Peut-être est-il possible de penser que la directive du CSP témoigne d'un accord difficile, d'une harmonisation laborieuse des réglementations et des médecines européennes.

Nous sommes en présence de deux systèmes qui ont chacun leurs partisans...

Les "Guidelines" FDA sont précis mais par là même peuvent conduire à des excès. L'évolution rapide des techniques d'examen risque de les rendre périmées à bref délai et le nombre de malades qui sont en mesure de satisfaire aux critères imposés sont réduits à un petit nombre.

Les directives du CSP sont vagues et laissent aux cliniciens beaucoup de liberté ; celle-ci peut inciter au laxisme. Par contre une telle directive permet d'utiliser les techniques nouvelles. Le nombre de malades qui peuvent entrer dans l'étude est plus large.

Comment les directives du CSP vont-elles évoluer au fur et à mesure de leur application ? Est-ce vers un modèle du type FDA ? Est-ce vers un modèle propre voisin du système Britannique CSM ?

Lequel des deux systèmes permet d'établir avec plus de précision et de sévérité les propriétés des nouveaux médicaments ? Beaucoup de questions restent sans réponse, ces journées en apporteront certainement.

II

POST MARKETING SAFETY ASSESSMENT

INTERET ET LIMITES DES METHODES D'EVALUATION CLINIQUE DES EFFETS INDESIRABLES DES MEDICAMENTS APRES MISE SUR LE MARCHE

PRESENT METHODS

METHODES ACTUELLES

Sécurité et médicaments (1982), pp. 73-82

Spontaneous Notification

J.E. IDÄNPÄÄN-HEIKKILÄ

National Board of Health, Siltasaarenkatu 18, 00530 Helsinki 53, Finland

Abstract — Spontaneous notification system of adverse drug reactions (ADRs) to a national register or center has been established in several countries. Since 1968 W.H.O. has supported an international monitoring system. Case reports from national centers form the basis of this program. Properly operating spontaneous, voluntary reporting is a useful early warning system of suspected ADRs especially connected with new chemical entities in postmarketing phase. It is cheap, easy and simple method to survey drug safety on a national level. It serves starting material for in-depth studies and collects additional, complementary information about already known ADRs. Its main disadvantages may be incomplete reporting, lack of incidence data of an ADR as well as difficulties in detection, diagnosis and evaluation of ADR. Lack of motivation to report and tendency to publish but not report my primary ADR case are other disadvantages. Feedback information to medical profession is necessary. In Finland a copy of ADR report is also provided to the manufacturer but without the name of patient or doctor.

Spontaneous reporting of ADRs have been utilized to verify and estimate the risks of several recent drug problems. Examples of these in Nordic and other European countries are untoward effects of hydralazine, oral contraceptives, clozapine, nitrofurantoin, biguanides, practolol and other betablockers, cimetidine, and halzion. Beside spontaneous notification other surveillance systems are needed.

After its discovery and synthesis a new chemical entity (a new drug, therapeutic substance) has to pass at first relevant toxicological studies in animals and then clinical trials (Table 1). Further, a product licence and registration issued by a health authority is required in most countries before marketing and prescribing of a new medicine. Although these pre-clinical and pre-marketing investigations are carefully performed and assessed, these tests of new medical products may not in every instance ensure the safety in patients.

DEFICIENCIES OF PRE-MARKETING TESTS

The experimental toxicity in animal studies sometimes eliminates otherwise promising therapeutic substances before clinical trials in man. Occasionally they have failed to show or predict toxicity that unfortunately occurs in some patients when the medicine is used in man. Thus laboratory tests on animals do not provide a reliable method of predicting human toxicity.

Phase I-III clinical trials are performed in well controlled conditions in which all effects — both therapeutic and side effects — are carefully recorded (Table 1). The conditions in trials may be too well controlled and too safe to mimic the actual situation

Table 1. Differences between patient conditions in clinical trials and routine prescribing

CLINICAL TRIALS :
- Well controlled conditions
- Highly selected cases, and diseases
- Limited number of patients
- Short-term therapies

ROUTINE PRESCRIBING :
- Less controlled conditions
- Less selected objects
- Associated diseases, drugs
- Individual features, rarities
- Variations in food, race, and environmental factors
- Long-term therapies
- High number of patients.

the patient has while taking his medicine at home. Further, only highly selected cases with clear, single and simple disease or symptoms are taken to these trials to prove primarily the efficacy. The number of cases is limited. Some hundreds of patients may be exposed and ADRs with frequencies lower than one per cent are not discovered. Clinical trials seldom explore the effects in long-term treatment and reactions that are long delayed remain undefined.

PRESCRIBING CONDITIONS

When the drugs are marketed and routinely prescribed to the patients several differences can be found in the proceedings if they are compared with clinical trials (Table 1). Patients' conditions and drug intake are not equally well controlled. Selection of patients is less evident, associated diseases and medications may cause interactions. Individual differences and rarities as well as rare responses may occur. Variations in food, use of herbs, genetic background and living environment are unavoidable. Often long-term treatments are applied and even gradually developing reactions may appear especially when a high number of patients (up to thousands or millions) are chronically exposed to the drug.

ADR REGISTERS IN PMS

The deficiencies in pre-marketing safety tests have promoted the significance of post-marketing surveillance of drug safety. In recent years several methods have been applied to PMS (Table 2). Since 1969 national systems for spontaneous notification of ADRs were established in Australia, the United Kingdom, West-Germany, the U.S.A.,

Table 2. Various methods used for post-marketing surveillance (PMS) of adverse drug reactions.

Monitored release
Restricted release
Recorded release
Population monitoring
Case control studies
Registered release
Intensive monitoring
Hospital monitoring
Spontaneous notification

Canada, the Netherlands, New Zealand and Sweden, followed by Czechoslovakia, Ireland, Finland, Norway, Japan and many other countries.

The spontaneous notification is based on voluntary co-operation of physicians with the ADR centre. The centre may be national as in most countries, or institutional. The words — spontaneous or voluntary — indicate that not all reactions may be notified.

Usually a very simple and easily filled form is used to report the ADR to the ADR centre. The preliminary notification may only contain the most essential data to encourage the busy physician to collaborate with the centre. These data may be completed if necessary with an additional inquiry to the physician.

ADVANTAGES AND DISADVANTAGES

Many discoveries have proved that spontaneous reporting (Table 3) operates as an early warning system of new unknown ADRs. This has been especially important when

Table 3. Main advantages of spontaneous notification system of ADRs

— Early warning system
— Simple, easy, and fast
— Cheap
— Enables comparisons
between drugs
between patients
between countries
— Starting material for in-depth studies
— Complementary data of rare drug disorders.

new, recently marketed medicines have caused unexpected, serious side effects. I shall give later some examples of these.

Spontaneous reporting is easy and simple to operate — both to the physician and to the centre. If the notification card is practical it saves the physician's time. The system is not expensive to establish and run, which is important to any government agency or institute.

The data collected may be used for comparisons of ADRs between various drugs, patients and countries. Many published investigations show that these data serve as useful starting material for in-depth studies. Cumulation of a high number of case reports collects sometimes valuable additional and complementary data of rare reactions to drugs (Table 3).

However, the reporting is seldom — if ever — quantitative (table 4). Studies in Sweden have revealed that only up to 5 to 10 % of all significant ADRs and about 30 to 40 % of serious ADRs may be reported[1]. This may be due to the inability to recognize the ADR especially if the disease is serious or close to the ADR. This was clearly seen in the oculomucocutaneous syndrome of practolol.

Some doctors are unwilling to co-operate with a governmental agency. Fear of involvement in litigation may decrease the motivation to report ADRs. Many physicians are anxious to publish their discoveries and they may then forget reporting. The mistaken belief that only safe drugs are allowed on the market or lack of interest or "time" are other reasons for failure to report suspected drug-induced reactions.

SPONTANEOUS REPORTING AND IDENTIFICATION OF A NEW HAZARD

Several discoveries have demonstrated that spontaneous reporting of ADRs provide a rapid and decisive confirmation of previously unsuspected drug reactions. There are usually three situations that are most likely to produce an hypothesis of a new ADR[2]. Sometimes the reports are more numerous than would be expected in the patient pop-

Table 4. Main difficulties of spontaneous reporting system of ADRs

— Seldom quantitative if ever
5-10 % of all and 30 % of serious ADRs reported ?
— Inability to recognize ADR
— Incomplete reports
— Unwilling to cooperate
— Fear of involvement in litigation,
big brother
— Guilty, harm to patient —
Anxious to publish first
— Lethargy.

Table 5. Spontaneous reports as early warning of new ADRs

Centre and drug	ADR	Outcome, conclusion
THE NETHERLANDS CENTRE (NARD)		Warning issued to physicians, and data sheet
— Glafenine (Glifanan) (Meyboom 1976)	Anaphylactic shocks	
Aprindine (Fiboran) (Leeuwen 1976)	Agranulocytosis	Warning issued
THE U S A		
— Tienilic acid (Tycrynafen) (FDA 1980)	Hepatic injuries	Withdrawal
THE FINNISH ADR CENTRE		
— Clozapine (Leponex) (Idänpään-Heikkilä & al. 1977)	Agranulocytosis, leucopenia	Withdrawal
— Bromocriptine (Parlodel) (Rinne 1981)	Pulmonary infiltrations, pleural effusions and thickening	Warning issued

ulation under treatment. Secondly, the reports may describe serious events or findings. And further, the ADR findings or events themselves may be of an unusual nature. In the following examples two or all three of these apply at the same time (Table 5).

In 1976 the Netherlands Bureau of Adverse Reaction Monitoring had received in about four years 32 reports of anaphylactic reactions attributed to the use of glafenine — an anti-inflammatory agent of anthranilic acid derivative[3]. Based on these findings a warning was issued to the physicians and the data sheet was accordingly revised. Since then over 100 similar cases have been reported to the same monitoring centre.

Six patients who developed agranulocytosis while taking aprindine — an anti-arrhythmic drug — were reported to the ADR register in the Netherlands[4]. Two patients died. Since aprindine had been available only for a relatively short time, it seemed likely that the drug induced an unacceptably high incidence of serious complication. A warning was issued. Later on more cases were reported and other equally or more efficacious and safer alternative drugs were recommended[5].

Tienilic acid, a new uricosuric diuretic was introduced in the USA in 1979. In 1980 it was withdrawn because more than 50 cases of liver damage, including at least four fatalities, had been reported in patients while taking the drug[6]. The causal link appeared very probable since liver changes re-appeared in cases re-exposed to the drug.

A promising anti-psychotic drug clozapine was registered in Finland in January 1975. Five months later the first case of fatal agranulocytosis in connection with the drug was reported[7]. Within about seven weeks seven cases of neutropenia and ten cases of agranulocytosis (eight fatal) were reported in Finland. The risk of agranulocytosis was estimated to be 0,5 — 0,7 % on the basis of drug utilization data. The risk was considered unacceptable and clozapine was withdrawn from the Finnish market.

In an open study of long-term efficacy and safety of high dose (from 20 to 90 mg daily) bromocriptine alone or with levodopa in Parkinson's disease among 123 patients seven developed pleurisy accompanied by effusion, pleural thickening and pulmonary infiltrations[8]. These discoveries have initiated further studies to judge on the relationship of the reports to therapy.

RELATIVE RISKS OF VARIOUS DRUGS

Between-drug comparisons of profiles or patterns of ADRs may reveal significant differences between alternative therapeutic agents. Because of underreporting the absolute incidence of ADRs cannot be measured by voluntary reporting system. In most instances the relevant information of comparative safety can be derived from an estimate of the reported incidence. If several similar drugs have been introduced to the market at about the same time and if there are no biases which account for selective reporting of ADRs to one or other of the drugs the comparisons between drugs may be of great value.

Inman used the "yellow card" system in the United Kingdom (Table 6) to study the correlation of morbidity and mortality trends with the various oestrogen content of oral contraceptives[10]. Using ADR and sales data from the U.K. and the Nordic Countries he concluded that there was a clear trend towards a greater risk of thromboembolism with the large doses of oestrogen. These findings early in 1970 contributed in an important way to the safety of oral contraceptive drugs. The high-dose preparations were withdrawn from the market in most countries and new preparations containing oestrogen of 30μg or less have been introduced. This ADR study showed also the need for international co-operation between ADR centres to gather sufficient material to permit statistical evaluation.

Table 6. Spontaneous reports and comparative safety of various drugs

Centre and drug	ADR	outcome, conclusion
THE UNITED KINGDOM		
— Oestrogen content of oral contraceptives[10]	Thromboembolitic complications	Move from high-dose to low-dose preparations
THE SWEDISH REGISTER		
— Biguanides = phenformin[11]	Lactic acidosis deaths	Phenformin withdrawn, replaced with metformin

The reported lactic acidosis cases and other ADRs to various biguanides in 1965-1975 were analysed in Sweden in relation to sales and prescriptions (Table 6). No differences in age and sex between patients receiving phenformin and metformin were discovered. In 1975-1977 both drugs were used in similar amounts in Sweden. Significantly more cases of lactic acidosis and deaths were reported for phenformin[11]. Phenformin was withdrawn but metformin was left to the Swedish market. The follow-up studies seem to prove that the risk of lactic acidosis has significantly decreased in the same patient population.

ADR'S AND IN-DEPTH STUDIES

Several studies on drug safety have been published based on ADR material of spontaneous reporting systems.

Australian Registry of Adverse Drug Reactions received in 1972-1973 a number of reports of a neurological syndrome possibly associated with the ingestion of bismuth subgallate powder[12]. The medical practitioners were invited to report details of any similar cases of which they were aware. Collected additional reports defined bismuth encephalopathy, earlier most evidently unrecognized and misdiagnosed syndrome.

Similarly an old well-known anticholinergic drug emepronium was recently discovered to cause ulceration of the œsophagus and widespread œsophagitis[13, 14]. This adverse reaction has been possibly misdiagnosed earlier as angina pectoris, œsophagitis or as an unknown chest pain.

Phenylpropanolamine (norephedrine) has been mainly used in mixtures with antihistamines to produce nasal decongestion. It is known to have a relatively little CNS-stimulant effect. Phenylpropanolamine preparations for pediatric use were increasingly reported in Sweden to cause in children psychic irritation, restlessness, aggressions, sleep disturbances and even psychoses[15]. These reactions may have been masked by the same kind of symptoms typical to pediatric infections.

The doctors activity to report nitrofurantoin induced eosinophilic lung reactions has offered a valuable material for in-depth studies of this syndrome both in Sweden[17] and Finland[16].

WHEN AND WHAT TO REPORT

The clear definitions of what to report and when to report are very difficult to describe. There seems to be a tendency to report more such adverse reactions which are already known. Especially when the drug is new it is important to know all possible reactions connected with the new substance. Therefore all suspected drug associated reactions may be reported. Several weak suspicions strengthen each other and taken together they may confirm a new earlier unknown adverse reaction. In many instances spontaneous reporting system has produced first suspected reactions. The same suspected reaction has been diagnosed independently by several doctors in several patients and the reaction has been associated in all cases with the same single drug. If the ADR cen-

Table 7. ADR reports as a starting material for in-depth studies

Centre and drug	Result of investigations
The Australian Registry	
— Bismuth subgallate (Lowe 1974)	Description of bismuth encephalopathy
The UK and Finnish Centre	
— Emepronium bromide (Hugues 1979, Puhahaka 1978)	Detection of oesophagial corrosions and ulcers
The Swedish Register	
— Phenylpropanolamine (Wilderlöw 1979)	Psychic reations, psychoses in children
The finnish and Swedish Register	
— Nitrofurantoin (Sovijärvi et al. 1977, (Holmgerg et al. 1980)	Descriptions of the clinical picture of eosinophilic lung reaction and other ADRs

tre is able to recognize this development in reporting, a new ADR may be easily found. Sometimes this is not easy as we remember in the case of practolol. In the table 8I have listed those medical situations which may be relevant to report to the ADR centre. Inman has proposed an event-reporting system (18). According to Inman the term "event" includes "any new diagnosis, unexpected deterioration in a pre-existing condition, accident or complaint of symptoms which were present before the treatment was started and which are of sufficient severity to be recorded in the patient's notes, or which lead to referral for a consultation or to hospital admission."

FEEDBACK OF INFORMATION

It is the duty of the ADR centre to disseminate relevant information of the reported cases to the collaborating doctors. In the Finnish ADR centre the evaluation of the single report is done by a group of three doctors (all pharmacologists) and using the W.H.O. causality grading and terminology. The reporting doctor receives this evaluation with a letter from the ADR centre. This is important to encourage the practitioner to collaborate with the centre and report his findings in the future.

Our national centre has tested over three years an information programme in which we release the individual reported ADR to the manufacturer of the drug but without the name of the reporting doctor and without the name of the patient. So far no "adverse experiences" have been found. We feel that the manufacturer should know everything about his product including suspected adverse reactions reported to the national ADR centre.

Table 8. Conditions in which it may be relevant to send a spontaneous notification

— When *suspected* to be ADR
— Drug younger than two years, all
— Fatal ADRs
— Disease prolonged or need to hospital admission
— Rare, less known ADRs
— New or strange to doctor
— Unexpected reactions
— "Any events", "advents"

The Finnish ADR centre reports back the main ADR discoveries to the doctors and health personnel annually via articles published in medical journals. We have several regular contacts with ADR centres in other Nordic Countries and we participate in the W.H.O. international ADR project.

Several clinics and university institutes have had research projects in common with our ADR centre to investigate in-depth some actual and important ADR problems.

CONCLUDING REMARKS

It is important to realize the advantages and limitations of the spontaneous reporting system. Among various PMS systems voluntary reporting has clearly shown its value to monitor the safety of a new drug on a national level. On the other hand, we can refer to instances like practolol, in which spontaneous reporting did report the ADR but the system itself could not detect and recognize this reaction early enough. To overcome the deficiencies of voluntary reporting scheme several other methods of PMS are necessary to monitor the drug safety.

REFERENCES

1. Böttiger L.-E. and B. Westerholm, *BMJ* **3**, 339, 1973.
2. Inman W.H.W., in : Monitoring for Drug Safety, W.H.W. Inman ed., MTP Press Limited, 1980, p. 24.
3. Meyboom R.H.B. and T. Ned., *Geneesk* **120**, 926, 1976.
4. Leeuwen R. van and R.H B. Meyboom, *Lancet* **2**, 1137, 1967.
5. Aronson J.K., *in : Side Effects of Drugs*, Annual 2, M.N.G. Dukes ed., Excerpta Medica, 1978, pp. 162-63.
6. *FDA Drug Bulletin* **10**, 3, 1980.
7. Idänpään-Heikkilä J. *et al.*, *Europ. J. Clin. Pharmacol.* **10**, 1, 1977.
8. Rinne U.K., *Lancet* **1**, 44, 1981.
9. Venulet J., *Progress Research* **21**, 233, 1977.
10. Inman B. *et al.*, *BMJ* **2**, 203, 1970.
11. Bergman U. *et al.*, *BMJ* **2**, 464, 1978.
12. Lowe D.J., *Med. J. Aust.* **2**, 664, 1974.

13. Puhakka H.J., *J. Laryng. Otol.* **42**, 927, 1978.
14. Hugues R., *BMJ* **2**, 132, 1979.
15. Widerlöw E., *Läkartidningen* **49**, 4529, 1979.
16. Sovijärvi A.R.A. *et al.*, *Scand. J. Resp. Dis.* **58**, 41, 1977.
17. Holmberg L. *et al.*, *Am. J. Med.* **69**, 733, 1980.
18. Inman B., *BMJ* **2**, 1216, 1981.

Sécurité et médicaments (1982), pp. 83-91

Assessment of the Cause and Effect Relationship of Suspected Adverse Drug Reactions

J. VENULET* and A.G. CIUCCI**

*Ciba-Geigy, Medical Department, 4002 Basle, Switzerland
**Medical Department, Clinical Drug Safety, Ciba Geigy Ltd, 4002 Basle, Switzerland

Abstract — Because of the variability of clinical judgement there is a growing interest in systems of causality assessment based on clearly defined operational criteria. In this connection, two basic questions arise :
1. What types of information are required for such an assessment ? And
2. What is the relative importance of these various types of information ?
Probably most important are data relative to the patient in whom the reported adverse event was seen (circumstances and course of the suspected event and his past adverse reaction history). The second major set of data is more closely related to the evaluator's experience and the existing epidemiological evidence. The relative importance and "proving power" of both types of data are frequently debated.
The system of Standardized Assessment (SA) developed by us is based on a set of questions with different numerical values according to their assumed "proving (or disproving) power". In addition to the usual evaluation by the medical expert, more than 2000 cases have also been assessed with SA. The procedure and results will be presented and discussed. The question arises whether further development in this direction is desired as a means for diminishing variability, improving quality (in certain cases) and communication. If so, a closer cooperation between interested parties would be required to arrive at a consensus on methods to be used.

The assessment of the causal relationship between the drug and the adverse event represents one of the most important goals in the evaluation of individual case reports and is essential before any more definitive views about the safety of a particular drug can be reached.

However, the desired degree of certainty about the correctness of the assessment will depend not only on the severity of the undesired event but also on the anticipated type of action. For example, for signalling purposes of the "early warning" type the assessment should be highly critical of the drug, to increase the sensitivity of the signal. In other words, the threshold level should be set rather low, thus accepting a rather high number of signals which during the follow-up would be recognized as false-positive.

Because of the well known variability of clinical judgement[6, 7, 9] there is a growing interest in systems of assessment based on clearly defined, operational criteria.

The first attempts at rationalizing this process were the various proposals to define the words and phrases commonly used in the cause-and-effect relationship, i.e. "possible", "probable", "not drug-related", etc.[1, 11, 12, 13, 14]. However, even on these seemingly modest proposals agreement has not been reached and some drug-monitoring centers seem to have concluded that the cause-effect relationship is simply either "probable", or "not excluded"[3]. Further progress has been made by Karch and Lasagna[8], and by Dangoumau, Evreux and Jouglard[2], Kramer *et al.*[10], Venulet *et al.*[15] who have developed algorithms for decision-making, i.e. an assessment of causal relationship based on the decision-making process.

In our approach, and I will use it here as an example, we have focused our attention on the following aspects of causality assessment :

1. Types of information required
2. Relative importance of various types of information.

The required information in the evaluation of a cause-and-effect relationship can be thought of as answers which the physician tries to give to a series of questions.

The questions are of two different types. The first set of questions concerns the observations made on the patient. Some of these are related to the present ADR, and some are related to the patient's drug history.

The second set of questions deals with information which is part of the knowledge and experience of the physician evaluating the case, referred to in this paper as the Evaluator.

It should be noted that while the first set of questions deals with the observed facts, the second deals with the Evaluator's experience and knowledge. This will differ from one Evaluator to another and may change with time. Part of this knowledge is derived from formal epidemiological studies, but all kinds of published evidence as well as the experience of the evaluating doctor fall into this category. However, epidemiological evidence is not a substitute for actual patient data and is of limited help to the Evaluator in assessing the individual ADR, no more than the knowledge that a patient with lung cancer is a heavy cigarette smoker helps the physician in deciding whether or not, in that particular case, cigarette smoking has *in fact* caused the lung cancer.

This type of knowledge may even bias the Evaluator, thus creating a vicious circle, since every incorrectly evaluated ADR will reinforce the observer's (or Evaluator's) bias. Nonetheless, it must be realistically accepted that this bias is present in the Evaluator and is not likely to remain inoperative, at least at a subconscious level. For instance, the smaller the amount of "hard facts" available in the single ADR case, the greater the importance that epidemiological evidence and past experience acquire in determining the Evaluator's opinion. If the only known facts are that the patient took the drug and a few weeks later suffered an aplastic anaemia, the suspicion will be greater for the drug if this were chloramphenicol than if it were, say, penicillin. Quite often the amount of patient data is insufficient, particularly in the case of spontaneous reporting, while the judgement on the most plausible degree of causal relationship may still be required. In such instances heavier reliance on epidemiological evidence and experience would be justified. However, the limitations of this approach should be recognized.

In practical terms the assessment of individual cases is based on a certain type and amount of information actively sought by the monitoring centres and selected for that purpose because it was considered essential for the type of judgement required. In most cases the requested data also represents a reasonable compromise between what one would like to know and what is feasible to collect.

In addition to answering the questions, the physician assigns, in his mind, a "weight" to each question. Some questions have almost always a considerable "weight". For instance an affirmative answer to the question of rechallenge (i.e. a positive rechallenge).

Many other questions are not and their importance is relative, i.e. their "weight" changes according to the clinical picture and the clinical judgement of the physician.

At the first step toward developing a less subjective evaluation procedure, a check-list of questions relevant to the causality assessment was developed in the Clinical Drug Safety Unit of CIBA-GEIGY in Basle with the aim of assuring some degree of uniformity of approach and analysis of all cases. They are divided into three subject areas:

1 Relative to the present ADR

2. Relative to patient's past ADR history;

these two groups of questions reflect the type of information actively sought by the Company in cases of suspected adverse reactions to our drugs. The third set of questions is

3. Relative to Evaluator's experience.

A special form including these questions (Fig. 1) is attached to every case report and is filled out by the Evaluator according to the information provided in the report and to his own experience. In order to make this more uniform a Guide including comments and definitions relative to all questions was prepared for use by the Evaluators. At the bottom of the form the most plausible opinion about the causal relationship between the suspected drug and the unwanted effect is given by checking one of the "causality" boxes.

It is difficult to express in quantitative terms the impact of the check-list. It was very well received by all Evaluators and considered a useful tool for a systematic assessment by most of them as it increased the chances that the most relevant aspects are considered.

At this point an empirical system of "weights", expressed numerically for each question in the form was, developed. All the answers speaking *in favour of* a causal relationship were given a positive value and those speaking *against* such a relationship a negative value. The absolute value depended on the strength of the evidence that the item was thought to carry. The actual values are given in figure 2. These are based on the preceding considerations relative to actual data, past history, and Evaluator's experience. The algebraic summation of all the positive and negative values gives one value (positive or negative) for the case.

Values falling within certain ranges were assigned to one of the five categories: not-related to the reported drug, unlikely, possible, probable or definite. The currently used ranges are indicated in figure 2.

The cut-off points for various ranges were assigned in an empirical way, but in accordance with the general aim that the resulting ranges should allow for grouping of cases according to the pre-established characteristics of each causality level.

There is also a category "insufficient amount of information to assess" but it was decided that because the main objective of the system is clearly signalling, this category should be used only in extreme situations.

The detailed results achieved with this procedure have been published elsewhere but in essence in 61 % of cases the results of our standardized approach were identical with the judgement of the Evaluator and in 35 % they differed by no more than one step of our scale (e.g. possible, probable, definite). Thus in 4 % of cases there was a major difference of opinion.

In most cases of discrepancy between the Evaluator's judgement and the standardized approach, the standardized approach was more critical, suggesting a higher degree of causal relationship.

MEDICAL DEPARTMENT Date : ....
CDS/PH 3.51 CDS Monitor : ....

Check List and Assessment Form for Case Report No.: ....

Suspected drug: Adverse reaction (A.R.):

UNLESS OTHERWISE SPECIFIED, ALL QUESTIONS REFER TO THE SUSPECTED DRUG.	Y (yes), N (no) or "–" check one
I. – **History of present adverse reaction**	
1. THERAPEUTIC DOSE EXCEEDED? (as per Vademecum)	Y N "–"
2. DRUG GIVEN PRIOR TO EVENT? (as per dates)	Y N "–"
3. CONCOMITANT OR PRECEDING DRUG THERAPY?	Y N "–"
4. REACTION AT SITE OF APPLICATION? (inj., supp., sublingual and topical)	Y N "–"
5. DRUG/A.R. INTERVAL COMPATIBLE WITH THE EVENT?	Y N "–"
6. A.R. IMMEDIATELY FOLLOWS THE DRUG AND OF ACUTE ONSET?	Y N "–"
7. RECHALLENGE ATTEMPTED?	Y N "–"
8. RECHALLENGE POSITIVE? (only if 7 = Y) (Skin test positive?)	Y N "–"
9. DECHALLENGE ATTEMPTED? (drug stopped or dose reduced)	Y N "–"
10. DECHALLENGE POSITIVE? (only if 9 = Y) Without treatment = YY; with treatment = Y	YY Y N "–"
11. WERE CONCOMITANT DRUGS STOPPED AT THE SAME TIME (only if 3 = Y)	Y N "–"
II. – **Patient's past adverse reaction history**	
12. SUSPECTED DRUG TAKEN IN THE PAST?	Y N "–"
13. SAME A.R. TO THIS DRUG BEFORE? (only if 12 = Y)	Y N "–"
14. OTHER A.R. TO THIS DRUG BEFORE? (only if 12 = Y)	Y N "–"
15. SIMILAR SYMPTOMS IN THE PAST? (in the absence of established disease [s])	Y N "–"
16. SIMILAR A.R. WITH OTHER DRUGS IN THE PAST?	Y N "–"
If acute (Type I) allergic mechanism of A.R. strongly suspected, check ☐	

III. – **Monitor's experience**

17. ADVERSE EVENT OF RARE SONTANEOUS OCCURRENCE (Y or N only)	Y N
18. SIMILAR EVENTS KNOWN TO OCCUR WITH THE DISEASE TREATED?	Y N "–"
19. A.R. OCCURRENCE FACILITATED BY DISEASE (S)? (:concomitant disease)	Y N "–"
20. CONTRIBUTORY ROLE OF NON-DRUG THERAPIES?	Y N "–"
21. OTHER CONTRIBUTORY FACTORS (HABITS, ENVIRONMENT, ETC.)?	Y N "–"
22. A.R. KNOWN WITH THE SUSPECTED DRUG? (Y or N only) (Put YY if A.R. well known)	YY Y N "–"
23. A.R. EXPLAINABLE BY THE PHARMACOLOGICAL PROPERTIES OF THE SUSPECTED DRUG?	Y N "–"
24. A.R. KNOWN WITH CHEMICALLY-RELATED DRUGS?	Y N "–"
25. A.R. KNOWN WITH PHARMACOLOGICALLY-RELATED DRUGS?	Y N "–"
26. A.R. KNOWN WITH CONCOMITANT OR PRECEDING DRUG THERAPY? (only if 3 = Y)	Y N "–"
27. DRUG INTERACTION AS A POSSIBLE CAUSE OF A.R. (only if 3 = Y)	Y N "–"

YOUR VERDICT: (check one): Insufficient amount of data to assess ☐

Not related to susp. drug ☐

Causality: unlikely ☐

possible ☐

probable ☐

definite ☐

0 ——————————————————————— 100

Fig. 1.

A closer analysis of the few cases where the opposite was true indicated that these were in general poorly documented cases in which the occurrence of the reported drug adverse reaction association was accepted by the Evaluator on the basis of experience. However, as already stressed, we should assess the case on the basis of its merits.

There is of course the more basic question of the pros and cons of standardization.

Results achieved with any method of standardized assessment of ADRs should be consistent, in that cases with the same amount and type of information should lead to an identical end result. However, not only is this not true but, a fortiori, as demonstrated by Begaud *et al.*[1], the results vary according to the method used : in only 25 % of 100 cases were the results obtained with the four methods under comparison identical.

Consistency of assessment, though difficult, is essential but not sufficient *for correctness of assessment*. Generally accepted and well defined points of reference for assessing the correctness of assessments do not exist. The mere existence of a consistent consensus of judgement does not ensure, though it may imply, the correctness of a judgement.

Standardized Assessment addresses the problem of consistency as a prerequisite for correctness by providing a point of reference, or defining a yardstick.

The correctness of the measurements will depend upon the extent to which the

MEDICAL DEPARTMENT

CDS/PH 3.51

Standardized Assessment - Assessment Key

		Weighting of answers Y	N
I. – **History of present adverse reaction**			
1. THERAPEUTIC DOSE EXCEEDED? If A.R. is drug dependence Y = + 10		excluded	cont.
2. DRUG GIVEN PRIOR TO EVENT?		cont.	excluded
3. CONCOMITANT OR PRECEDING DRUG THERAPY?		— 5	+ 5
4. REACTION AT SITE OF APPLICATION?		+ 35	—
5. DRUG/A.R. INTERVAL COMPATIBLE WITH THE EVENT?		+ 5	— 5
6. A.R. IMMEDIATELY FOLLOWS THE DRUG AND OF ACUTE ONSET?		+ 30	—
7. RECHALLENGE ATTEMPTED?			
8. RECHALLENGE POSITIVE?		+ 30	— 25
9. DECHALLENGE ATTEMPTED?			
10. DECHALLENGE POSITIVE?	YY without treatment	YY = + 20	— 15
	Y with treatment	Y = + 10	
11. WERE CONCOMITANT DRUGS STOPPED AT THE SAME TIME	If 8 or 10 = Y	— 5	+ 5
	If 8 or 10 = N	+ 5	— 5
II. – **Patient's past adverse reaction history**			
12. SUSPECTED DRUG TAKEN IN THE PAST?	If 4 = Y quest. 12-14		
13. SAME A.R. TO THIS DRUG BEFORE?	are valid if route the same	+ 15	— 10
14. OTHER A.R. TO THIS DRUG BEFORE?	Only if 13 = N or "–"	+ 10	— 5
15. SIMILAR SYMPTOMS IN THE PAST?	Only if	— 10/+ 10*	+ 5/"–"*
16. SIMILAR A.R. WITH OTHER DRUGS IN THE PAST?	18 = N "–"	— 5/+ 5*	+ 5/"–"*

* If A.R. is an acute allergic reaction

III. – **Monitor's experience**

17. ADVERSE EVENT OF RARE SONTANEOUS OCCURRENCE ?		+ 5	— 5
18. SIMILAR EVENTS KNOWN TO OCCUR WITH THE DISEASE TREATED?	Y only if 15 = N or "–"	— 5	+ 5
19. A.R. OCCURRENCE FACILITATED BY DISEASE (S)?		— 5	
20. CONTRIBUTORY ROLE OF NON-DRUG THERAPIES?		— 5	
21. OTHER CONTRIBUTORY FACTORS (HABITS, ENVIRONMENT, ETC.)?		— 5	
22. A.R. KNOWN WITH THE SUSPECTED DRUG?	YY if A.R. "well known" Y if A.R. "known"	YY = + 10 Y = + 5	— 5
23. A.R. EXPLAINABLE BY THE PHARMACOLOGICAL PROPERTIES OF THE SUSPECTED DRUG?		+ 5	— 5
24. A.R. KNOWN WITH CHEMICALLY-RELATED DRUGS? 23-25 consider only if 22 = N; maximum		+ 5	— 5
25. A.R. KNOWN WITH PHARMACOLOGICALLY-RELATED DRUIGS? negative points allowed for 23-25:–10		+ 5	— 5
26. A.R. KNOWN WITH CONCOMITANT OR PRECEDING DRUG THERAPY?		— 5	+ 10
27. DRUG INTERACTION AS A POSSIBLE CAUSE OF A.R. ?		+ 5	

Causality levels currently assigned to different ranges of case values:

Not related to susp. drug ≤ — 30

— 25 ≤ Unlikely ≤ — 5

0 ≤ Possible ≤ 30

35 ≤ Probable ≤ 50

55 ≤ Definite

Fig. 2.

yardstick approaches the "truth" and, as Begaud *et al.*[1] have demonstrated, the quality (in this sense) of the four yardsticks they compared is not the same. They were of course not able to tell us which is the "true" one. The correctness of the assessment still remains to be conjured up by some magician !

Whatever the result of the standardized assessment, it clearly means that the case met certain clearly defined although arbitrary criteria allowing its assignment to a certain level of probability (e.g. "definite" or "unlikely") and not that the assigned degree of causal relationship was really proved beyond doubt. A problem that requires discussion is that of expressing confidence in judgement, whether of expert opinion or of formal methodologies, both as a question in itself and in relation to actions that may be taken in consequence.

There could, however, be cases in which the Standardized Assessment, at least in its present form, would underestimate the degree of causal relationship.

Standardization usually involves simplification and paying more attention to those items of information that are more readily available. For example, drug concentration in blood or results of elaborate immunological tests may be conclusive but are rarely available and therefore of subordinate importance in practice.

Procedure of Standardized Assessment, or at least those in current usage, are applied to all drugs and to all reactions in the same way. However, certain acute reactions occuring within a short period of time after the administration of a specific drug are so well known that the occurence of this sequence of events is considered sufficient to prove the definite relationship between them, as for example with an attack of asthma after taking a Non-Steroid Anti-Inflammatory Drug (NSAID) in a patient known to be an ASA (acetylsalicylic acid)-sensitive asthmatic subject.

If these or other observations of similar importance are available in a given case report, a method of Standardized Assessment that omits them is clearly inadequate for that case. Many of these "out-of-pattern" reactions are potentially life-threatening and as such they would in any case generate a signal because of the severity of the outcome.

Probably no general system of causality assessment could handle such cases in a completely satisfactory way.

Standardized Assessment of drug adverse event relationships represent relatively new developments and the currently used methodologies will certainly undergo considerable modifications as more practical experience is gained.

If one of the main objectives of standardized assessment is to improve communications between various users, the time has also come to discuss ways and means of developing a common approach — otherwise we risk facing several entrenched and incompatible systems in the near future as it has happened so many times before.

REFERENCES

1. Adverse Drug Reactions in the United States, published by : Medicine in the Public Interest, Washington, D.C., USA.
2. Dangoumau J., J.-C. Evreux and J. Jouglard , Méthode d'imputabilité des effets indésirables des médicaments, *Thérapie* **33** (1978), 373-81.
3. Bötiger L.A., A.K. Furhoff and L. Holmberg, Drug-induced blood discrasias, *Acta Med. Scand.* **205** (1979), 457-61.
4. Hutchinson T.A., J.M. Leventhal, M.S. Kramer, F.E. Karch, A.G. Lipman and A.R. Feinstein, An Algorithm for the Operational Assessment of Adverse Drug Reactions, II. Demonstration of Reproducibility and Validity, *JAMA* **242** (1979), 633-38.
5. Irey N.S., Tissue Reactions to Drugs, *Amer. J. Path.* **82** (1976), 617-47.
6. James D., E. Haller, G. Rosselet, E.M. Brooke and J.L. Schelling, Fréquence des prescriptions de médicaments et de leurs effets indésirables dans un département de médecine, *Schweiz. Med. Wschr.* **108** (1978), 1270-77.
7. Karch F.E., C.L. Smith, B. Kerzner, J. Mazzullo, M. Weintraub and L. Lasagna, Adverse Drug Reactions — A Matter of Opinion, *Clin. Pharmacol. Ther.* **19** (1976), 489-92.
8. Karch F.E. and L. Lasagna, Towards the Operational Identification of Adverse Drug Reactions, *Clin. Pharmacol. Ther.* **21** (1977), 247-54.
9. Koch-Weser J., E.M. Sellers and R. Zacest, The Ambiguity of Adverse Drug Reactions, *Europ. J. Clin. Pharmacol.* **11** (1977), 75-78.

10. Kramer M.S., J.M. Leventhal, T.A. Hutchinson and A.R. Feinstein, An Algorithm of the Operational Assessment of Adverse Drug Reactions, I. Background, description and introduction for use, *JAMA* **242** (1979), 623-32.

11. Meddelande fran Läkemeddsbiverknings Kommitten, *Meddelande* **20** (1974), in Swedish.

12. Report of Suspected Adverse Drug Reactions No. 4, p. V, Australian Drug Evaluation Committee, Australian Government Publishing Service, Canberra, 1978.

13. Seidl L.G., G.F. Thornton and L.E. Cluff, Epidemiological Studies of Adverse Drug Reactions, *Amer. J. Publ. Hlth.* **55** (1965), 1170-75.

14. Venulet J., "Methods of Monitoring Adverse Reactions to Drugs" *in : Progress in Drug Research*, E. Jucker ed., Basel, Birkhäuser Verlag, 1977, v. 21, pp. 233-92.

15. Venulet J., A. Ciucci and G.C. Berneker, Standardized Assessment of Drug-adverse Reaction Associations — rationale and experience, *Int. J. Clin. Pharmacol.* **18** (1980), 381-88.

Sécurité et médicaments (1982), pp. 93-103

Experiences of Registers in Drug Safety Assessment in Sweden

B. WESTERHOLM* and B. E. WIHOLM**

* General Director, National Board of Health and Welfare, Linnégatan 87, S-106 30 Stockholm, Sweden
** National Board of Health and Welfare, Linnégatan 87, S-106 30 Stockholm, Sweden

Abstract — In addition to the ADR-register (1965), the NBH have access to many other patient, disease or drug oriented registers for drug safety assessment. Some examples will be given. 1. The mortality is published yearly (1911) by sex, age and cause (ICD). No proven drug induced change was found in the incidence of fatal myocardial infarction among fertile women between 1961-63 (before oral contraceptives, OC), 1966-68 (high-oestrogen OC) and 1975-77 (low-oestrogen OC). 2. From computerised hospital registers of discharge diagnoses (1964) the yearly incidence of thrombo-embolism in OC users was significantly higher than in non-users in all but the lowest age group. Incidence and causes of blood dyscrasias and the Stevens-Johnson syndrome has also been studied. The Cancer Register (1959) was useful for excluding an increased incidence of thyroid cancers after diagnostic and therapeutic doses of I-131. 4. The Malformation Register (1965) and the Medical Register of Births (1973) have been used to exclude suspicions of Mb Down from OC and CNS malformations from hexachlorophene and phenoxy-acids. 5. The amounts of drugs sold since 1970 to pharmacies and hospitals by region are computerised and stored as the number of defined daily doses (DDD). For antidiabetics 15-33 DDD/1000 inhabitants/day gives a rough estimate of regional differences in the drug treatment of diabetes. 6. The number of prescriptions/patient/year ($\overline{m} = 5$) by age and sex and the mean prescribed daily dose can be found in a continous survey of a random sample (1 : 288) of all 39 × 10^6 prescriptions. By combining sales and prescription data with ADR-reports it was possible to show that the relative risk of inducing lactic acidosis was significantly higher for phenformin than for metformin. By use of these registers it is possible to obtain valuable information about drug safety. The raw data must however be interpreted with care and often be supplemented with in depth studies of the various problems.

The first suspicions about new adverse reactions usually originate from observations made by single physicians who report them as case reports in the literature. In spite of enormous efforts put into different "early warning" systems, this generally holds true. As soon as the suspicion has arisen, the next step is to prove or disprove a cause-effect relationship, to establish incidence, identify mechanisms and find special risk groups. In this work different epidemiological techniques can be applied, depending on the nature of the problem[1].

Here, we will discuss the usefullness and limitations of various registers available in Sweden by means of which drug safety can be assessed.

REGISTERS, CLASSIFICATIONS AND CODES

Table 1 depicts a summary of the available registers. Generally, the patients are regis tered with a unique ten-digit birth-number and the diseases in accordance with the Nordic version of the International. Classification of Diseases (ICD). In the Nordic ver-

Table 1. Registers available in sweden for drug safety assessment*

I.	Adverse drug reaction oriented
	1. Spontaneous reporting system
	(2. Intensive hospital monitoring)
II.	Patient & disease oriented
	1. Mortality register
	2. Cancer register
	3. Patient register
	4. Malformation register
	Medical birth record register
III.	Drug utilisation oriented
	1. :Sales register
	2. Prescription surveys
	3. Medical index of sweden

*Only one limited study

sion, the ICD code is further specified by a fifth digit. The drugs are identified by a special number which is widely used in Sweden and can be found in the official Swedish drug list and in the Physicians Desk Reference. This code number identifies single drugs — but not synonyms.

We will not go into the adverse drug reaction registers in detail as these are presented by others.

THE MORTALITY REGISTER

The Mortality Register is based on information from death certificates and has been published annually since 1911. As the quality of the diagnoses (ICD-code) in some respects are unsatisfactory, especially for patients who do not die in hospital, it has only been used once, and with limited value, to assess adverse drug reactions[2].

CANCER REGISTER

The Swedish Cancer Register (SCR) started in 1959 and has recently been updated to 1976[3]. In addition to patient data and diagnoses (ICD) it contains information on histology and outcome. It is possible to search this register for cancer which might be drug induced and then go back to the patients or their case-records. The Cancer Register has recently been used to investigate the significance of ^{131}I used in diagnostic and therapeutic doses for causing thyroid tumors[4]. The birth-numbers of 10,133 patients given diagnostic doses of Iodine 131 between 1952-65 in one hospital were run against the Cancer Register. The average follow up time was 17 years. Nine of the patients were found to have developed a malignancy and the expected number — computed from data for all of Sweden was 8.3. Similarly, no increased incidence of malignant thyroid

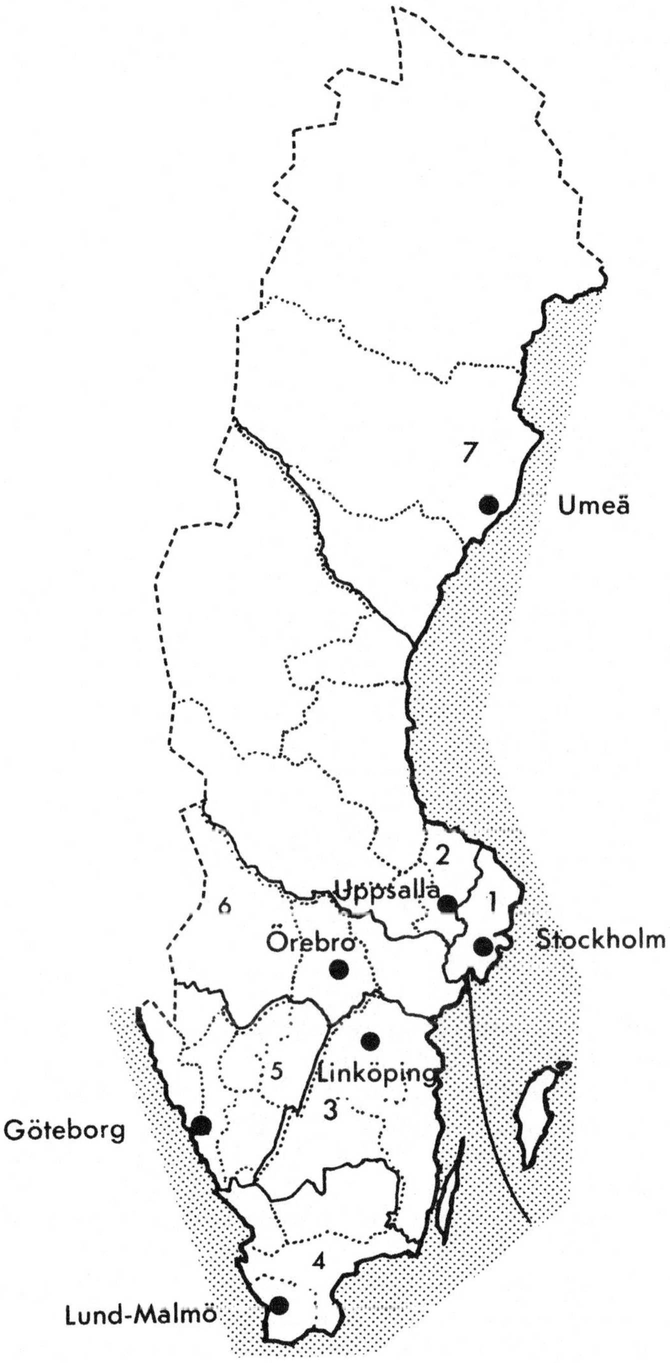

Fig. 1. Sweden has 7 health care regions. Each of these is centered by a regional hospital and in all but number 6 this a university hospital.

Table 2. Blood Dyscrasias in the Uppsala Region 1964-1968*

Disease	Yearly All	incidence per 10^6 Drug induced	Drug induced %	Causative drug(s)
Aplastic anemia	13.2	0.7	5.3	butazones, chloramphenicol
Agranulocytosis	12.8	2.5	19.3	dipyrone, antithyroid, sulfonamides
Thrombocytopenia	59.0	3.1	5.3	thiazides, quinidine
Hæmolytic anemia	26.6	1.1	4.1	methyldopa, sulfonamides

*Data derived from ref 5.

tumors was found in 3,000 patients given therapeutic doses of Iodine 131 for hyperthyroidism or cardiac disease between 1951 and 1965. The average follow up time was 13 and 6 years respectively. An induction time of malignancies of over 20 years has been reported and therefore this patient material is followed up continuously. A reevaluation of 200 cases reported to the SCR revealed a low incidence (10 %) of overdiagnosing. In view of a near total (>95 %) reporting this indicates that the incidence data in the Cancer Register can be used for epidemiological studies.

PATIENT REGISTER

Most hospitals in Sweden have a computerised register of discharge diagnoses which allows a retrieval of medical records according to specific diseases. The system has existed for the longest period of time in the Uppsala region, which comprises 1.2 million inhabitants or about 15 per cent of the Swedish population (Fig. 1).

The patient register from the Uppsala region has been used in order to study to what extent drugs have induced blood dyscrasias[5]. The yearly incidence per million inhabitants, the per cent drug induced cases and the main causative drugs for the blood discrasias are shown in table 2.

In two more recent investigations conducted in the same way in the Stockholm area during 1973-1977, the mean annual incidence of drug induced neutropenia was of the same order but there was a change in drugs pattern[6, 7]. The most common causative drugs were then tenalidine, sulfonamides and antithyroid drugs.

By comparing the incidence of drug induced thrombocytopenias in the Uppsala region with the percentage of consumers of diuretics from the continuous survey of drug purchases in part of the region (Jämtland county) a certain parallellism in the age relation was seen[5]. However, when the incidence was calculated by age, patients over 45 years appeared to have a doubled risk of developing thrombocytopenia (Table 3).

A retrospective evaluation of 89 patients treated for Stevens-Johnson's syndrome[8] disclosed that 77 cases (87 %) had received drugs. In 40 cases sulfonamides were incriminated.

Thromboembolic complications during use of oral contraceptives have been the

Table 3.
Estimated risk for thrombocytopenia*
induced by diuretics

Total	1 : 15,000
Risk vs Age	
over 45 years	1 : 14,100
under 45 years	1 : 27,200
Risk vs sex	
men	1 : 14,400
women	1 : 15,100

* Data derived from ref 5.

cause of constant concern. In a previous study the risk of getting a thromboembolic episode had been calculated at 1 : 3,600 in users as compared to 1 :23,000 in non users[9]. Parallel with the introduction of low oestrogen pills on the market the number of thromboembolic episodes reported to the ADR-Committee fell drastically from an average of 26 per 100,000 users in 1966-1970 to 7 in 1974-1977[2]. A comparison of the morbidity rate in the Uppsala region between periods with predominantly high oestrogen and low oestrogen pills[2] showed that the incidence of hospitalisation due to thromboembolic disease was significantly higher for oral contraceptive users during both periods (Table 4). Moreover, there seemed to be a decreased risk during the latter period (risk ratio 15 vs 11) but in this restricted material the difference did not reach statistical significance. The risk of thromboembolic complications during use of oral contraceptives increased markedly with age, from about 20/100,000 women aged 15-24 years to 90/100,000 women aged 35-44.

MALFORMATION REGISTER AND MEDICAL BIRTH RECORD REGISTER

Since 1965 children born with serious malformations are reported to the Malformation Register. The malformations are classified according to a more specified and detailed classification than the ICD-code.

This register was primarily intended for the detection of drug-induced malformations. As such it is relatively sensitive. Had it been functioning in 1960 it would only have taken four months of reporting to detect the thalidomide malformations[10]. Since 1973 the outcome of all pregnancies are also registered in the Medical Birth Record Register in accordance with the ICD-code. These two registers are presently being integrated.

In 1974 the Adverse Drug Reaction Committee received a report maintaining that the use of hexachlorophene-containing soaps by pregnant women would lead to an increased risk of malformations in their offspring[11]. To investigate this suspicion information was sought from the Medical Birth Record Register on the outcome of births by women working in long time care hospitals in relation to the extent of hexachlorophene used in these hospitals[12]. Only crude data on hexachlorophene use were available.

Table 4. Women admitted to hopital with thromboembolic disease in relation to use of oral contraceptives with different estrogen content.

	High estrogen pills	Low estrogen pills
No. of users with disease	46	35
Incidence+	1:2,300	1:5,300
No. of non-users with disease	20	9
Incidence+	1:34,900	1:80,000
Risk ratio	15	11
Level of significance	$P < 0.001$	$P < 0.001$

+) Estimated from sales and prescription data for the whole of Sweden
Data derived from ref 2.

From Table 5 it can be seen that no increase was found in the rate of perinatal deaths or malformations which could be attributed to the use of hexachlorophene.

DRUG SALES AND PRESCRIPTION REGISTERS

For an evaluation of the risk/benefit ratio of drugs it is also important to know how much different drugs are used, on what indications and to whom they are prescribed. During the last ten-year period various drug-oriented registers have been established in Sweden which are useful in providing these important background data.

Table 5. Perinatal death and malformation rates 1973 and 1975 in hospitals where soaps containing hexachlorophene were generally or rarely used.*

	Hexachlorophene generally used in hospital	
	Yes	No
Number of hospitals	31	18
Number of births	3007	1653
Perinatal deaths:		
No. found	45	17
No expected	45	18
Malformed infants		
No. found	157	101
No. expected	152	86

*Data derived from ref 12.

WHOLESALE LEVEL

The total amount of drugs delivered from the National Corporation of Swedish Pharmacies[13] to different pharmacies since 1970 and hospitals since 1976 by region are computerised and stored as the number of so called defined daily doses (DDD)[14]. For antidiabetic drugs a range of 15-33 DDD per thousand inhabitants per day gives a rough estimate of the large regional difference in the drug treatment of diabetes[13]. In-

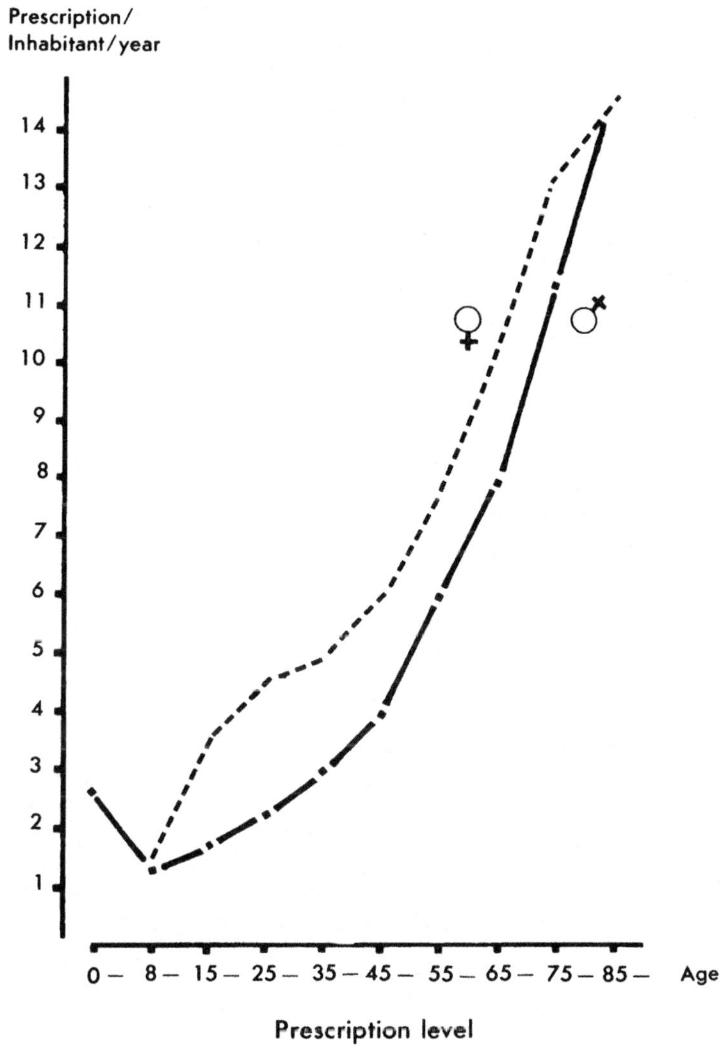

Fig. 2. Average number of prescriptions per inhabitant and year by age in Sweden during 1975-77. Derived from the continuos 1:288 prescription sample (17).

ternational comparisons based on this unit of measurement have shown that five times as much oral anti-diabetics are used in Sweden as in Iceland[15].

PRESCRIPTION LEVEL

Since 1974 a random sample of 1 : 288 prescriptions is picked out in the pharmacies[16]. Information about age and sex of the patient, the name, amount and daily dosage of the drug is coded and computerised. In Fig. 2 it is shown that the number of prescriptions per patient increases markedly with age and that women tend to get more prescriptions than men[17]. In the county of Jämtland a continuous individual register of drug purchases for 1/7 of the population has been recorded in a similar way since 1970[18]. Since 1978 the Medical Index of Sweden has been run in collaboration between the drug industry, the National Corporation of Swedish Pharmacies, the Swedish Medical Association and the National Board of Health and Welfare. In this survey a random sample of physicians each week registers all prescriptions on special forms which also state the indication for each drug treatment. From this survey it has been possible, for example, to disclose to what extent diuretics and beta-blockers are used for hypertension and other indications[19].

An example of how a combination of various pieces of information from different registers has been useful is the problem of biguanides and lactic acidosis (LA). Be-

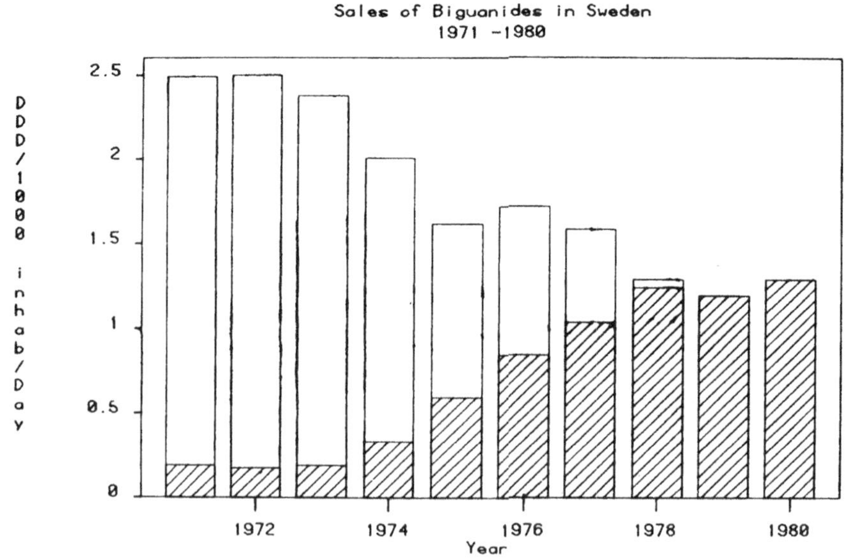

Fig. 3. Sales of biguanides in Sweden 1971-79, expressed as the number of defined daily doses (DDD) per 1000 inhabitants and day. Open bars = phenformin, DDD = 100 mg.
Striped bars = metformin DDD = 2.0g. In 1976 the average prescribed daily doses were 74 mg and 1.5 g respectively. Data derived from ref's 13, and 20.

Table 6. Numbers of adverse reactions to phenformin and metformin reported in Sweden during 1975-77 and relation to sales.

	Phenformin	Metformin	P
Sales (x 10^6 DDDs)	7.37	7.50	
Adverse reactions:			
Reported	16	12	NS
Probable and not excluted	14	7	NS
Lactic acidosis:			
Reported	13	2	0.01
Probable and not excluded	13	1	0.001
Fatal reactions			
Reported	6		0.02
Probable and not excluded	6		0.02

DDD = Defined daily dose. NS = Not significant.
Data from ref 20.

tween 1970-1974 an increasing number of cases of LA associated with the use of phenformin were reported to the Swedish Adverse Drug Reaction Committee. The situation prompted a series of warnings against an indiscriminate use of phenformin and the indications for its use were restricted. At that time (Fig. 3) the use of metformin in Sweden was low and no comparisons of the relative risk of inducing LA could be made. Moreover, very few cases of LA were reported in the literature during use of metformin. After these warnings, there was a shift in the use of biguanides from phenformin to metformin and parallel to the increased use, adverse reactions to metformin were reported in increasing frequency.

In 1978[20] a comparison of the total number of ADRs reported for phenformin and metformin in relation to the sales showed no significant difference (Table 6). However, the number of LA and thereby also fatal reactions were significantly higher for phenformin than for metformin. From the prescription survey no difference in age and sex could be found between patients treated with the two biguanides. The relation between the DDD and the average prescribed daily dose (p=74 mg, m=1.5 g) from the prescription survey was also comparable. Thus, confounding of the results in these respects could be ruled out. This information formed a relatively solid ground for the decision in October 1978. Since then the situation has been closely monitored. A metabolic study on patients with LA did not indicate that a genetic impairment of hydroxylative capacity was a major reason for the LA in survivors of this adverse reaction[21]. A few cases of metformin induced LA have been reported since 1978. The incidence has been calculated at about 1 reported LA in 10,000 patients per year.

CONCLUDING REMARKS

By use of different registers, much valuable information has been gathered on safety problems with different drugs. However the raw data must be interpreted with care and often be supplemented by in-depth studies of the various problems. Although this presentation is restricted to the use of Swedish registers, we dare the presumption that similar experience has been encountered also in other countries.

The advantage of all the registers is that they comprise the whole population and that the reporting routines are fairly simple. With the help of the registers it is possible to trace the cases with diseases which might be drug induced and to make estimations of frequency. Since the information (the Malformation Register excepted) is collected nevertheless for other purposes (like health care planning), the cost for the information is almost negligible.

The greatest disadvantage with all the sources of information (except for the Malformation Register) is the inaccuracy of the diagnoses. Since the physicians are not aware of the fact that the diagnoses are being used for other purposes than the production of diagrams, enough effort is not put into accurate recording. Besides, the ICD-code is not always suitable for the recording of adverse reactions. Thus, a single diagnosis according to ICD may cover a group of diseases only one of which may be caused by a drug. If the drug code is left out of the discharge diagnosis the analysis of individual medical records is required. This can only be done for some rare diseases.

A disadvantage may also be the delay in the appearance of the data. In Sweden the drug utilisation registers are the quickest with a delay of about three months, followed by the Malformation Register with a delay of six months. The Cancer Register is the slowest with five years' delay at present which is not acceptable from an epidemiological point of view. The other registers have a delay of about a year.

To improve this situation we must therefore educate the physicians in order to make them write proper discharge diagnoses. We should adapt the ICD-code to the needs in drug monitoring. We should convince the administrators about the necessity of quick updating of the registers. Since these registers contain information which for the individual patient might be very sensitive we should finally see to it that confidentiality of the data is assured.

Acknowledgments — Grants were received from the National Corporation of Swedish Parmacies and the Karolinska Institute.

REFERENCES

1. Jick H., The discovery of drug-induced illness, *New Engl. J. Med.* **296** (1977), 481-85.

2. Böttiger L.E., G. Boman, G. Eklund and B. Westerholm, Oral contraceptives and thromboembolic disease. Effects of lowering oestrogen content, *Lancet* **1** (1980), 1097-1101.

3. Cancer Incidence in Sweden 1975 and 1976, National Board of Health and Welfare, The Cancer Registry, S-106 30 Stockholm Sweden, Liber Förlag, 1980.

4. Holm L.E., Incidence of malignant thyroid tumors in man after diagnostic and therapeutic doses of Iodine 131, Epidemiologic and histopathologic study, Medical thesis (1980), Karolinska Institutet, S-104 01, Stockholm, Sweden.

5. Böttiger L.E. and B. Westerholm, Drug induced blood dyscrasias in Sweden, *Br. J. Med.* **3** (1979), 339-43.

6. Arneborn P. and J. Palmblad, Drug-induced neutropenia in the Stockholm area 1973-75 : frequency and causes, *Acta Med. Scand.* **204** (1978), 283-86.

7. Arneborn P. and J. Palmblad, Drug-induced neutropenia in the Stockholm region 1976-77, *Acta Med. Scand.* **206** (1979), 241-43.

8. Böttiger L.E., J. Strandberg and B. Westerholm, Drug-induced febrile mucocutaneous syndrome, *Acta Med. Scand.* **198** (1975), 229-33.

Sécurité et médicaments (1982), pp. 105-110

Méthodes actuelles pour évaluer l'innocuité des médicaments : enquêtes prospectives

C. RUMEAU-ROUQUETTE

Unité 149 de l'INSERM, 44 chemin de ronde, 78110 Le Vésinet. France

Résumé — La surveillance d'une cohorte de sujets, pour enregistrer les effets indésirables des médicaments, peut être envisagée dans différentes situations en allant du plus simple au plus complexe.

La surveillance d'un produit ou d'un petit nombre de produits utilisés chez des malades hospitalisés pour étudier des effets à court terme représente la forme la plus simple. Elle nécessite cependant la mise en place d'une structure d'enquête dont un exemple sera donné (femmes enceintes traitées pour menace d'accouchement prématuré).

On envisagera ensuite la surveillance à long terme d'individus prenant un type précis de produit (contraceptifs par exemple), dans différents contextes médicaux.

Les formes plus complexes d'enquêtes prospectives visant à suivre les effets de thérapeutiques multiples avec des effets indésirables à court terme et à long terme seront enfin examinées sous l'angle du coût et de l'efficacité.

Le bilan des avantages et des inconvénients de ces enquêtes est extrêmement variable selon la situation envisagée, le système de santé et selon qu'existent dans le pays considéré des systèmes d'information sanitaire plus ou moins développés.

Au cours des trente dernières années, les épidémiologistes se sont d'abord attachés à étudier l'efficacité des médicaments dans le cadre d'essais comparatifs contrôlés, dont la méthodologie a été longuement définie. Ce faisant, ils s'intéressaient davantage aux effets bénéfiques des produits qu'aux complications liées à leur usage. Le contexte dans lequel se faisaient ces essais explique sans doute cette lacune, il s'agissait en général de maladies graves, telles que le cancer, et les inconvénients apparaissaient moindre que les bénéfices attendus. Ces inconvénients étaient d'ailleurs limités en raison de la haute qualification des services dans lesquels ces essais étaient réalisés.

En France, les épidémiologistes ont été sensibilisés au problème de la pharmacovigilance, à partir des années 60, par quelques "affaires" ayant un large retentissement : malformations liées à l'usage du thalidomide, complications cardio-vasculaires des contraceptifs oraux... C'est dans ce cadre que sont nées des enquêtes prospectives conduisant à suivre une cohorte de sujets pendant une période plus ou moins longue afin de détecter les complications. Nous en examinerons quelques exemples en allant du plus simple au plus complexe.

Le terme médicament sera pris dans son sens large : «toute substance ou produit utilisé ou destiné à être utilisé en vue de modifier ou d'étudier un système physiologique ou un état pathologique, dans l'intérêt du sujet auquel il est administré»[1].

CAS RELATIVEMENT SIMPLES

On se propose de suivre, pendant une période relativement courte, des sujets recevant un médicament ou un petit nombre de médicaments pour étudier la fréquence de complications dont la nature est connue. Ces enquêtes sont particulièrement faciles à mener si elles sont conduites dans un cadre hospitalier. Elles comportent toutefois deux difficultés.

– La première est fondamentale, elle concerne le *choix d'une situation de référence*. Si l'on administre un produit à un malade hospitalisé pour une maladie donnée, il est difficile en l'absence de témoin de savoir si certaines complications sont dues à l'administration du médicament, à la maladie, aux autres traitements ou tout simplement à l'hospitalisation. Sans doute peut-on objecter que certains effets adverses sont spécifiques d'un produit donné et n'existent jamais en son absence. Ces cas sont assez rares et ils ne sont pas toujours les plus intéressants. La plupart du temps, il est nécessaire de suivre deux groupes de sujets atteints de la même affection dont l'un reçoit le produit surveillé et l'autre un produit différent. Dans la pratique médicale courante, ces deux groupes ne sont pas comparables, car l'attribution d'un traitement est évidemment lié à la gravité de la maladie, à l'âge des sujets... D'où l'intérêt des essais contrôlés dans lesquels l'attribution du traitement est aléatoire parmi les individus reconnus bons pour l'essai. Il nous semble important de rappeler très nettement que *les essais contrôlés entrent dans les techniques classiques d'évaluation de l'innocuité des médicaments*. Ils permettent non seulement de comparer l'efficacité de deux produits (dont l'un peut être un placebo), mais aussi de comparer leurs effets adverses dans un bilan coût/efficacité dont D. Schwartz a décrit les modalités[2].

– La deuxième difficulté réside dans l'organisation de la surveillance prospective des individus. Même dans les cas les plus favorables (malades hospitalisés), elle nécessite la mise en place d'un *protocole* qui doit être soigneusement préparé tant en ce qui concerne la définition des objectifs, que celle de la population, des modalités d'examen et des méthodes d'analyse.

A titre d'exemple, nous examinerons brièvement une étude portant sur les complications liées à l'usage d'un ß mimétique dans la prévention de l'accouchement prématuré.

La première phase a consisté en un essai comparatif : 58 femmes présentant une menace d'accouchement prématuré entre 20 et 36 semaines d'aménorrhée, ont été réparties en deux groupes de façon aléatoire ; le premier recevait de l'ifenprodil et le second un ß mimétique la ritodrine. Nous n'insisterons pas sur les modalités de l'essai qui était de type séquentiel et qui ont été décrites en détail par ailleurs[3]. Les résultats ont montré la supériorité de la ritodrine (la ritodrine a entraîné l'arrêt des contractions dans 90 % des cas et l'ifenprodil dans 45 % des cas), mais aussi la fréquence plus élevée des complications (69 % pour la ritodrine et 17 % pour l'ifenprodil). Il a donc été décidé, par le service hospitalier concerné, d'arrêter l'utilisation de l'ifenprodil, mais aussi d'instituer une surveillance des cas traités par ß mimétique.

C'est l'objet d'une deuxième enquête actuellement en cours. Elle a pour but de surveiller, dans un centre hospitalier, l'efficacité et les réactions adverses aux ß mimétiques pris en cours de grossesse. Il s'agit des effets à court terme et à moyen terme observés pendant la grossesse ou à la naissance (signes d'intolérance : hypotension, tachycardie, troubles digestifs... ; effets sur le nouveau-né : troubles cardiaques, troubles de la glycorégulation...). Ce système de pharmacovigilance intensive se limite actuellement aux femmes hospitalisées pour menace d'accouchement prématuré, mais le système peut être étendu ultérieurement aux traitements ambulatoires. Toutes les femmes font l'objet, à leur entrée dans le service, d'un interrogatoire systématique portant sur les médicaments pris avant l'hospitalisation et les réactions adverses déjà constatées, de façon à pouvoir interpréter les résultats en fonction des médications antérieures et en particulier d'étudier les problèmes d'interaction. Pendant la durée de l'hospitalisation, un enquêteur établit un relevé quotidien des médicaments présents et réellement pris par la femme. Il recherche par interrogatoire et examens, les effets indésirables connus et suspectés, il enregistre également les troubles déclarés spontanément par la femme.

CAS DE COMPLEXITE MOYENNE

Dans le schéma précédent, la difficulté peut être accrue par le fait qu'il s'agit de sujets non hospitalisés donc difficiles à suivre, par la longueur de la surveillance ou par la nature des complications. Les cas les plus difficiles étant ceux où l'on étudie des complications rares et relativement tardives.

Nous supposerons toutefois, et ceci est un élément très favorable, que le problème est nettement posé : il s'agit d'un type de produits bien spécifié et l'on a une idée sur la nature des complications et leur délai d'apparition. Les enquêtes prospectives portant sur les contraceptifs oraux entrent dans ce cadre. Deux cas sont à distinguer selon qu'il s'agit de réactions précoces et relativement fréquentes, ou de réactions tardives et rares.

a) *Dans les enquêtes visant à rechercher des complications précoces*, il s'agit de suivre quelques centaines, voire quelques milliers de femmes pendant 1 ou 2 ans. Elles ne présentent pas de très grandes difficultés dans les pays où la clientèle des médecins est relativement stable. Il n'en va pas de même en France. De 1970 à 1975, nous avons réalisé une enquête prospective en collaboration avec 10 médecins volontaires (gynécologues pour la plupart), 4 000 femmes commençant à utiliser une méthode de contraception (pilule, DIU, diaphragme) sont entrées dans l'enquête[4]. La durée théorique de la surveillance variait de 2 à 5 ans et toutes les femmes auraient dû être suivies pendant au moins 1 an. Au cours de la première année, 50 % des femmes environ ont été perdues de vue par le médecin qui a prescrit la contraception. Dns ces conditions, il devient très difficile d'étudier valablement les complications. Sans doute, le problème des durées inégales de surveillance peut être résolu par des méthodes mathématiques tout à fait classiques (méthode actuarielle, calcul du nombre de personnes-années suivies ou du nombre total de cycles enregistrés), mais ces méthodes reposent sur l'hypothèse que la période de la surveillance est homogène quant à la fréquence d'apparition des réactions adverses, or il n'en est rien. De plus, les femmes perdues de vue ne sont certainement pas comparables aux autres et sont à l'origine d'erreur dans l'interprétation des résultats.

b) *Les vastes enquêtes destinées à rechercher les complications tardives et rares* présentent encore plus de difficultés. Ceci explique sans doute que les premières enquêtes prospectives n'aient pu mettre en évidence une relation existant entre les contraceptifs oraux et les thromboses[5]. Depuis, quelques grandes enquêtes prospectives ont affirmé cette liaison. On ne sera pas surpris que deux d'entre elles soient anglaises, compte tenu des particularités de la médecine dans ce pays. L'une est l'enquête du Royal College of General Practitioners[6], réalisée par 14 000 médecins praticiens, portant sur 23 000 utilisatrices de pilules, de 15 à 49 ans, qui ont été comparées à 23 000 témoins utilisant une autre méthode ou pas de contraception ; l'autre est l'enquête de l'Oxford University Family Planning Association[7] portant sur 17000 femmes, de 25 à 39 ans, utilisatrices des contraceptifs oraux, des DIU ou des diaphragmes. Vessey a récemment fait le point des résultats de ces deux études[8].

Compte tenu de ces difficultés, il est absolument indispensable d'établir avant le début de l'enquête l'ordre de grandeur de la population à suivre. Shapiro a envisagé ce problème à partir de l'exemple de l'agranulocytose ; il suppose que sa probabilité est de 1/100 000 personne-année, dans une population non exposée. Si la fréquence dans la population exposée est de 1/500 personne-année (risque relatif = 200), il est nécessaire de suivre 4 000 personnes pendant 1 an ; si la fréquence est de 1/1 000 il faut suivre 8 000 personnes-année ; si la fréquence est de 1/20 000, il faut en suivre 245 000... De même doivent être spécifiées la longueur de la surveillance et ses modalités.

On conçoit que de telles enquêtes soient rares et qu'on les réalise seulement lorsqu'un certain nombre de conditions favorables sont réunies.

CAS TRES DIFFICILES

Il s'agit des cas où les hypothèses sont mal spécifiées : on se propose à l'extrême de rechercher les complications pouvant être liées à l'usage de n'importe quel médicament, sans avoir d'idée précise sur la nature exacte des complications. Ce type de problème est mal accepté par les épidémiologistes qui refusent souvent d'appliquer des techniques difficiles à mettre en œuvre pour répondre à une question mal posée. Et c'est pourtant là un problème très fréquent dans le domaine de la pharmacovigilance.

En dépit des difficultés, le schéma classique des enquêtes prospectives peut s'appliquer, en présence de circonstances favorables.

Tel est le cas de la grossesse en raison de la surveillance médicale exercée sur les femmes et de la durée limitée de la surveillance. Ceci explique la multiplication des enquêtes et notamment des grandes enquêtes prospectives destinées à étudier l'effet tératogène possible des médicaments.

En France, une enquête prospective s'est déroulée entre 1963 et 1969[9] et elle a été complétée depuis par une enquête plus limitée en 1975-1977. Dans la première enquête, 18 275 femmes ont été interrogées sur leur consommation de médicaments pendant les trois premiers mois de leur grossesse, dans 12 maternités d'hôpitaux publics de Paris et de la région parisienne. L'enquête comportait outre l'interrogatoire et l'examen de la femme enceinte au 3e mois, une étude sérologique, un examen de l'enfant à la période néonatale, une surveillance ultérieure des enfants dont l'examen néonatal avait montré ou fait soupçonner qu'ils étaient atteints d'une malformation et d'un groupe d'enfants normaux.

La deuxième enquête portait sur 4 000 femmes enceintes dans quatre maternités à Lille et à Paris[10]. Les principales difficultés rencontrées ont été les suivantes :
– difficultés de l'interrogatoire liées aux oublis portant sur la consommation des médicaments, en dépit d'un protocole très élaboré comportant une description des produits usuels, des vérifications faites à partir des ordonnances...
– nombre élevé de produits consommés (1 500 spécialités dans la première enquête, 400 dans la deuxième) ; il alourdit l'exploitation des résultats et conduit à un petit nombre de femmes exposées (100 à 500 pour les produits moyennement consommés).
– nombre élevé de femmes perdues de vue au cours de la grossesse (1/3 environ) ; si la disparition de ces femmes entraîne peu de biais lorsqu'elle a lieu avant le diagnostic porté sur l'enfant, elle contribue à réduire le nombre de cas.

Ces difficultés se trouvent multipliées lorsqu'on souhaite prolonger la surveillance au-delà de la naissance pour étudier par exemple la relation existant entre l'exposition fœtale aux médicaments et le cancer chez le jeune. Compte tenu de la rareté de la maladie, il y aurait lieu de suivre plusieurs dizaines, voire plusieurs centaines de milliers d'enfants. Devant un tel problème, les enquêtes prospectives classiques s'avèrent le plus souvent impossibles et des solutions nouvelles doivent être envisagées. Dans le cas du cancer, on pourrait imaginer une région comportant un nombre assez élevé de naissances, où seraient concentrés :
– des enregistrements systématiques et informatisés dans les principales maternités ;
– un système de pharmacovigilance au cours de la grossesse ;
– un enregistrement des malformations congénitales ;
– un enregistrement des cancers de l'enfant et du jeune.

La coordination des deux premiers systèmes pourrait conduire à l'enregistrement d'un certain nombre de médicaments pris au cours de la grossesse, celui-ci devrait sans doute être limité pour que l'enregistrement reste fiable. Il serait ensuite possible d'établir une relation entre les produits et les cas de malformations et de cancers. En dépit d'une apparente simplicité, un tel système requiert des efforts considérables, mais il a été mené avec succès en Finlande en ce qui concerne les malformations.

En conclusion

Il nous semble que l'usage des enquêtes prospectives et des essais contrôlés classiques est tout à fait justifié dans les cas simples où la surveillance peut s'exercer en milieu hospitalier à partir d'hypothèses bien définies sur la nature des médicaments et des complications.

A l'inverse, ces enquêtes s'appliquent mal à la surveillance en population des complications rares liées à l'usage de médicaments plus ou moins bien définis. A cet échelon, de nouvelles méthodes doivent être imaginées.

Entre ces deux situations extrêmes existent des états intermédiaires où l'application des enquêtes prospectives dépend à la fois de la nature du problème, du système de soins et de prévention.

REFERENCES

1. O.M.S., Série des rapports techniques, N° 341, 1966, Principes applicables à l'étude préclinique de l'innocuité des médicaments : rapport d'un groupe scientifique de l'O.M.S., p. 7.

2. Schwartz D., R. Flamant et J. Lellouch, *Essais thérapeutiques chez l'homme*, Paris, Flammarion, 1981, 2e édition.

3. Breat G., C. Sureau et C. Rumeau-Rouquette, Etude de l'efficacité comparée de l'ifenprodil et de la ritodrine pour le traitement de la menace d'accouchement prématuré, *J. Gyn. Obst. Repr.* **8** (1979), 261-63.

4. Feinerman D., Y. Rabarison et J. Cohen, Enquête de surveillance des femmes sous contraception, *Fert. Orth.* **4** (1972), 33-44.

5. Drill V.A., Oral contraceptive and thromboembolic disease. Prospective and retrospective studies, *J. am. Med. Assoc.* **219**, 583-92.

6. Kay C.R., Oral contraceptives and health : the Royal College of General Practitioners Study, *Am. J. Epid.* **102** (1975).

7. Vessey M.P., R. Doll, R. Peto *et al.*, A long-term follow-up study of women using different methods of contraception : an interim report, *J. Biosoc. Sci.* **8** (1976), 373.

8. Vessey M.P., Contraceptive methods : risk and benefits, *Brit. Med. J.* **2** (1978), 721-22.

9. Rumeau-Rouquette C., J. Goujard, G. Huel et M. Kaminski, Malformations congénitales risques périnatals, Paris, INSERM, 1978, 1 vol.

10. Goujard J., C. Rumeau-Rouquette et M.J. Saurel-Cubizolles, Tests hormonaux de grossesse et malformations congénitales, *J. Gyn. Obst. Biol. Repr.* **8** (1979), 489-96.

Sécurité et médicaments (1982), pp. 111-121

Case-Control Studies in the Evaluation of Drug Safety

M.P. VESSEY

University, Department of Community Medicine and General Practice, 8 Keble Road, Oxford, OX1 3 QN. United Kingdom

Abstract — In a case-control study, the basic approach is to identify a group of subjects newly presenting with the illness of interest and to discover how many of them were exposed to the suspected cause (i.e. within the context of the present meeting, a particular drug or group of drugs). The frequency of exposure in these cases is then compared with that in a series of control subjects free from the illness under investigation.

Many of the epidemiological studies of drug induced illness now appearing in the literature are of the case-control type, principally because such studies are usually easy to set up, reasonably cheap, and can often be completed within 1-2 years.

The paper will consider the main areas of methodological importance in carrying out a case-control study of the effects of drugs, i.e. selection of cases, selection of controls, identification of exposure to the drugs under study, influence of confounding factors, analysis of the data and interpretation of the results.

Usually, a case-control study is set up to test a hypothesis which has been suggested by animal studies, clinical observation, etc. Brief reference will also be made to so-called 'case-control surveillance', which has as one objective the discovery of drug induction of serious illness.

In a case-control study, the basic approach is to identify a group of subjects with the illness of interest and to determine how many of them were exposed to the suspected cause (i.e. within the context of the present paper, a particular drug or a member of a group of drugs). The frequency of exposure in these cases is then compared with that in a series of control subjects free from the illness under investigation. The control series is, of course, intended to provide an estimate of the exposure rate which would have been seen in the case series if, in fact, the exposure and the illness were unrelated.

An important limitation of case-control studies is that usually they can provide only very limited information about the size of any risk (or benefit) that they demonstrate. It is, in fact, often possible to obtain an estimate of *relative risk* from a well designed case-control study, e.g. to be able to estimate that myocardial infarction occurs, say, three times more frequently in oral contraceptive users than in other women, but in general, no estimate can be provided of the *absolute risk* in terms of incidence or mortality rates. Relative risks are, of course, of great interest to the epidemiologist because they indicate the strength of the association. Those concerned with the public health are, however, likely to be much more concerned about absolute risks.

The main advantage of the case-control approach is that studies can often be done quickly and inexpensively.

Table 1. Case-control study

Cases — those *with* disease of interest (e.g. breast cancer)
Contrôls — those *without* disease of interest (otherwise similar to cases)
History of exposure to suspected cause (e.g. oral contraceptive use) obtained from cases and controls and frequency of exposure compared in the two groups.

For this reason, many of the epidemiological studies of illnesses suspected of being caused by drugs now appearing in the literature are of the case-control type. Unfortunately, however, case-control studies may be subject to biases which are hard to control while, in addition, information obtained retrospectively may be incomplete and unreliable. Accordingly, a proper understanding of the design and interpretation of case-control studies is essential both for those conducting this type of research and for those responsible for assessing the importance of published reports.

When studying the role of drugs in the causation of illness, it is important to remember that drug exposure differs in important ways from the exposures traditionally evaluated in case-control studies. The latter (e.g. ethnic group, country of residence, occupation, cigarette smoking) are either inborn or determined fairly early in life and are usually unrelated to any medical problem at the time they are determined. Drug exposure, on the other hand, may occur at any time and is almost always in response to some symptom or illness. It is therefore of great importance when studying the role of drug exposure in the aetiology of disease to consider whether any medical condition providing a particular drug indication (or contraindication) might be related to the illness under study. To give a very simple example — is the apparent association between the use of anticonvulsant drugs in pregnancy and the occurrence of birth defects in the offspring attributable to an adverse effect of the drugs or is it the result of an innate tendency for epileptic women to bear malformed children ?

There are seven major areas of methodological importance in any case-control study, namely 1. determining the size of the study, 2. selecting the cases, 3. selecting the controls, 4. identifying the exposure, 5. controlling confounding factors, 6. analysing the data, and 7. interpreting the results. In the following paragraphs, some of the

Table 2. Estimating risk in case-control studies

Case-control studies can usually provide an estimate of *relative risk*, but in general no estimate can be provided of the *absolute risk* in terms of incidence on mortality rates.

Table 3. Case-control studies involving drugs

Drug exposure differs in important ways from exposures traditionally evaluated in case-control studies (e.g. ethnic group, occupation, smoking). In particular, it is almost always in response to some symptom or illness. Accordingly it is important to consider whether any medical condition providing a particular drug indication (or contra-indication) might be related to the disease under study.

important principles under each of these headings are briefly summarised. Problems that particularly apply to studies involving drugs are considered in more detail.

Determining the size of the study

The factors which have to be taken into account are : 1. the size of relative risk that would be considered of clinical or public health importance ; 2. how certain it is necessary to be that a detected association is not attributable to chance (alpha-error) ; 3. how much risk of failing to detect a real association is acceptable (beta-error) ; 4. the level of exposure to the suspected cause in the population under study.

These matters are considered in detail in a paper by Schlesselman[1], an author who has also prepared a valuable set of tables to help in determining sample size. A point of particular importance is that case-control studies are unlikely to be of much help in assessing possible adverse effects of drugs which are uncommonly used unless the relative risk is substantial. This fact is illustrated in Table 6. It is because of this difficulty that the present author has been unable to pursue the adverse effects of hormone replacement therapy in the United Kingdom, a country in which this particular approach to the management of problems in middle aged women has never really caught on.

Table 4. Case-control studies. Areas of methodological importance.

1) Determining the size of the study
2) Selecting the cases
3) Selecting the controls
4) Identifying the exposure (to the suspected drug)
5) Controlling confounding factors
6) Analysing the data
7) Interpreting the results

Table 5. Case-control studies — deciding on size

Need to consider:
1) Magnitude of difference (in terms of relative risk) which would be of clinical importance
2) How certain it is necessary to be that a detected association is not due to chance
3) How much risk of failing to detect a real association is acceptable
4) Level of exposure to suspected cause in population

Selecting the cases

The following considerations should be kept in mind : the illness under study should be as clearly defined and as accurately diagnosed as possible ; where feasible, the cases should be derived from a defined population ; the cases should be newly presenting ones and should represent a consecutive series.

While the above points are all fairly obvious ones, increasing attention has been paid in recent years to the more subtle problem of selection bias in case-control studies. Such bias is particularly likely when the hypothesis under study has already been widely entertained or where subjects exposed to the suspected cause are under increased medical surveillance. Vessey and Doll[2], for example, in their study of venous thromboembolism were concerned in case doctors had diagnosed thromboembolism more readily or had admitted patients to hospital more readily, when they had obtained a history of the use of oral contraceptives than when they had not. Vessey and Doll[2] argued that if this had been so, the association between oral contraceptive use and the disease would have been strongest in those for whom the physical basis for the diagno-

Table 6. Sample size requirements for case-control studies designed to detect the stated relative risks at the stated levels of use the drug under suspicion in the population. All sample sizes assume a test of significance at the 5% level and a power of 90%.

Frequency of use of drug under suspicion in population (%)	Relative risk to be detected		
	1.2	2.0	5.0
1	58429	3206	406
5	12269	689	92
10	6536	378	54
20	3746	229	37

Note: The sample size is that required for *each* group (cases and controls)

Table 7. Case-control studies — selecting the cases

the following should be considered :
1) Illness under study should be clearly defined and accurately diagnosed
2) Cases should if possible, be derived from defined population
3) Cases should be newly presenting ones and should represent a consecutive series
4) Attention should be paid to selection Bias

sis was least certain. In the event, the association was strongest among those in whom the diagnosis was most firmly established (and the disease most severe). More recently, Horwitz and Feinstein[3] have suggested that the association between œstrogen therapy and endometrial cancer is explicable in terms of detection bias. They have postulated that the administration of œstrogens may cause occult endometrial cancers to bleed, thus leading to the diagnosis of neoplasms in œstrogen users which would otherwise have gone unrecognised. Convincing arguments against this explanation have been put forward, among others, by Jick *et al*[4] and Shapiro *et al*[5].

From the above, it will be apparent thet selection bias is potentially of great importance in case-control studies, especially those concerned with the effects of drugs. It must always be taken into consideration during planning, analysis and interpretation. Feinstein has been particularly concerned (perhaps over-concerned) with this problem and an advanced discussion of some of the issues will be found in a recent paper by this author[6].

Selecting the controls

"The series of control subjects should be chosen in such a way that when a proper analysis is made, i.e. statistical adjustment is made for confounding factors, they are comparable with the cases in all relevant ways except that they do not have the illness under study"[7].

Table 8. Case-control studies — Selection Bias

Selection Bias is particularly likely to occur when the hypothesis under study has already been widely entertained or when subjects exposed to the suspected cause are under increased medical surveillance

Table 9. Case-control studies — Selecting the controls

If *hospital controls* are used, it is essential to exclude subjects admitted for conditions known to be related in any way (either positively or negatively) to the drug of interest.
If community controls are used, care is necessary to ensure that they are comparable with the cases with respect to the likelihood of being admitted to hospital and being drug users.

Since in many case-control studies, the cases represent hospital inpatients, it is common practice to select hospital inpatients as controls as well. If this is done, it is essential to exclude from among the controls any admitted for conditions which are known to be related in any way (either positively or negatively) to the drug of interest. For example, in studying the possible relationship between oral contraceptives and breast cancer, it woud obviously be absurd to include patients with thromboembolism, myocardial infarction or stroke among the controls. In practice, many conditions are potentially related to oral contraceptive use in one way or another and the choice of acceptable diagnoses for hospital controls in studies of the effects of oral contraceptives is rather limited. When hospital controls are used, they should, of course, be drawn from as many diagnostic groups as possible to minimise the impact of including an admitting illness which (unbeknown to the investigator) is associated with the exposure under study.

In some case-control studies, the controls may be selected from the community at large. There are many ways of doing this, but in the United Kingdom, the simplest method is to use general practitioners patient lists (which, collectively, cover about 95 % of the British population). This approach was used, for example, in both the Brit-

Table 10. Case-control studies — Identifying the exposure

1) Data may be obtained from records, by interview, by post or by examination
2) Method of obtaining information must be identical for cases and controls
3) Ideally, recording of exposure Data should be done "blind"
4) Information should be obtained about other drug esposures and about other relevant variables (e.g. smoking)

Table 11. Case-control studies — Controlling confounding factors

A variable is said to confound a relationship when it is associated both with the exposure of interest and with the illness under study
Confounding may be dealt with by appropriate *matching* of cases and controls or by methods of statistical analysis which take confounding into account

ish case-control studies of the relationship between fatal cardiovascular disease and the pill[8,9]. Although the idea of selecting "community controls" is intuitively attractive, care has to be taken if the cases were identified through the hospital services. It may then, for example, be difficult to obtain information from cases and controls by exactly the same means (see below). Other factors influencing comparability may also be important. Accordingly, when community controls are used, care should be taken to ensure that they are comparable with the cases with respect to the likelihood of 1. being admitted to hospital, 2. being drug users and 3. encompassing the range of relevant confounding factors.

Identifying the exposure

Information about exposure to the suspected drug may be obtained from medical records, by post, by telephone, by personal interview or by examination. It is most important that the source of information should be equally complete for the cases and controls ; the methods used for obtaining the information should also be the same. Ideally, the recording of the drug exposure data should be done "blind" (i.e. the recorder should be unaware of the hypothesis under test and of which subjects are cases and which controls). Often, however, this is not feasible.

In addition to obtaining information about the suspected drug, data should be collected on the use of other medicines. Such data enable cases and controls to be com-

Table 12. Case-control studies — Analysing the Data

1) Method used must be appropriate
2) Confounding must be controlled
3) Relative risks as well as significance levels should be estimated
4) Subgroup analyses may be important

pared with regard to the level of use of drugs in general. Data about other relevant variables (e.g. alcohol consumption, cigarette smoking) will often be required as well.

Controlling confounding factors

"A factor or variable is said to confound a relationship when that factor is associated both with the exposure of interest and with the illness being studied"[7]. Confounding factors are dealt with by matching of cases and controls and/or by statistical analyses which take confounding into account.

A recent paper on the association between oral contraceptives and breast cancer provides good examples of the use of both techniques[10]. Confounding by age, parity, marital status, hospital of admission and date of admission was dealt with by matching, while possible confounding by other factors such as social class, age at first term birth and past history of benign breast disease was considered during the analysis.

In general, it is feasible to match cases and controls on only two or three characteristics ; these should always be variables known to have a major confounding influence — in drug studies age and sex will usually be among them. It is most important to remember that no assessment of the effect of a matched variable is possible in the analysis of a case-control study ; accordingly, no matching should be undertaken for a variable which might prove to be of importance in itself.

Sometimes il is important not merely to match for or to adjust for differences between cases and controls in the distribution of confounding factors, but also to assess differences in risk in various subgroups. For example, in the study of hepato-cellular adenoma recently reported by Rooks *et al.* [11], the relative risk associated with oral contraceptive use in women up to 30 years of age was around 30, but in older women, the relative risk was much higher. In this investigation, age was a major modifier of the ef-

Table 13. Questions to be asked in deciding whether an association is causal

1) Is relative risk large?
2) Have similar results been obtained in other studies by different investigators
3) Is there a dose-response and/or duration response relationship?
4) Do the results of laboratory research and animal experiments support the association?
5) Is the association consistent with known facts about the disease?
The ultimate test will often be intervention

fects of the pill, and important information would have been lost if Rooks and her colleagues had merely calculated and overall "age-adjusted" relative risk.

Analysing the data

The correct analysis of data collected in a case-control study is essential ; clearly it is appropriate to make only some general points here.

While the approach to the analysis of unmatched studies is straightforward[12] matched designs present more complex problems. Sophisticated new methods of analysis have been developed during recent years by a number of authors, but notably by Breslow *et al.*[13]. These methods, however, require access to an electronic computer and help from a statistician familiar with the techniques.

At its simplest level, statistical analysis will enable the "significance" of differences between cases and controls to be tested and allowance to be made for the influence of confounding factors. In addition, however, relative risks should be computed. "Confidence limits" should always be attached to the relative risks to indicate how statistically reliable they ae likely to be[14].

Interpreting the results

Proper interpretation of the results of an observational study involves careful consideration of the adequacy of the design, conduct and analysis of the investigation along the lines already discussed. If, after careful consideration an association in an observational study does not seem to be attributable to chance or to the shortcomings of the investigation, a causal interpretation may be considered. Under these circumstances, the more of the following questions that can be answered affirmatively, the more likely is the association to be causal.

1. Is the relative risk large ? (It is always difficult to be sure that bias and/or confounding are not the explanation for relative risks close to unity. Unfortunately, for common serious diseases like breast cancer, small increases in relative risk, which are so hard to assess, are potentially very important).
2. Have similar findings been obtained by different investigators in other studies ?
3. Is there a dose-response and/or duration response relationship ?
4. Do the results of laboratory research and experiments in animals support the findings ?
5. Is the association consistent with known facts about the disease ?

The ultimate test will often be intervention — i.e. the change in practice suggested by the study will be implemented and appropriate observations will be made to see if the expected effect occurs.

A detailed discussion of the factors to be considered in interpreting an association will be found in a classical paper by Hill[15].

Conclusion

The case-control method in common with all other scientific methods, has occasionally led to erroneous conclusions due either to faulty technique or to misinterpretation of the results. On the other hand, on many occasions it has led to discoveries which have been confirmed by other types of investigation and have been used in practice to prevent disease. Sometimes it is impossible to reach a rapid conclusion by any other means and practical decisions have to be taken on the basis of case-control studies alone interpreted in the light of other existing circumstantial and biological evidence.

Usually, a case-control study is set up to test a hypothesis which has been suggested by animal studies, clinical observation, etc. Slone *et al.*[16] have also described the use of case-control methods to provide a system for monitoring serious illnesses in relation to exposure to drugs. Basically, this involves interviewing large numbers of hospital inpatients with a variety of diseases which might be drug induced together with other hospital inpatients with diagnoses such as disc disease, trauma, appendicitis and haemorrhoids as controls. While this approach has been of considerable value in providing detailed information about drug-disease associations already recognised by other means, it does not appear to have been very fruitful in discovering previously unsuspectd drug induced illness.

REFERENCES

1. Schlesselman J.J., Sample size requirements in cohort and case-control studies of disease, *Am. J. Epidem.* **99** (1974), 381-84.

2. Vessey M.P. and R. Doll, Investigation of relation between use of oral contraceptives and thromboembolic disease, *Brit. Med. J.* **2** (1968), 199-205.

3. Horwitz R.I. and A.R. Feinstein, Alternative analytic methods for case-control studies of estrogens and endometrial cancer, *New Engl. J. Med.* **299** (1978), 1089-94.

4. Jick H., R.N. Watkins, K.J. Rothma and A.M. Walker, Estrogens and endometrial cancer, *New Engl. J. Med.* **300** (1979), 1334.

5. Shapiro S., D.W. Kaufman, D. Slone, L. Rosenberg, O.S. Miettinen, P.D. Stolley *et al.*, Recent and past use of conjugated estrogens in relation to adenocarcinoma of the endometrium, *New Engl. J. Med.* **303** (1980), 485-89.

6. Feinstein A.R., Methodologic problems and standards in case-control studies, *Am. J. Epidem.* **108** (1979), 299-307.

7. Jick H. and M.P. Vessey, Case-control studies in the evaluation of drug-induced illness, *Am. J. Epidem.* **107** (1978), 1-7.

8. Inman W.H.W. and M.P. Vessey, Investigation of deaths from pulmonary, coronary and cerebral thrombosis and embolism in women of childbearing age, *Brit. Med. J.* **2** (1968), 193-99.

9. Mann J.I. and W.H.W. Inman, Oral contraceptives and death from myocardial infarction, *Brit. Med. J.* **2** (1975), 245-48.

10. Vessey M.P., R. Doll, L. Jones, K. McPherson and D. Yeates, An epidemiological study of oral contraceptives and breast cancer, *Brit. Med. J.* **1** (1979), 1755-58.

11. Rooks J.B., H.W. Ory, K.G. Ishak, L.T. Strauss, J.R. Greenspan, A.P. Hill and C.W. Tyler, Epidemiology of hepato-cellular adenoma. The role of oral contraceptive use, *J. Am. Med. Ass.* **242** (1979), 644-48.

12. Mantel N. and W. Haenszel, Statistical aspects of the analysis of data from retrospective studies of disease, *J. Nat. Cancer Inst.* **22** (1959), 719-48.

13. Breslow N.E., N.E. Day, K.T. Halvorsen, R.L. Prentice and C. Sabai, Estimation of multiple relative risk functions in matched case-control studies, *Am. J. Epidem.* **108**(1978), 299-307.

14. Rothman K.J., A show of confidence, *New Engl. J. Med.* **299** (1978), 1362-63.

15. Hill A.B., The environment and disease : association or causation, *Proc. Roy. Soc. Med.* **58** (1965), 295-300.

16. Slone D., S. Shapiro and O.S. Miettinen, Case-control surveillance of serious illnesses attributable to ambulatory drug use, *in : Epidemiological Evaluation of Drugs*, F. Colombo, S. Shapiro, D. Slone and G. Tognoni eds, Amsterdam, Elsevier-North Holland, 1977, pp. 59-70.

Sécurité et médicaments (1982), pp. 123-125

Hospital Surveys

H. JICK

Boston Collaborative Drug Surveillance Program, 400 Totten Pond Road, Waltham, Massachusetts, 02154 USA

Hospital survey studies have been utilized extensively in the past primarily to identify and quantitate the acute toxicity of drugs used in medical practice. The methods applied also allow for the evaluation of factors such as age, sex, and renal function which may influence toxicity. Such studies for acute toxicity may involve a single drug or a few drugs, or it may be designed to evaluate simultaneously all of the drugs commonly used in hospital[1].

The results of many studies which use the technique of intensive monitoring of only one or a few drugs have been reported[2, 5]. In this setting, the method has the advantage that specific questions for the drug or drugs of interest may be explored in detail. This type of research has an important role to play in the quantitation of acute clinical drug toxicity, particularly for drugs which have been recently approved for general use. Its limitation is, of course, that it provides information on a limited number of drugs and, since there are literally thousands of drugs in clinical use, a large number of studies would be required to cover the entire area of clinical therapeutics.

A program of intensive inhospital monitoring of drug effects which is designed to evaluate the acute toxicity of all drugs simultaneously has been functioning since 1966 and is known as the Boston Collaborative Drug Surveillance Program (BCDSP)[1]. The BCDSP has, during these past 15 years, involved over forty hospitals in seven countries. As of January 1, 1981, working together with our colleagues abroad, we have collected data on acute drug effects in some 40,000 medical and 4,000 surgical inpatients.

The methodology and many of the results of this research program have been published in a book[6] and a series of some 140 publications[7].

We are quite satisfied that the data that have been collected are comprehensive and generally of good quality. They provide an opportunity to obtain reasonably valid quantitation of acute drug toxicity and factors which influence toxicity, for virtually all commonly used drugs which have been marketed for many years.

We already have for some time had sufficient amounts of data for most of the job to be done and have, over the past few years, put less emphasis on data collection and more on organizing and refining for publication the data collected during the earlier years of the program.

We do not feel that a repetition of a large-scale monitoring program for *marketed drugs,* based on or similar to the methods of the BCDSP, is indicated. Rather, we believe that the data already gathered are sufficient to satisfy the needs for quantifying the acute toxicity of drugs which have been marketed for years. These data are fully and freely available to all responsible members of the world health care community.

There remains the matter of providing information for newly marketed drugs. In our judgment, the intensive monitoring system of the BCDSP, which is designed to study all drugs, is far too expensive to employ for the relatively few new drugs which become available. These drugs should be studied individually. As mentioned before, efficient techniques for such studies have been utilized in the past[2, 5] and can be used in the future.

Inhospital monitoring may also be used to evaluate long-term drug toxicity which leads to hospitalization. Once again, the technique may be applied to a single drug or few drugs or to all drugs at large.

The Royal College of General Practitioners[8] and Professor Vessey and his associates[9] have provided extremely valuable information on the toxicity of oral contraceptives and other forms of contraception. These are excellent examples of intensive monitoring of a few treatments for long-term toxicity.

As to the monitoring of large numbers of drugs simultaneously, the BCDSP has certain information on regular drug use prior to admission, as well as diagnosis information for over 50,000 medical inpatients and over 15,000 surgical inpatients. This has allowed us to evaluate the relationship of regular drug use to many illnesses, and we have, to date, published over a dozen papers in this area[7]. These data also provide the necessary background for the development of a substantive, quantitative insight into the nature and frequency of illnesses which require further study in terms of drug etiology and to understand the strategy which is required to most efficiently achieve important goals in this research area.

Our views on this subject have been presented in detail in an article in the March 3, 1977 New England Journal of Medicine[10]. I would here like to summarize our conclusions concerning research work which we believe still needs to be done.

Our analysis of the problem of potential undiscovered drug-illness relations indicates that the areas of concern are well defined and relatively small in scope. We believe that the following research policy and strategy is called for.

1. Unrecognized effects of established, marketed drugs in causing rare but serious illness, such as aplastic anemia, can be discovered most efficiently by the use of case-control studies. Systematic study of selected illnesses of this kind may be called for, insofar as there is reason to suspect that such side effects may have escaped clinical detection. Since we refer to rare illnesses, it is understood that such information could not be obtained by routine monitoring, such as was carried out by the BCDSP in 1972 and has been ongoing since 1968 in medical patients and now in surgical patients. The general survey study of 1972 provided virtually no data on rare illnesses. In order to study such illnesses efficiently, one must identify a source for these rare cases, as is done in Sweden and Britain where much excellent work has been done, and having identified the source, carry out separate studies for each illness. It should be noted that for drugs which have been marketed for many years, it is possible, but quite unlikely, that rare, serious side effects have remained unrecognized. It is, therefore, unlikely that much

new, unanticipated information will result from such research, and its main value may lie in providing more precise quantitation of drug toxicity that we know exists.

2. From the multipurpose case-control studies already carried out over the past decade, vast amounts of information are now available on the relationship of *drugs marketed for some years* to reasonably common illness. Therefore, there is no need for further data collection of this type. Hypotheses which have not arisen from the extensive data already analyzed are very unlikely to arise from additional multipurpose data collection of this type.

3. Newly marketed drugs should be routinely and systematically monitored for serious toxicity through registration and follow-up study of the earliest users. Such monitoring — properly designed and implemented — could be expected to identify practolol-type problems within the first dozen cases. Where such studies are designed to be multipurpose, automated recording of drug exposures and outcomes is essential.

REFERENCES

1. Jick H., O.S. Miettinen, S. Shapiro, G.P. Lewis, V. Siskind and D. Slone, Comprehensive drug surveillance, *JAMA* **213** (1970), 1455-60.
2. Wood A.J.J., D.C. Moir, C. Campbell, J.F. Davidson, S.C. Gallon, E. Henney and S. McAllion, Medicines Evaluation and Monitoring Group : Central nervous system effects of pentazocine, *Br. Med. J.* **1** (1974), 305-07.
3. Paddock R., E.G. Beer, J.W. Bellville, B.J. Ciliberti, W.H. Forrest and E.V. Miller, Analgesic and side effects of pentazocine and morphine in a large population of postoperative patients, *Clin. Pharmacol. Ther.* **10** (1969), 355-65.
4. Koch-Weser J., V.W. Sidel, M. Dexter, C. Parish, D.C. Finer and P. Kanarek, Adverse reactions to sulfisoxazole, sulfamethoxazole and nitrofurantoin, *Arch. Intern. Med.* **128** (1971), 399-404.
5. Koch-Weser J., V.W. Sidel, E.B. Federman, P. Kanarek, D.C. Finer and A.E. Eaton, Adverse effects of sodium colistimethate : Manifestations and specific reaction rates during 317 courses of therapy, *Ann. Intern. Med.* **72** (1970), 857-68.
6. Miller R.R. and D.J. Greenblatt eds, *Drug Effects in Hospitalized Patients. Experiences of the Boston Collaborative Drug Surveillance Program*, New York, John Wiley & Sons, 1976.
7. Cohen M.R., A compilation of abstracts and an index of articles published by the Boston Collaborative Drug Surveillance Program, *Hosp. Pharm.* **12** (1977), 455-92.
8. Royal College of General Practitioners' Oral Contraception Study : Mortality among oral-contraceptive users, *Lancet* **2** (1977), 727-31.
9. Vessey M.P., K. McPherson and B. Johnson, Mortality among women participating in the Oxford-/Family planning Assicuatuib Contraceptive Study, *Lancet* **2** (1977), 731-33.
10. Jick H, The discovery of drug-induced illness, *N. Engl. J. Med.* , **296** (1977), 481-85.

Sécurité et médicaments (1982), p. 127

Cost and Effectiveness of Post-marketing Surveillance

P.E. LUCCHELLI

Direttore Medico, Smith Kline & French S. p. A., Viale Ortles, 12, 20139 Milano, Italy

Abstract — Health is considered a primary good ; for keeping or promote health any expenditure, re gardless of entity, appears justified. Decision-makers are bound however to allocate the limited available re sources on a benefits versus costs maximization basis.

In presence of strong emotional elements, choices are sometimes irrational. To a confuse picture adds a widespread ignorance by doctors and even public health administrators of the economic impact of health op erations. Waste of resources is common. On the other hand, cost-benefit analysis methodology has not ye received an entirely satisfactory application to the health care. Very few, if any, examples of application are known in post-marketing surveillance, where balancing benefits versus costs is essential : post-marketing surveillance techniques in fact can vary in cost manyfold, cost being often unrelated to results. Being in last instance the cost borne by the community, a rational approach to the problem is necessary.

III

POST MARKETING SAFETY ASSESSMENT

INTERET ET LIMITES DES METHODES D'EVALUATION CLINIQUE DES EFFETS INDESIRABLES DES MEDICAMENTS APRES MISE SUR LE MARCHE

NEW METHODS

MÉTHODES NOUVELLES

Sécurité et médicaments (1982), p. 131

Scientific Obstacles to Overcome in Establishing Systematic Post-marketing Surveillance

K.L. MELMON

Standford University Medical Center, Department of Medicine S102D, Standford, California 94305, USA

Abstract — After three years of study, the Joint Commission on Prescription Drug Use unequivocally and unanimously supported the need for extending post-marketing surveillance beyond what presently exists in the United States. A Center for Drug Surveillance was requested. The Center was not to focus on regulatory implications or requirements of a post-marketing surveillance system rather it was to develop information that would encourage optimal medical decisions. The Center was to be a private, non-profit organization capable of generating support and research funds from industry, academia, and government. It was charged with the responsability for the development and dissemination of therapeutic information that could be applied to the optimal use of drugs. The dominant functions of the Center would include education of physicians about drug related effects ; the development of new methodology for post-marketing surveillance activities ; and the training of physicians in epidemiology applicable to post-marketing surveillance requirements. The Commission stressed the need for the determination of rates of anticipated and unanticipated efficacy to be developed on the same patient population in whom incidences of adverse drug effects were determined. The feasibility for and approach to such studies of efficacy was stressed. The Commission found that even non-experimental techniques could be used for the estimation of anticipated efficacy in a large percentage of situations of actual practice use of the drugs. The Commission also indicated the requirement that data on the epidemiology of prescription drug use in the United States could be acquired and would be useful to practitioners and the public. The academic challenges that present themselves in developing an effective PMS will be discussed.

Sécurité et médicaments (1982), pp. 133-135

Cohorts From Data Banks

H. JICK

Boston Collaborative Drug Surveillance Program, 400 Totten Pond Road, Waltham, Massachusetts, 02154, USA

Abstract — Group Health Cooperative of Puget Sound is a comprehensive care consumer-owned health maintenance organization which has placed all prescriptions filled at its pharmacy onto computer files. Also available on computer files are discharge diagnoses for all hospitalizations. The availability of computer records of prescriptions filled provides a cohort of users for each drug which can be used for follow up. This system appears to be ideally suited for postmarketing follow-up. Studies have already been completed utilizing this resource on the drug etiology of endometrial cancer, breast cancer, moving vehicle accidents, and congenital disorders. These studies can be done rapidly and at low cost. The quality of the information is excellent.

In considering the optimum circumstance for studying adverse drug effects after marketing, it is helpful to keep in mind the key ingredients in such studies : accurate identification of drug exposures, accurate identification of illness outcomes, and control of confounding factors.

The ideal circumstance in terms of data quality and cost would be one where all prescriptions in a known, fixed population are recorded on automated equipment and can be linked to automated recording of major illnesses in the population. Such a system has existed for about five years at Group Health Cooperative of Puget Sound, a consumer-owned health maintenance organization with a membership of over 250 000 people.

The Group Health resource allows for the study of all drugs used in the population in terms of any serious illness which might be induced. Large cohorts of users are now available for follow-up for almost all important drugs. Table 1 lists a number of important drugs, together with the number of people at Group Health who have filled at least one prescription for that drug. It can be seen that there is already a vast experience with many of these drugs.

To date, we have completed a number of studies utilizing this uniquely valuable resource.

DESCRIPTION OF THE RESOURCE

Group Health Cooperative is a consumer-owned cooperative founded in Seattle in 1947. As of 1980, there were about 280 000 members. The plan provides virtually complete prepaid medical coverage for outpatient care, drugs, and hospital services. Members are hospitalized at Seattle-area hospitals maintained by the Cooperative, with the exception of about 10 % of members who live in the Olympia, Washington, area, some 95 km southwest of Seattle. Olympia members are sometimes hospitalized locally.

Information on all discharges from Group Health hospitals has been recorded and computerized by the Commission on Professional and Hospital Activities-Professional Activity Study (CPHA-PAS) in Ann Arbor, Michigan, since 1972. This information includes discharge diagnoses and surgical procedures performed, together with routine demographic data. The CPHA-PAS records provide for ready identification of cases of cancer. Among Olympia members of Group Health admitted to the local hospital, cases of cancer may be identified by reference to a local tumor registry.

In July 1975, Group Health began to computerize records of prescriptions filled in its nine regional outpatient pharmacies. This data automation was accomplished in stages by the phasing in of one regional pharmacy at a time, yielding an increasing proportion of the pharmacy use of the population. It was completed by July 1, 1976.

Information on outpatient drug exposure and on hospital diagnosis is received each six months at a nominal cost. Files are updated at that time. Curretly, we have full information on four years of experience, representing over 1 000 000 patient years. These data include drug exposures in pregnant women and children.

We have already completed some dozen studies of the cohort type. These include evaluation of the relation of estrogens to endometrial cancer and breast cancer,[1-3] drugs taken during pregnancy to congenital disorders[4], triamterene to renal stone[5], and ibuprofen to liver, bone marrow, and kidney disease.

Table 1. Number of Users of Particular Drugs (1975-1979)

	Number of Users
Ampicillin	52,229
Oral contraceptives	>30,000
Erythromycin stearate	30,675
Diazepam	29,764
Phenylbutazone	29,057
Hydrochlorothiazide	25,130
Dicyclomine	20,183
Metronidazole	15,402
Conjugated estrogens	13,661
Propranolol	11,146
Bendectin	7,334
Furosemide	6,021
Amitriptyline	3,315
Reserpine	980
Lithium carbonate	824

These studies may be done quickly at little expense. The quality of the information is excellent. Such a system is ideal for postmarketing follow-up of drugs for unsuspected adverse effects.

REFERENCES

1. Jick H., R.N. Watkins, J.R. Hunter, B.J. Dinan, S. Madsen, K.J. Rothman and A.M. Walker, Replacement estrogens and endometrial cancer, *New Engl. J. Med.* **300** (1979), 218-22.
2. Jick H., A.M. Walker, R.N. Watkins, D.C. D'Ewart, J.R. Hunter, A. Danford, S. Madsen, B.J. Dinan and K.J. Rothman, Oral contraceptives and breast cancer, *Am. J. Epidemiol.* **112** (1980), 577-85.
3. Jick H., A.M. Walker, R.N. Watkins, D.C. D'Ewart, J.R. Hunter, A. Danford, S. Madsen, B.J. Dinan and K.J. Rothman, Replacement estrogens and breast cancer, *Am. J. Epidemiol.* **112** (1980), 586-94.
4. Jick H., L.B. Holmes, A.M. Walker, R.N. Watkins, K.J. Rothman, D.C. D'Ewart, J.R. Hunter, A. Danford and S. Madsen, Vaginal spermicides and congenital disorders, *JAMA* (in press).
5. Jick H., B.J. Dinan and J.R. Hunter, Triamterene and renal stones, *JAMA* (submitted for publication).

Sécurité et médicaments (1982), pp. 137-142

The Drug Surveillance Research Unit (DSRU)

W.H.W. INMAN

Drug Surveillance Research Unit, the University of Southampton, 34 Bassett Crescent East, Southampton, England S023FL, United Kingdom

Abstract — An independent, non-governmental, non-regulatory and multidisciplinary resarch unit was set up at the University of Southampton, England, in June 1980, under the direction of Dr. W.H.W. Inman, formely the Principal Medical Officer in charge of adverse drug-reaction monitoring for the U.K. Committee on the Safety of Medecines. It has four principle objectives —

1. to develop new methods for post-marketing drug surveillance ;
2. to utilise existing expertise in the solution of safety problems ;
3. to provide an educational programme which will include training in the skills of drug monitoring ;
4. to conduct research into improvements in communication of information about the safety and efficacy of drugs.

A major exercise in prescription-based monitoring in general practice is planned for 1981.

The Drug Surveillance Research Unit (DSRU) was set up within the Faculty of Medecine at the Universtiy of Southampton in 1980. It is an independent, non-governemental and non-regulatory unit totally dedicated to the study of the safety of drugs after they have been released for marketing. It's objectives include the development of new methods for the detection of potential hazards (hypothesis testing) and the provision of an environment in which people may obtain the skills needed in post-marketing drug surveillence (PMS). The DSRU also aims to improve communications by arranging frequent meetings to review the state of the art, by providing facilities for consultation and by encouraging progress towards a better understanding between the professions, the public and the industry, with special emphasis on the need for more responsible reporting by the media.

This paper will describe the first of the DSRU's major research programmes which is directed towards the earlier detection and investigation of previously unsuspected hazards with new drugs.

BACKGROUND

For the past 17 years we have, in the United Kingdom, relied largely on the voluntary yellow-card reporting system as a means of early warning of potential drug hazards. Similar systems have been operated in many other countries, most of which pass information on to the World Health Organisation's central collecting agency in Sweden. Voluntary reporting has brought many new hazards to light but, on occasions, it has been slow to do so. The most important recent example of failure in early detection was the Practolol incident. Nearly 4 years after marketing, only a single report of conjuctivitis had reached the Commitee on Safety of Medicines. However, once the oculo-muco-cutaneous syndrome had been identified in the medical journals, the yellow cards proved to be an invaluable method by which the extent of the disaster could be measured.

Voluntary reporting of adverse drug reactions (ADR's) is hindered by the fact that nearly all reactions are indistinguishable clinically and in the laboratory from conditions that can occur spontanously or as a response to non-drug factors. The observer of the reaction may not know which drugs have been taken or he may fail to report the reaction even when he suspects a drug to be its cause.

In the past 4 or 5 years, our attention has focused on the concept of "event-reporting" in which no medical opinion need be given about the cause of an adverse drug reaction (ADR). Event-reporting of an event should be less likley to have medicolegal consequences, since the reporter need not admit that his prescription might have been responsible. The chances that events, which at first sight appear to be totally independent of treatment, will be reported are considerably increased. Event-reporting may also reveal unexpected beneficial effects of drugs.

A number of schemes have been proposed for prospective event-monitoring in general practice such as Recorded Release[1] or Registered Release[2] and the Committee on Safety of Medicines has recently proposed a method known as Retrospective Assessment of Drug Safety (RADS) which has been set aside because of economic difficulties. The DSRU is currently conducting a rather similar experiment making use of the fact that most drug prescriptions issued to patients in the United Kingdom are processed centrally by the Prescription Pricing Authority (PPA) for the purposes of remunerating retail pharmacists for drug dispensed by the National Health Service.

INCIDENCE OF ADR'S

Before describing the DSRU's scheme it is important to define the level of toxicity that it will measure. It is sometimes possible to determine a level of risk associated with treatment which may be regarded as acceptable. Various people will have different ideas about what this level should be but the general principle (Fig. 1) is that the more serious the disease the greater the acceptable risk. We require more patients to detect small risks than we need to detect large risks. Rare but serious ADR's produced by medicines which are sold for the treatment of coughs, colds and headaches might only be detected in studies involving thousands or even millions of patients. More frequent events, on the other hand, may come to light in clinical trials in a few hundred patients. The number of patients, and therefore the cost of the study is inversely proportional to the level of acceptable risk. The enthusiasm of doctors who cooperate in the study, is generally greater when they are asked to investigate drugs used for the treatment of serious disease. They may be less likely to cooperate in the very large studies which would be necessary to determine acceptable levels of toxicity of a treatment for minor

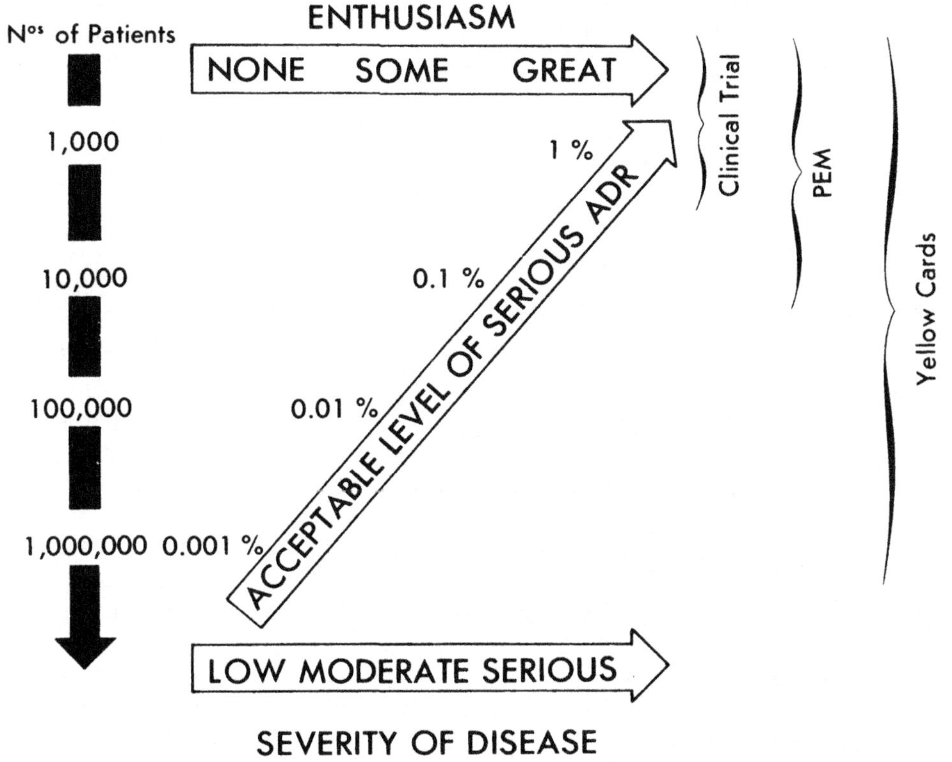

Fig. 1.

complaints. In practical terms it is unlikely that we could ever afford the massive studies that would be needed to identify rare, but important hazards with the many thousands of minor remedies which are marketed and we believe that a realistic target will be to devise a system capable of detecting adverse events that affect one in every 1,000 patients who receive a new drug. This means that we will probably need to study groups of up to 10,000 patients.

Because nearly all patients with disease or symptoms tend to be treated with drugs, it will rarely be possible to obtain information about the absolute prevalence of events in untreated patients. All judgements will tend to be relative and to make them we will need to study groupes of patients receiving alternative treatments.

PRESCRIPTION-EVENT MONITORING (PEM)

The prescription pricing system in the United Kingdom affords a unique opportunity to identify large populations of patients. The DSRU is currently collecting all the prescriptions for four drugs and it should be stressed that we have selected them, not because of any particular concern about their safety, but on the estimated volume of their sales. With comparitively limited resources it is necessary to ensure that we obtain a useful sample without swamping the system with prescriptions that cannot be handled. It is likely that the pilot study will involve processing 500,000 prescriptions or roughly one out of every 600 prescriptions issued in England. The prescriptions are identified by the 2,000 pricing clerks and photocopied for transmission to the DSRU. Bundles of photocopies, correspondint to 90 areas covered by the 11 English divisions of the PPA, will be processed in monthly batches. Wales and Scotland are not included for the very simple reason that in these countries there are abnormally large numbers of people who share the same name (eg. Jones, MacDonald). In England, on the other hand, the chances that more than a handful of patients with the same name will be treated by a single doctor with the same drug are small enough to allow rapid identification of the great majority of patients included in the study.

Unfortunately the prescription does not tell us whether the patient has received earlier prescriptions for the same drug. If we commence PEM before a new drug is marketed, all patients who appear in the first sample will be "new" patients. In order to obtain contemporary controls who start treatment with an "old" drug at the same time, we will need to monitor prescriptions for several months and identify patients who are "new to the system". Having done this we can then commence the second phase of PEM in which a simple questionnaire will be sent to the prescribing doctors. We will ask for a note of any "events" which may have occurred whether they are thought to be accidental, a change for better or worse in the patient's condition, a new diagnosis or a suspected ADR, which may have been reported to the doctor or which may have led to referal to hospital. We also hope that doctors will record the date of birth and the National Health Service number so that the records may be linked with the death or cancer registers.

Finally, once the completed questionnaires have been assembled, in phase 3, we will compare the patterns of events experienced by patients taking the test and control drugs in the light of ADR experience from other systems (eg. the yellow cards) and with morbidity and mortality statistics obtained in a variety of other ways. If, at this stage, one or more classes of event appear to be unexpectantly frequent, the large pool of identified patients that will have already been created during the first phase of the study will be used as the starting point for more detailed investigation. The records will have been collected under conditions which are entirely free from selection bias because the doctors will not have been aware at the time the prescriptions were written that the drug was being monitored. Thus PEM makes it possible both to generate and test hypotheses.

BARRIERS TO PROGRESS

Most of the barriers to progress in post-marketing surveillance are medico-political rather than technical. Firstly there is considerable concern about confidentiality and the need to obtain patient-consent before transmitting the data required for epidemiological research. Research workers involved in PMS are perhaps the least likely of all people to misuse the data they obtain. The identities of patients are required only for record linkage purpose and work is invariably conducted in such a way that neither the identity of the patient nor the doctor are revealed to people who are not involved in the study. Recently it has been suggested that a patient should always give written consent to the transmission of personal information. The procedure for seeking consent would, however, almost certainly deter the majority of doctors from collaborating in studies of this kind and would cause unnecessary concern to patients, who might imagine that the drugs they were taking were suspected to be producing serious reactions of which they were unaware.

A second barrier has arisen because of popular misconception about drug safety and efficacy. The public still believes that all drugs should be totally effective and completely safe, neither of which will ever be true. There is also a false belief that improved monitoring methods will prevent accidents. All we can ever hope is that improved methods will enable us to detect serious hazards at an earlier stage and will reduce the scale of the accidents which will inevitably happen from time to time. Thirdly, there is increasing involvement in litigation and compensation. Whether injured by drugs, by accidents or by disease, patients require the same high standard of care irrespective of the cause of their injury. This care must start from the time of their injury and not after years of struggle in the courts. Insurance rather than litigation should provide for their care. We must not create an elite of drug-damaged patients who are entitled to sums of money which are enormously greater than those obtained in other types of injury. Finally it should be remembered that the greatest danger is the risk of premature publicity. This can lead to unjustifiable alarm, to illness resulting from withdrawal of treatment, to the false belief that injury has been caused by a drug and can also make epidemiological studies, which might otherwise confirm or refute the hazard, difficult or impossible to carry out.

Table 1. 100,000 Patients have disease with 5 % annual mortality. Drug is 80 % effective but causes fatal side-effects in 1 per 1,000.

	Deaths/Year
No drug	5,000
All on drug: —	
disease	1,000
side-effects	100
Total	1,100
Publicity causes 1 in 5 to stop drug	
20,000 untreated	1,000
80,000 treated: —	
disease	800
side-effects	80
Total	1,880

Deaths due to publicity 1,880 — 1,100 = 780

Table 1 represents a hypothetical example of the magnitude of the damage to patients receiving treatment with an effective drug which could result from adverse publicity.

Let us suppose that 100,000 patients suffering from a disease which has an annual mortality of 5 % are being treated with a drug which is 80 % effective. Let us further suppose that the drug itself carries the unusually large risk of producing fatal side effects in 1 per 1,000 patients per year. Without the drug, 5,000 patients would die each year from the disease. If all 100,000 patients are treated, this mortality will be reduced to 1,000 patients, but a further 100 will die from side-effects.

Let us now see what happens if a scare story in a newspaper leads as few as one in five patients to stop taking the drug. We now have two sub-populations. 20,000 who stopped the drug will be subject to the full 5 % annual mortality and 1,000 will die. The remaining 80,000 patients who continue to take the drug will suffer 800 deaths from the disease and 80 due to side-effects. Note that the publicity has saved 20 deaths from the drug, but if we subtract 1,880 post-publicity deaths from the 1,100 which would have occurred without it, we see that the publicity was responsible for 780 deaths.

As an independent institution, the DSRU is well placed to resist the pressures which may lead to premature publicity, but at the same time it is well aware of the need to improve communications, to take the media into its confidence at the right time and to ensure that stories of alleged hazards are placed in their proper perspective.

SUMMARY AND CONCLUSIONS

Because more than 80 % of drugs are presribed by general practitioners, future improvements in post-marketing surveillance are likely to occur mainly in their speciality. A new type of event-monitoring is being developed by the DSRU which should enable the first 10,000 or more patients who receive a new drug to be monitored by methods which are not burdensome to doctors. The identification of large populations of patients treated with a varity of drugs allows comparisons of the relative frequency of events and earlier recognition of hazards. The same populations will be used for testing hypotheses raised in PEM or by other schemes.

The great advantage of PEM is that it does not modify prescribing practice or patient-selection and thus avoids much of the bias inherent in prospective methods.

Sécurité et médicaments (1982), pp. 143-150

Post-marketing Safety Assessment New Zealand Experience

J. S. PHILLIPS

Division of Clinical Services, Department of Health, P O BOX 5013, Wellington, New Zealand

Abstract — Following discussion over several years and consideration of more expensive monitoring systems New Zealand implemented its present Intensified Adverse Drug Reaction Reporting Scheme in early 1977. The Scheme is an intensification of ordinary volontary adverse drug reaction reporting whereby selected medicines are accepted in the Scheme and by continuing publicity directly to doctors and pharmacists reports of adverse drug reactions and unexpected events are solicited. Usage is provided by manufacturers, and pharmacists supply regular lists of users of these medicines. This data is collated by Committee on Adversed Drug Reactions.

Reponse from doctors has been encouraging although to date no dramatic findings have resulted. Dramatic results do not appear from postmarketing monitoring unless the medicines being monitored have dramatic dangers. Earlier distribution of possibly dangerous medicines is made possible. Rare and unexpected problems may still be missed for some time. Building up of cohorts of users in a number of collaborating countries has immense future potential.

Discussion on the need for post-marketing surveillance commenced in New Zealand in about 1975 and was first discussed at the Drug Assessment Advisory Committee which assesses new drug applications. This is an advisory committee to the Minister of Health composed of practising physicians but with a Department of Health chairman. The interest first arose from the point of view of releasing, at an earlier stage, new medicines with a known or suspected, but not unduly dangerous problem. The practolol experience also increased interest in finding unexpected problems.

Various types of monitoring were discussed including close monitoring of medicines at the expense of the pharmaceutical firms and payment of doctors for reporting. New Zealand is a small country of just over 3 million people with a perpetual shortage of money for fresh schemes. The administrative costs of more complex methods of post-marketing surveillence rapidly became apparent and by 1976, with the co-operation of the Department of Health and the Committee on Adverse Drug Reactions, a much simpler and less expensive scheme was decided upon and this scheme was launched early in 1977, being one of the first in the world to get under way. It is noteworthy that this exercise was a combined Government and non Government exercise and was agreed to by the Pharmaceutical Manufacturers Association.

The scheme is called the Intensified Adverse Drug Reaction Reporting Scheme and is, as the name suggests, an intensification of the normal voluntary adverse drug reaction reporting scheme operating in New Zealand. Those medicines to be included in the scheme (no more than ten at any one time) are selected by the Drug Assessment Advisory Committee and the list of names is constantly publicised to medical practitioners and pharmacists. Mention that a medicine is included in the scheme is also required on all advertising of the medicines involved.

REPORTING

Reporting cards are distributed to doctors by representatives of the pharmaceutical firms concerned and are also enclosed in the New Ethicals Drug Catalogue provided free to doctors three times a year, so that an ample supply is available in each doctor's surgery. They are the same cards as are used for ordinary ADR reporting. Desk reminder cards listing the medicines involved are also circulated to medical practitioners, dentists and pharmacists. Letters and editorials have been written to the New Zealand Medical Journal, Pharmacy Journals and Nursing Journals, stressing the requirements of reporting.

Doctors are asked to report not only adverse drug reactions, but also all untoward or unexpected events befalling patients receiving the particular medicines. Reports are sent to the Medical Assessor of the Committee on Adverse Drug Reactions (Professor E. G. McQueen) whose unit collates the reports with other recorded data.

RELATING TO USAGE

It became apparent at an early stage, that there was little point in a list of adverse reactions and unusual events is they could not in some way be related to usage.

Manufacturers of the products concerned in the scheme have been co-operative. Indeed, appearance of the product name on the list of products being monitored has appeared to increase sales, presumably by drawing the name of the product to notice. The firms have all supplied sales figures as requested and have ensured that their representatives promote the scheme.

However, more precise data was also required and pharmacits are now asked to return lists of all patients to whom they have dispensed the medicines involved in the scheme. These returns are made four monthly and include the name and address of patient, the date of dispensing, dose and the name of the prescribing practitioner. More recently the age of the patient is also being sought.

All this data is stored and has enabled a comparison of usage and adverse reactions and events to be produced with a fair degree of accuracy. It has also enabled a list to be compiled of those patients who ceased therapy for any reason.

The accuracy is, of course, dependent on the degree of voluntary response to the intensive pusblicity, but this has been pleasing. An interesting reaction to the implementation of the scheme was an increase in normal voluntary adverse drug reaction reporting outside the intensified scheme, which increased some twofold in the first year. More difficulty is, however, being experienced in maintaining the original enthusiasm although a resurgence is expeeted with the recent addition of new medicines to the list being monitored.

Overall, this scheme has proven to be particularly suitable for a small country like New Zealand with limited resources and where it is practical to maintain a close scrutiny of what is happening. The data available on the computer now allows follow-up of individual cases and further questioning where this is considered necessary.

MEDICINES

The list of medicines which have been included in the scheme since its inception are

Acebutolol
Atenolol
Metoprolol
Labetalol
Perhexiline Maleate
Sodium Valproate
Cimetidine
Nifedipine

Currently, the last four are in the scheme and a recent addition is Captopril.

SALES

The effect on sales can be clearly seen in the following slide.

Table 1. Drug Sales by 6-Month Periods

	Perhexiline	S. valproate (tab. equiv.)	Cimetidine
April – September, 1977	125,300	389,200	Nil
October 1977 – March 1978	185,600	500,600	281,850
April 1978 – September 1978	276,600	656,460	571,950
October 1978 – March 1979	255,900	805,220	717,450
April 1979 – September 1979	424,500	1,088,660	1,156,650
October 1979 – March 1980	352,700	1,341,260	1,220,550
April – September 1980	362,500	1,446,720	1,768,050

The passing drop in sales of perhexiline maleate followed a published warning about possible dangers. Sales of the beta blockers prospered even more clearly during the period of monitoring.

NUMBER OF REPORTS

The number of reports received is schown in the next slide. The drop in reporting from December 1979 followed the removal of the beta blockers from the scheme.

Table 3. I.A.D.R.R.S.

Repors per month: April 1977 to October 1980

April 1977	6	April 1978	35
May	11	May	37
June	8	June	30
July	16	July	19
August	13	August	33
September	20	September	28
October	13	October	29
November	26	November	18
December	37	December	19
January 1978	22	January 1979	13
February	26	February	7
March	40	March	19
	238		287

April 1979	7	April 1980	2	(2 for B-blockers)
May	16	May	7	(3 ")
June	17	June	1	(3 ")
July	21	(+3 nifedipine)		
August	13	July	3	(5 ")
September	15	August	2	(3 ")
October	28	September	9	(7 ")
November	25	October	5	(6 ")
December	18			

CIMETIDINE, PERHEXILINE AND SODIUM VALPROATE ONLY:

January 1980	2	(9 for B-blockers now off list)
February	3	(9 ")
March	9	(4 ")
	165	

RESULTS

The reported side effects have not shown any dramatic unexpected results. This has underlined the truism that dramatic results do not appear from post-marketing monitoring unless the medicines being monitored have dramatic dangers. Il you are going to set up a post-marketing monitoring scheme and you wish it to be very successful you must select very dangerous medicines to monitor.

BETA BLOCKING AGENTS

The next slide shows the results of monitoring usage of the newer beta blockers.

Table 2. I.A.D.R.R.S. Events reported with beta blockers

	% of total for drugs in each category							
	No. of Events	"Immunological" *	Neurological	Cardiac	Periph. vascular	Respiratory	Alimentary	Unclass.
Acebutolol	105	20.0	36.2	4.8	3.8**	8.6	13.3	13.3
Atenolol	132	15.2	31.1	8.3	9.8**	5.3	22.7	7.6
Metoprolol	280	17.5	39.6	4.3	8.9**	10.0	13.9	5.7
Labetalol	82	31.7	34.1	4.9	2.4***	4.9	14.6	7.3

* "Immunological" includes all skin rashes and all processus possibly having an immunological basis ;
** Peripheral ischaemia, Raynaud's phenomenon ;
*** Peripheral vasodilatation.

You will note the slightly higher number of immunological problems with acebutolol, but still well below the level experienced in New Zealand with practolol. There is a relatively high number of alimentary symptoms with all beta blockers.

OTHER MEDICINES

In the case of cimetidine and valproate, reactions were mostly of the type now well known to be associated with these medicines. In the case of perhexiline, many of the adverse effects were of considerable severity and included two deaths, one of which was a case of gross peripheral neuropathy and myopathy with papilloedema.
The patient died after vertebral angiography performed to exclude a space occupying intracranial lesion.

CESSATION OF THERAPY

358 doctors were sent lists of their patients who appeared to have ceased therapy with the following findings: —

Table 4. Reasons for cessation of therapy

	Perhexiline	Valproate	Labetalol
Total confirmed ceased	89	52	53
Deaths	22 (25%)	8 (15%)	5 (9%)
Other events	18 (20%)	8 (15%)	23 (43%)
Other reasons	49	36	25

Doctors circulated 358; Number responding 289 (81 %)
Information was unavailable to doctors in 42 patients on perhexiline, 52 on valproate and 23 on labetalol.
Because of the high proportion of deaths with perhexiline a further questionnaire was sent to doctors asking for the cause of death. The results are in the next slide.

Table 5. Deaths

Perhexiline: Total 22		Sodium valproate: Total 8	
Myocdardial infarction	7	Myocardial infarction	1
Sudden death	3	Asphyxia during a fit	1
Ventricular tachycardia	1	Familial nervous disease	1
Resp/cardiac failure	1	Cause not given	5
Cerebrovasc. accident	1	Labetatol: Total 5	
Multiple myeloma	1	Ruptured aortic aneurysm	1
Cause not given	8	Tetanus	1
		Cause not given	3

As can be seen, most deaths from perhexiline resulted, as would be expected, from myocardial ischaemia. These results draw to attention, in comparison to the two deaths spontaneously reported on adverse effect of perhexiline, the fact that death is often not reported as being associated with drug usage.
You will note that hepatic failure, hyperammonaemia and pancreatitis were not noted

in New Zealand at that stage as a cause of cessation of valproate therapy. A closer survey is currently taking place making specific enquiries in this respect.

UNUSUAL ASSOCIATIONS

Another use, which has been made of the data, is more detailed investigation of unusual associations.

Early reports on labetalol drew attention to the occurrence of five cases of scalp tingling, three of polyuria, one of polydipsia and one of polyuria and polydipsia.

In this case a questionnaire was sent to the patients concerned, and also to a group of patients on metropol who served as a control. Over 80 % of the questionnaires were returned. A significant association of scalp tingling and a greater degree of thirst were demonstrated. The main importance of this is in demonstrating a possible type of use of the data collected. Such an exercise would not previously have been possible.

SODIUM VALPROATE FOLLOW-UP

Only one case with abnormal liver function tests had been reported in New Zealand, but because of overseas reports, a questionnaire has recently been sent to doctors of 1906 patients who had used valproate. To date 1192 returns, representing 66 % have been received.

These have revealed two cases of pancreatic disturbances, one fatal and one with abnormal amylase. Fifteen cases of abnormal liver function have been revealed but many were marginal and there were no cases of severe liver failure. A number of miscellaneous reports have been received such as pancytopenia, neutropenia, thrombocytopenia, haemorrhagic proctitis, rashes, aching and weak legs, unwanted pregnancy and loss of hair. There have been two sudden deaths. This data has yet to be fully collated but it once again demonstrates the immense potential of having ready access to lists of users of medicines.

ADVANTAGES OF AN INTENSIFIED VOLUNTARY TYPE OF MONITORING SCHEME

In summary, the type of scheme which has been used in New Zealand is of particular importance to the smaller, less wealthy type of country without the resources to run a major computerised and closely monitored type of system which may be possible in a larger country. New Zealand has demonstrated that sufficient co-operation both in Government and non Government areas can be engendered to make such a scheme well worth-while.

The particular advantage is that, for instance, there now exists in New Zealand on computer, a complete list of users of the newer types of beta blockers over a known period of time. Should any unexpected problems with these medicines turn up in the future, it will be possible to rapidly contact these patients.

If other smaller countries should adopt a similar type of scheme and build up similar lists of cohorts of users, immense future potential is envisaged. Liaison between countries would add greatly to the value of post-marketing surveillance.

Rare and unexpected problems may still only be discovered in the large comprehensive type of scheme and even then may elude discovery for some considerable time. Post-marketing surveillance allows confidence for distribution of new medicines at an earlier stage. It does not guarantee safety.

Sécurité et médicaments (1982), p. 151

Post-marketing Surveillance in U. K. : A Study of Cimetidine Recipients

P.H. Lawson

Dept. of Clinical, Pharmacology, Wards 4/5 Royal Infirmary, Glasgow G 4 OSF, Scotland Kingdom

Abstract — A study of 10,000 cimetidine recipients seen in four centres in U. K. (Glasgow, Nottingham, Oxford & Portsmouth) is currently underway. Primary aims are to look for serious events occurring at low frequency, quantitate known effects and generate a cohort for further study if the need arises. Secondary aims are to assess methods of identifying and following such patients. Details of prescriptions for cimetidine are obtained and a research worker then visits the prescriber twice to determine the reason for prescription of cimetidine together with details of whether patient died, was hospitalized or attended as an out-patient during the ensuing 18 months. On the initial visit a comparison subject is also enrolled and followed (this patient being age- and sex-matched with the recipients).

Detailed analyses of the resulting information will be undertaken once the study is complete. Preliminary analyses indicate that the methods adopted are feasible and practical. A substantial body of information has accumulated both about cimetidine usage and subsequent hospitalizations of recipients. Cooperation of pharmacists and prescribers in this study has been excellent.

Sécurité et médicaments (1982), p. 153

Post-marketing Surveillance Experience Gained with an Orally Active Asthma Prophylactic Agent

P. KRUPP* and D. CROWDER**

*Sandoz Ltd. Pharmaceutical Division Clinical Research, Drug Monitoring Centre, 4002 Basle, Switzerland
**Sandoz Products Ltd, Feltham, United Kingdom

Abstract — The prophylactic treatment of asthma requires long-term medication ; therefore, a post-marketing surveillance (PMS) was initiated with the introduction of ketotifen, an orally active drug. A pilot study was performed in CH with the objective of looking for a methodology suitable for identifying adverse events and for monitoring efficacy in actual practice with the ultimate goal of establishing a risk/benefit profile. The main investigation was set up in the UK and aimed at recruiting a cohort of 10,000 patients treated for one year. Interim information is available on 16,164, 8,913, 4,801 and 1,721 patients respectively treated for 3, 6, 9 and 12 months. The results obtained by this PMS approach confirm the pre-marketing studies, although, as expected, some slight differences are to be recognized. Furthermore, new insight has been gained with respect to patients at special risk usually not encountered in controlled clinical trials, namely small children and pregnant women.

Sécurité et médicaments (1982), pp. 155-159

La sécurité passe par l'information sur le médicament. Role du médecin de l'industrie pharmaceutique

J.F. SCHLUMBERGER

Pharmuka, 35, quai du Moulin de Cage, 92231 Gennevilliers Cedex, France

Résumé — L'industrie pharmaceutique se trouve à un carrefour privilégié entre le médecin qui prescrit le médicament, le pharmacien qui le délivre, le patient qui le prend. Sa responsabilité dans l'information délivrée à chacun de ces protagonistes est entière.

– L'industrie doit donc s'assurer de la fiabilité de cette information et la divulguer sans rétention mais en l'adaptant à chacun des protagonistes.

– Le médecin de l'industrie pharmaceutique a là un rôle fondamental à jouer. C'est lui qui est responsable de la fiabilité de l'information recueillie par ses soins et ce à tous les stades de développement du produit. C'est lui qui doit contrôler que l'information divulguée aux médecins prescripteurs, aux pharmaciens et aux patients est conforme à l'information recueillie, sans omission, sans déformation. Il serait donc souhaitable, pour que cet objectif puisse être atteint, que dans chaque société pharmaceutique un médecin puisse jouer le rôle de contrôle.

Si la sécurité du malade dépend de la bonne information de son médecin sur le produit qui lui sera prescrit, elle dépend également de l'adhérence du malade à ce traitement et du respect des précautions d'emploi qui lui auront été données.

Je voudrais, dans cette introduction, insister sur quatre points qui me paraissent fondamentaux en matière d'information :

1. L'information, pour être source de sécurité pour le malade, doit être fiable : elle dépend donc de la qualité des essais pré-cliniques et cliniques.
2. L'information doit parvenir intacte aux médecins prescripteurs à travers les exigences commerciales propres à toute industrie.
3. L'information doit être en permanence réactualisée, c'est le rôle de la pharmacovigilance.
4. L'information passe par la notion de responsabilité, puisqu'il ne peut y avoir de responsabilité sans information.

Nous avons choisi, pour réfléchir au rôle du médecin de l'Industrie pharmaceutique dans l'information, de suivre le développement puis la commercialisation d'un produit, ce qui nous permettra, à chaque étape, de décrire la nature de l'information à divulguer et les partenaires impliqués.

LA PREMIERE ETAPE est le passage en clinique.
Le médecin de l'Industrie pharmaceutique doit préparer ce passage en rédigeant une brochure décrivant les caractéristiques du produit. Cette brochure a pour objet de renseigner le clinicien sur l'ensemble des travaux qui ont été faits et de ceux qui sont en cours. Elle doit être périodiquement mise à jour. Elle permet d'avoir une vue d'ensemble du dossier pré-clinique (chimie, galénique, pharmaco, toxico, térato, mutagenèse, fertilité, métabolisme, etc.) et du dossier clinique au fur et à mesure que les résultats rentrent.

Le médecin de l'Industrie pharmaceutique joue là un rôle d'intermédiaire, de trait d'union, entre les chercheurs du laboratoire et les cliniciens. Il doit faire connaître à l'extérieur l'information scientifique dont le laboratoire est détenteur et ce sans rien omettre ni déformer sous prétexte de rendre plus accessibles aux cliniciens des données qui ne sont pas toujours claires pour tout le monde.

Certes, les rapports rédigés par les pharmacologues, analystes, biochimistes ou toxicologues sont à la disposition des expérimentateurs cliniques mais l'expérience montre que peu d'entre eux les lisent intégralement. C'est pourquoi il me paraît fondamental que tous ces rapports scientifiques soient lus et analysés par le médecin de l'Industrie pharmaceutique afin d'en faire un rapport de synthèse précis et adapté à l'usage du clinicien. On voit combien, dès ce stade, le rôle du médecin de l'Industrie pharmaceutique est important. Il est évident que pour bien remplir cette mission le médecin de l'Industrie pharmaceutique doit avoir de très bonnes connaissances scientifiques.

LA DEUXIEME ETAPE est celle qui sépare la précédente du dépôt du dossier en vue de son enregistrement.

Pendant toute cette période, le médecin de l'Industrie pharmaceutique aura pour tâche de veiller :

1. à la qualité de l'information recueillie.
2. à ce que le niveau d'information des expérimentateurs soit identique.
3. à ce que les chercheurs de la société soient tenus au courant des résultats obtenus chez l'homme.

Dans le cadre de cet exposé seul le premier point sera abordé, à savoir la qualité de l'information.

La sécurité passe, certes, par l'information sur le médicament, mais pas n'importe quelle information. Notre souci constant doit être de pouvoir mettre à la disposition de nos interlocuteurs quels qu'ils soient une information fiable. C'est pourquoi je vais insister sur les conditions nécessaires à l'obtention d'une information fiable.

– la première est la conception rigoureuse d'un plan de développement adapté au produit, tenant compte :
  . des impératifs de la recherche puis de l'administration de tutelle,
  . des spécificités propres du produit.

– La deuxième est la mise au point, pour chaque étude, d'un protocole extrêmement précis ayant pour objet de répondre à une question.

– La troisième est de veiller ensuite à ce que ce protocole soit scrupuleusement observé par l'expérimentateur, la meilleure façon de s'en assurer étant de recueillir les observations une par une pour les contrôler en vérifiant notamment que :

. les critères d'inclusion et d'exclusion sont respectés,

. les examens demandés, cliniques ou paracliniques, ont été faits aux temps prescrits,

ce qui n'est pas toujours facilement accepté par les experts !

C'est ainsi que le médecin de l'Industrie pharmaceutique peut, surtout en phase III, contrôler le correct déroulement de l'ensemble des essais qui peuvent s'étendre sur plusieurs années ; dépister précocement l'apparition d'effets indésirables ; en apprécier l'importance, la fréquence.

Ce n'est que si ces conditions sont respectées que l'on pourra recueillir une information fiable, cette information étant tout aussi indispensable pour la compagnie que pour l'administraton.

Le rôle du médecin de l'Industrie pharmaceutique durant toute cette longue période apparaît capital, interface privilégiée et obligatoire entre la société et les experts cliniciens travaillant hors de la société dans les hôpitaux.

Interface entre ces cliniciens, les chercheurs et la direction générale, il devrait être pour l'administration un interlocuteur privilégié.

LA TROISIEME ETAPE est celle qui débute avec la commercialisation du produit et se prolonge durant toute sa vie.

L'Industrie pharmaceutique se doit :

. de faire connaître son nouveau médicament

. en poursuivre l'étude

. mettre en place un processus de recueil de l'information auprès des médecins et des pharmaciens.

Faire connaître son nouveau médicament

C'est mettre à la disposition des médecins, des pharmaciens et du malade une information adaptée à chacune de ces catégories. Cette information peut prendre différentes formes, être véhiculée par différentes voies, mais sa qualité doit être identique.

Dans la règle, cette information est élaborée par le marketing qui choisit également les moyens de diffusion : brochure, articles dans la presse spécialisée, encart publicitaire dans les revues, visite médicale, symposium, etc. Les hommes de marketing sont soit des médecins, soit des pharmaciens, soit des commerciaux. En règle, il s'agit d'équipes pluridisciplinaires dans lesquelles travaillent des hommes de marketing, des publicistes et des médecins.

Leur objectif est certes de faire connaître le nouveau médicament ; il est aussi de le faire vendre. Chacun a une éthique et toute éthique est respectable, ce qui ne veut pas dire identique. Il peut y avoir des conflits d'intérêts entre commerciaux et médecins. Il y a là un difficile problème. Nos collègues américains l'ont résolu en faisant en sorte que toute information médicale sortant du Laboratoire soit contrôlée par un comité d'éthique dans lequel le médecin joue un rôle important. Je pense que cette façon de procéder est souhaitable et devrait être adoptée.

Poursuivre l'étude du médicament

Ceci est indispensable. En effet, quelle que soit la qualité du dossier d'enregistrement, il faut bien reconnaître qu'il présente deux faiblesses obligées, je dirai structurelles.

La première porte sur le faible nombre de patients traités eu égard à ceux qui seront traités durant toute la vie du produit.

La deuxième porte sur l'environnement. Avant la commercialisation, le produit était étudié essentiellement en milieu hospitalier, ce qui implique sur un certain type de malades par une certaine catégorie de médecins. La vente du médicament en officine va avoir pour conséquence d'élargir l'éventail des prescripteurs et des patients et un risque de voir apparaître des associations médicamenteuses non prévues ou non souhaitables et qui, donc, n'ont pas été préalablement étudiées.

C'est pourquoi durant toute cette période le médecin de l'Industrie pharmaceutique doit poursuivre les études cliniques auprès des médecins de ville, généralistes ou spécialistes, afin de connaître l'acceptabilité du médicament sur un échantillonnage de malades plus vaste et souvent différent.

Mettre en place un processus de recueil de l'information

auprès des médecins prescripteurs et des pharmaciens afin de dépister les effets secondaires nouveaux, d'en apprécier la gravité et la fréquence.

Tous ces problèmes de surveillance thérapeutique ont été abordés ces jours-ci et je n'y reviendrai pas, mais il est clair que le médecin de l'Industrie pharmaceutique a un rôle important à jouer dans ce processus de recueil puis de contrôle de l'information venant du prescripteur, du pharmacien ou du malade. Il a, de même, un rôle à jouer vis-à-vis des comités de pharmaco-vigilance, des pouvoirs publics, des prescripteurs en les informant de l'apparition de nouveaux effets secondaires ou de la modification de fréquence d'effets déjà connus.

Reste l'information délivrée au malade. La part du médecin de l'Industrie pharmaceutique est discrète puisqu'il n'est pas en contact direct avec le malade. Celui-ci doit recevoir l'information dont il a besoin de son médecin et/ou de son pharmacien. Il n'en reste pas moins que le médecin de l'Industrie pharmaceutique peut jouer un rôle dans la rédaction de la notice à l'usage du patient, notice incluse dans chaque boîte. Le malade doit être informé, non alarmé ; c'est dire que la plus grande prudence doit présider à la conception de cette notice. Lorsque l'on voit ce qui se passe aux U.S.A. où le patient hospitalisé doit à tout moment signer une décharge avant tout examen, toute opération, toute prescription, décharge dans laquelle sont précisés, statistiques à l'appui, les risques qu'il encourt, on peut légitimement se demander si cette façon de faire est un progrès pour le confort du malade ou pour celui du médecin. N'est-ce pas plutôt un transfert de responsabilité ?

Ce sujet information et responsabilité mériterait à lui seul un long développement débordant du cadre de cet exposé introductif. On peut dire cependant qu'il ne peut y avoir de responsabilité sans information, que l'information du médecin doit être aussi complète que possible car sa responsabilité est entière lorsqu'il prescrit un médicament à son malade. Mais pour ce dernier, où doit se situer son niveau d'information ? Quelle est sa part de responsabilité dans l'acceptation du traitement prescrit par son médecin ? Doit-on désirer que le malade ayant un niveau voisin de celui du médecin participe au choix de la thérapeutique qui lui serait la mieux adaptée ? Mais dans ce cas il y aurait partage de responsabilité, co-responsabilité. Est-ce ce que souhaite le malade ?

Je pense, pour ma part, que le niveau d'information, partant de responsabilité, ne peut être le même chez le médecin et le malade mais que c'est au médecin de s'assurer que son malade a une connaissance suffisante de sa prescription pour qu'elle soit suivie avec le maximum de sécurité possible pour lui.

Il ne faut pas, en effet, perdre de vue que le succès d'un traitement passe certes par la bonne information du malade mais aussi par sa bonne adhérence au traitement qui lui aura été prescrit. Or, il ne faut pas perdre de vue, aussi, qu'une information trop axée sur les effets secondaires potentiels, les précautions d'emploi, etc. peut inquiéter un patient qui sera tenté soit de diminuer les doses prescrites soit, même, de ne pas suivre le traitement. Il est bien évident que dans ces cas le risque pour la santé du patient peut être autrement plus préjudiciable que d'hypothétiques effets secondaires dans le sens où ces effets secondaires étant appréciés statistiquement rien ne permet de dire au préalable si ce malade aurait eu à en souffrir.

Il me paraît donc capital d'informer, certes, mais pas d'alarmer, et de s'assurer en fin de compte que le malade a bien compris et suivra la prescription qui lui aura été faite.

Pour conclure, je dirai :

— que *l'information doit être fiable*, ce qui implique que les essais cliniques de phase I, II, III et IV soient non critiquables sur le plan méthodologique,

— que l'information doit parvenir intacte aux médecins, ce qui implique un contrôle par un comité d'éthique de toute information émise par le laboratoire,

— que l'information doit être en permanence réactualisée d'où l'importance des études de pharmaco-vigilance,

— que l'information passe par la notion de responsabilité, que le principal responsable est le médecin-prescripteur dont l'information doit être aussi parfaite que possible ; que, surtout, je trouve dangereux tout comportement visant à faire glisser du médecin vers le malade la responsabilité des actes thérapeutiques.

IV

INFORMING THE PRESCRIBER

L'INFORMATION AU NIVEAU DU PRESCRIPTEUR

Sécurité et médicaments (1982), pp. 163-167

The Liability of Manufacturers in Respect of Known Effects of Medical Products

G.C. TUCK

Miles Laboratories Ltd., Stoke Court – Stoke Poges, Slough Bershire, United Kingdom

This morning's session is devoted to "Product Information and Drug Safety" and, in considering how we should deal with the question of Product Liability, Madame Martel and I felt that we could best contribute to your session by confining our remarks to a consideration of the liability that a manufacturer might incur in relation to the communication or rather, the failure to communicate information about a medicinal product.

We further decided to divide our remarks into two parts, the first dealing with liability in respect of the known and the second dealing with liability in respect of the unknown — by which, of course, we mean liability in respect of what was not known when the product was introduced to the market, but what has become known about it subsequently. That takes us into the realms of "strict liability" and "state of the art of defence" and Madame Martel will deal with this second part.

Turning to my part of this section, I propose to look first at what the EEC Commission's draft of a proposed Directive on Product Liability seems to be proposing in this area, and of course I want to deal specifically with the question of warnings, and then to compare and contrast this with the position in one or two specific countries.

What then did the EEC draft say regarding the giving of information about a product ? The answer is that the original draft of 1976 said nothing specifically.
What it did say, was that over and above the liability that already exists (e.g. in contract) for damage caused by defective articles on other grounds, producers should be strictly liable for damage caused by a defect in a product and Article 4 provides that a product is "defective" for this purpose :

> When it does not provide for persons or property the safety which a person is entitled to expect.

According to the Explanatory Memorandum that accompanied this draft, the question whether a particular product is sufficiently safe so as not to be regarded as "defective" is one to be judged by the court according to objective criteria on the basis of the circumstances in each individual case.

According to the Commission, and I would not disagree with this, it is impossible to determine in advance for all conceivable products the measure of safety that the whole range of consumers is entitled to expect.

Thus, for example, said the Commission, "a producer is liable in respect of the risk of damage arising from the particular subjective tendency of a person to suffer injury, *such as allergies to medicinal products which are objectively harmless,* only where he has failed to point out such generally known risks in presenting, his product, in particular in the instructions for use".

This was the only direct reference in the Commission's first formal utterances to the question of warnings in relation to their 1976 proposals for defective product liability.

The years following 1976 saw an indescribable amount of activity and discussion about the Commission's proposals throughout Europe and indeed elsewhere. In due time, consideration was given to the proposals by the ECOSOC and the European Parliament and it was as a direct result of the views expressed by these bodies that the Commission late in 1979 introduced certain amendments into its draft. Two of these amendments occur in Article 4, which now reads :

> A product is defective when, *being used for the purpose for which it is apparently intended,* it does not provide for persons or property the safety which a person is entitled to expect, *taking into account all the circumstances, including its presentation and the time at which it was put into circulation.*

Article 4 is, of course, one of the crucial articles in the draft and, while they do not by any means resolve all of the difficulties of interpretation arising from the original draft and while they introduce interpretational difficulties of their own, there is no doubt that these two amendments have clarified one very important matter namely that, in deciding whether a product does provide the safety which a person is entitled to expect, the court must take account of the "presentation" of the product.

I shall not attempt to define that word for that must be the role of the Courts in the future, but I have no doubt that the "presentation" of a product includes its labelling and packaging. I would also expect that information communicated otherwise than with the product, for example, data sheets, promotional material, mailings and perhaps even salesmen's oral representations would constitute part of the presentation of the product.

So, under the EEC Commission's proposals the information "presented" about a product is legally relevant to the question of "defectiveness" and it may have one of two effects.

First, it may actually constitute or create the defect itself. Obviously, inaccurate, inappropriate, ambiguous or misleading information can lead to misunderstandings about the activity and safety of a product. Therein a "defect" may well be found to exist.

Second, it may have the effect of rendering non-defective a product which would otherwise be defective.

This, of course, brings us to the whole question of warnings and their place under the Commission's proposals. The draft text is still I am afraid, all too silent on this matter, but let me try to list some principles which I believe will or should be relevant to a consideration of the place of warnings under the Commission's proposals.

1. It seems to be an accepted premise that the producer's liability for injury arising from an adverse effect of medicine can be precluded by an adequate warning in the "presentation" of the product.

2. To be effective or "adequate" for this purpose the warning must have been
a) appropriately described as a contra-indication, a precaution, a side-effect or whatever it may be,
b) appropriate in communicating the nature and degree of risk so that a responsible and balanced decision could be made.
c) sufficiently prominent and readable not to be ignored. Lengthy and indescriminate lists of warnings which have marginal importance and dubious reliability would only serve to dilute the effect of important warnings and reduce their credibility (and effectiveness).
3. Promotional activities may undermine or even render ineffectual printed warnings.
4. Compliance with legislative or health agency labelling requirements is probably a minimum requirement, but by no means conclusive of the fact that the product was adequately labelled.

If these considerations are fulfilled, and adequate warning can well have the effect of preventing a medicinal product from being "defective".

But to whom does this warning have to be "presented" ? In the case of non-prescription products the answer to that question can only be that to be effective for this purpose, the warning must be "presented" with the product so that it is available to actual users of the product.

In the case of prescription products, the answer in law is that warnings and other product information must be presented to the physician, not to the patient.

It is well settled in most countries that the patient musy be regarded as having chosen to rely upon the skill and judgement of a particular physician and he is bound by the expertise of the person he has chosen. The physician is the patient's agent, not the manufacturer's.

That has been the established position in most countries from time immemorial and I find nothing in the Commission's proposals to change that principle.

How then, in respect of warnings of adverse effects, for example, would the Commission's proposals change the position that exists today ? Primarily, the answer is that under the Commission's proposals, once it has been established that a "defect" existed in the product (e.g. because an inadequate warning was presented) it would be immaterial whether the producer had been careless, negligent, blameworthy or faultless. As it is today, in most countries the injured patient will not succeed unless negligence is established.

Let me emphasise again that the Commission's proposals do not impose upon the producer an obligation to notify the patient of warnings, side-effects and so on. The producer's obligation would be fully discharged if an adequate and relevant warning had been given to the physician.

Does it follow then that, if a patient suffers drug related injury and the manufacturer could have given, but did not give, a relevant, adequate warning the producer must necessarily be liable ?

The answer to that question is, "No, because that failure on his part may not have been the cause (in law) of the injury.

Suppose, for example, that the doctor knew from other sources precesely what an adequate warning for that product would have stated. In those circumstances, while the product would be defective on an objective basis, that defect would not have been the legal cause of the injury because the physician's intervening knowledge and conduct would serve to break the chain of causation for which the producer might have been responsible.

Nor, in such a situation, would the physician necessarily be liable to the patient. The Commission's proposals regarding strict liability apply only to the producer and not to the medical practitioner. Thus, in the case I have envisaged, if the physician had in fact acted without any professional negligence, in most countries he would not be held liable and the patient would be without legal remedy. Damnum sine injuria.

Let me illustrate this by contrasting two very interesting decisions from the Supreme Court in Oregon.

Both cases involved oral contraceptives and thromboembolic episodes and in both cases the plaintiff sought damages against the manufacturer for not having adequately warned of the risks of thromboembolism during the use of oral contraceptives.

In one case*, the treating physician was aware that the plaintiff had complained of loss of vision and yet still prescribed oral contraceptives. The Court found that it was wrong to have done so and that, had the product information to the doctor included an adequate warning, the doctor would have followed a different course. Thus, the manufacturers were liable because their inadequate product information had led the physician to make a wrong decision.

Contrast this with the other case** in which the Court found that the prescribing physicians did know of the risks of thromboembolism during the use of oral contraceptives and that they were unaware of the plaintiff's loss of vision or any other factor which would justify discontinuance of oral contraceptives.

In this case the Court found that there had been no "mis-prescription" on the part of the physician and that his course of conduct would not have been different even if the manufacturer's information had included an adequate warning. Thus the manufacturers were not liable because their act or omission had not been the legal cause of the injury.

What I have tried to do so far is to consider some general principles in relation to the Commission's proposals for defective product liability. I would like to conclude with a brief reference to the relevance of warnings in one or two other countries.

In Sweden, as you probably know, a compensation scheme for drug related injury has been operating for a few years now. This scheme is based on a separation of the question of compensation from the question of liability. In other words, the entitlement to compensation is not itself affected by such matters as mistakes in dispensing, negligence by the doctor or defects in the medicinal product. Thus, the giving or withholding of warnings or other product information is not relevant to the question of entitlement to compensation — but if in fact there has been some fault on the part of the dispenser, the doctor, the producer, the insurance firm may seek indemnity or contribution from them.

The scheme has not been operating long enough for considered judgements to be

* McEwan v. Ortho Pharmaceutical Corporation (1974).

** Vaughn v. G.D. Searle & Co. 1975).

made, but perhaps I should emphasise that there are quite significant limitations on the payment of compensation. For example, the nature and seriousness of the illness is considered and the compensation authority can decide that the injured party should reasonably have endured the injury as a side effect of the drug's use.

In Germany, the Medicines Act of 1976, established a system of strict liability for drug related injury so that the "manufacturer" of a licensed medecine which causes the death of or considerably damages the body or health of a person must make good the harm done by paying damages. However, this obligation arises only if the harm done

a) exceeded the bounds considered acceptable in the light of available medical knowledge and

b) arose from the development or production processes or from inadequate labelling or instructions for use.

Unlike the Swedish scheme, the German system is still one in which compensation and liability are interependent. Like the Commission's proposals, the German system is based on strict liability on the part of the producer, but unlike the Commission's proposals not all drug induced injury is compensated.

In Norway, the proposals that have recently been made for a new product liability law contain special provisions for drug liability. It is now doubtful whether these proposals will be adopted without substantial changes, but at present the proposal is that, unless he is a member of a Drug Liability Association, the manufacturer or importer of a drug will be liable for injury caused by it irrespective of fault and irrespective of the fact that the product contained no safety defect. However, if the injury was caused (inter alia) by use contrary to legitimate and specific warning, improper use through negligence on the part of a doctor then the producer will not be liable. Thus under the envisaged Norwegian scheme, adequate warnings will be relevant and effective to exclude a producer's liability.

Ladies and Gentlemen, I have confined my remarks to the question of *liability* for product defect — in other words, to the question of when may the producer be liable. One can, with equal merit and difficulty, approach the question of drug related injury from the point of view of *compensation* and ask when should the injured patient be compensated.

A consideration of both is fundamental and desirable. What, in my view, is not acceptable is to determine the answer to the latter question (about compensation) and then impose it in terms of the first. This I believe is the basic and almost insoluble problem presented by the Commission's proposals. Tort law is not and should not be used as a compensation system similar to Social Security or Workers Compensation. To ignore this precept leads to the problems and difficulties of fixing liability for the "unknowable" — which Madame Martel will now consider.

Sécurité et médicaments (1982), pp. 169-175

La responsabilité stricte des laboratoires pour tous les risques même imprévisibles

F. Martel

Rhône-Poulenc, Secrétariat Général, 22, avenue Montaigne, 75008 Paris, France

Nous connaissons les différents aspects de la responsabilité que les fabricants de produits médicaux sont susceptibles d'encourir pour des risques prévisibles.

Il est à remarquer que la nature même de ces produits, entraîne pour le fabricant une responsabilité très accentuée par rapport à celle qui est à la charge des autres fabricants, et le soumet à des contraintes extrêmement sévères tant dans la conception et les essais que dans la fabrication, la présentation et la diffusion.

Or, si l'on songe que le produit médical est destiné à modifier les processus physiologiques du corps qui sont eux-mêmes variables, on conçoit aisément que ce produit peut présenter des risques d'effets contraires malgré toutes les précautions et tous les moyens scientifiques et médicaux mis en œuvre pour les éviter.

Bien entendu, on peut toujours imaginer que certains effets contraires seraient prévisibles et reconnus, et en ce cas on se trouverait dans les hypothèses de responsabilité pour faute qui ont été précédemment traitées.

Mon propos est maintenant d'étudier les risques d'effets contraires plus ou moins nocifs qui sont imprévisibles compte-tenu des connaissances scientifiques et médicales du moment : ce sont les risques dits de développement.

Devra-t-on pour ces risques ou défauts de développement, retenir la responsabilité du fabricant alors même qu'on ne peut lui reprocher une négligeance ?

C'est le problème de l'appréciation du caractère défectueux d'un produit dans le temps.

Cette appréciation peut se faire selon divers paramètres, mais le type même du défaut de développement est celui qui résulte de l'apparition d'un effet insoupçonné découlant d'une utilisation répétée du produit et qui sera, lui, la cause de l'évolution des connaissances parce que précisément on voudra en comprendre la raison.

Je donnerai pour exemple les effets contraires insoupçonnés du bismuth, produit devenu d'usage courant.

Ainsi donc l'existence d'un danger, notamment en ce qui concerne le produit médical, peut n'apparaître qu'après plusieurs années, de surcroît le rapport de causalité entre ce danger et une lésion peut n'être jamais clairement établi. Il apparaît bien malaisé dans ces conditions d'établir une responsabilité quelconque du fabricant.

J'en veux pour preuves que très peu de décisions de justice ont fait état de défauts de développement.

On peut évidemment songer au cas de la thalidomide mais les opinions divergent et il est difficile d'affirmer si c'est un risque de développement qui est à l'origine de cet accident. Les victimes furent pourtant indemnisées, du moins partiellement, car cette affaire n'est pas encore terminée.

Le problème ainsi posé, comment en est-on arrivé à évoquer le principe même de la responsabilité du fabricant pour les risques de développement ?

— Indéniablement les procédés actuels de production et de distribution de masse ont suscité dans l'opinion publique une prise de conscience et la volonté qu'une protection croissante des consommateurs soit établie.

— Ainsi est apparue cette notion fondamentale de sécurité à laquelle tout individu a droit et le fabricant est devenu redevable d'une véritable obligation d'innocuité du produit et ceci que son intervention ait été fautive ou non.

— Sous cette pression constante, une évolution générale de la responsabilité mise à la charge du fabricant s'est opérée vers une stricte responsabilité objective liée aux risques du produit et détachée de la preuve d'une faute positive d'abstention, ou de simple négligence du fabricant.

Qu'est-ce qu'une responsabilité objective ?

C'est une responsabilité de plein droit par le fait qu'elle est engagée dès que la participation du produit à la création du dommage est démontrée. Elle ne suppose pas la preuve d'une faute ni même une faute présumée.

Ce n'est plus désormais la conduite du fabricant qui est en jeu, mais la performance du produit car le consommateur est considéré comme étant légitimement en droit de penser que les connaissances scientifiques actuelles sont suffisamment poussées pour lui assurer l'innocuité du produit.

Il s'est opéré tant sur le plan des droits internes que sur le plan des législations internationales, un glissement d'une responsabilité pour faute vers une responsabilité objective pour vice du produit.

Ainsi l'appréciation du caractère fautif ou négligent de la conduite du fabricant dans l'élaboration et la diffusion du produit n'est plus la condition de sa responsabilité.

Dès lors se trouve levé l'obstacle à l'application d'un principe de responsabilité objective pour le risque de développement :

La responsabilité est attachée au résultat néfaste qu'entraîne le produit même si ce résultat était imprévisible en l'état des connaissances.

Ce nouveau principe de responsabilité sera tout d'abord illustré par quelques exemples pris dans les droits internes.

Puis les projets de textes élaborés au sein des instances communautaires européennes montreront comment il est envisagé de traiter les risques de développement au sein de la C.E.E.

EXEMPLES DE DROITS INTERNES

La situation aux Etats-Unis

J'ai choisi de vous exposer la situation actuelle aux Etats-Unis à l'égard de la responsabilité mise à la charge du fabricant car elle est relativement complexe et de ce fait mal comprise, notamment par les pays européens, et elle tend à susciter une réaction de rejet en bloc face au danger extrême que semble représenter ce régime spécifique de la responsabilité.

Aux Etats-Unis la victime à plusieurs voies pour rechercher la responsabilité du fabricant. Ces voies s'interpénètrent et aboutissent à une responsabilité stricte du fabricant à l'égard de n'importe quelle victime, en raison des dommages physiques causés par des produits défectueux et dangereux.

Ces régimes sont :

— La responsabilité pour négligence dont l'appréciation est très large.

— La responsabilité pour non respect d'une garantie écrite qui ne se limite plus aux parties contractantes. En effet, désormais par le truchement des annonces publicitaires, il existe une relation personnelle entre le producteur et le consommateur et il en résulte une responsabilité stricte des producteurs pour renseignement inexact.

— La responsabilité pour non respect d'une garantie implicite du vendeur quant à la qualité commerciale et l'aptitude à l'usage de ses produits.

A ce titre, de nombreux jugements ont condamné des fabricants en évoquant le caractère "déraisonnablement" dangereux du produit.

— Enfin la responsabilité délictuelle stricte définie au paragraphe 402 A du "second restatement of torts" (en 1965).

Cependant contrairement à une opinion couramment répandue, il ne s'agit pas d'une responsabilité absolue car si elle ne suppose plus la faute du fabricant il faut néanmoins que le produit ait été défectueux lors de sa mise en vente et qu'en outre cette défectuosité l'ait rendu dangereux.

Il en résulte qu'un produit intrinsèquement dangereux mais sans présenter de défaut, ne répond pas aux critères requis au titre du paragraphe 402 A second restatement et ne permet pas en conséquence de retenir la responsabilité du fabricant.

Or, c'est à quelque chose près le même raisonnement qui a été adopté pour exonérer le fabricant d'une responsabilité pour risques de développement.

Il a été en effet admis que le produit, alors reconnu comme dangereux à l'usage, ne pouvait être considéré comme défectueux lorsqu'il fut mis en vente car le défaut était inconnu et indécelable à l'époque.

Ainsi, alors que le droit américian fait figure de précurseur en matière de responsabilité du fait des produits et apparaît comme le plus achevé. Des problèmes importants demeurent néanmoins en suspens.

Face au développement plus ou moins anarchique de ces régimes de responsabilité qui ont conduit à des indemnisations fréquentes et très importantes et pour répondre à l'inquiétude croissante des industriels et des assureurs, le gouvernement américain nomma en 1976 la commission «Interagency task force» chargée d'enquêter sur l'aspect juridique et économique de la question.

Je rappelle ici qu'aux Etats-Unis la victime peut faire appel à un Jury lorsqu'elle intente une action en responsabilité civile. Celui-ci bien évidemment apprécie la réalité de la responsabilité du défendeur et du montant des dommages et intérêts dus, non pas sur la base de critères juridiques qu'il ignore mais en fonction d'arguments "émotionnels" que les avocats ne manquent pas de faire ressortir.

De surcroît, les avocats étant rémunérés au prorata des indemnités accordées à la victime, ils n'hésitent pas à surévaluer le préjudice subi.

Enfin un autre élément qui a également contribué à l'ampleur du problème est l'accès du prétoire aux groupements d'intérêts tels les associations de consommateurs.

Enfin, pour conclure, l'enquête effectuée par l'Interagency task force a permis de détecter les "failles" du système américain et de préconiser des réformes. Or parmi ces mesures, la task force envisage d'intégrer dans le régime de responsabilité stricte la responsabilité du fabricant pour les risques de développement.

La situation en France

En France, la jurisprudence a la charge du fabricant, une obligation de compétence absolue, considérant que ce qui peut «scientifiquement être expliqué est scientifiquement prévisible.» En conséquence le seul fait de livrer un produit défectueux, créé par lui-même, une présomption irréfragable de mauvaise foi et de responsabilité entraînant l'obligation de réparer la totalité du préjudice en résultant. Cette rigueur est absolue à l'égard du fabricant pharmacien dont toute l'activité est régie par le principe du respect dû à l'intégralité de la personne humaine.

Ce fabricant, en raison de la spécificité de son secteur d'activité, doit être doué d'une science sans défaut.

On peut prétendre qu'il s'agit en définitive d'une véritable obligation de résultat mise à la charge de tout fabricant, et donc susceptible d'intégrer les risques de développement.

Nous allons maintenant étudier très rapidement les nouveaux régimes qui furent adoptés par l'Allemagne et la Suède en matière de responsabilité du fabricant du fait des produits pharmaceutiques.

Il faut en effet rappeler que dans l'ensemble des droits internes, la responsabilité du fabricant du fait des produits pharmaceutiques est déterminée par les règles générales de droit commun qui régissent la responsabilité de tout fabricant de produits, quels qu'ils soient.

La situation en Allemagne

En quoi consiste la nouvelle loi allemande du 24 août 1976, entrée en vigueur le 1er janvier 1978 sur les spécialités pharmaceutiques ?

Il s'agit principalement d'une loi de police sanitaire, plus ou moins similaire à celles qui existent en la matière dans la majorité des pays.

Mais en revanche, d'où son originalité, elle crée en outre une responsabilité spécifique du fabricant de spécialités pharmaceutiques.

— En effet, jusqu'à cette loi, le fabricant de produits pharmaceutique n'est reconnu responsable que sur la base d'une faute qu'il aurait commise à l'un des stades de l'élaboration et de la fabrication du produit.

— Or le droit allemand ne retient pas la responsabilité du fabricant si le produit a été conçu et fabriqué conformément au niveau le plus récent des connaissances scientifiques et techniques et s'il a été accompagné de l'information appropriée. Et de ce fait, les défauts de développement n'engagent pas la responsabilité.

Mais l'opinion publique, fortement alarmée par des sinistres graves comme ceux dus à la thalidomide, au stalinon, au mer 29 etc., considérant en outre que le médicament est le type même du produit qui peut avoir à long terme un effet nocif insoupçonné, exerça des pressions sur le gouvernement en vue d'obtenir une meilleure protection financière du consommateur.

C'est ce que réalisa cette loi en imposant au fabricant d'indemniser toute personne qui souffrirait d'un dommage (mort ou lésions corporelles importantes) à la suite de la consommation d'un médicament, et en l'obligeant à fournir des garanties, en principe d'assurances, pour faire face, le moment venu à son obligation de paiement.

Seule désormais l'action dommageable du produit est requise. Il suffit que les troubles physiologiques causés par l'usage d'un médicament excédent ce qui était connu ou prévu par le corps médical, que le produit soit ou non reconnu défectueux.

De ce fait, tel que ce texte est conçu, rien ne s'oppose à ce qui la garantie joue pour les risques de développement puisque seul le caractère dommageable du produit est exigé.

Je terminerai en précisant que les plafonds d'indemnités prévus, sont extrêmement élevés puisqu'ils peuvent atteindre 200 millions de D.M. en capital pour l'ensemble des dommages causés par un médicament.

La situation en Suède

A l'inverse de l'Allemagne, la Suède n'a édicté aucun texte légal modifiant le régime juridique de la responsabilité du fabricant, laquelle reste liée à la notion de négligence, entendue au sens le plus large.

Un accord est intervenu en 1976 à l'initiative du parlement, entre la profession pharmaceutique et les pouvoirs publics, sur l'indemnisation des victimes d'un médicament.

Au terme de cet accord un fond d'assurance a été créé, financé par les laboratoires pharmaceutiques et géré par un consortium des quatre plus grandes compagnies d'assurance du pays.

Les médicaments sont divisés en 2 classes, et seules les substances pouvant entraîner des effets secondaires corporels sérieux et imprévisibles sont couvertes (2 millions de couronnes par an et intervention financière de l'Etat au-delà).

Ainsi il suffit que le dommage ait été causé par le médicament avec une probabilité prédominante pour que la garantie intervienne.

En conséquence les dommages consécutifs aux risques de développement, du fait même de leur caractère imprévisible sont couverts sans restriction.

Cette démarche est très spécifique, car, par le biais d'une couverture d'assurance, un régime d'indemnisation automatique est instauré en faisant peser sur le fabricant une stricte responsabilité objective pour risques.

Il s'agit en réalité beaucoup plus d'un système d'assurances sociales que d'un régime de responsabilité civile.

LES PROJETS DE TEXTES COMMUNAUTAIRES

Je vais maintenant vous exposer brièvement et sous le seul angle des risques de développement, les 2 projets de textes qui sont à l'heure actuelle à l'étude au sein des instances communautaires européennes.

Il s'agit :

— du projet de convention européenne sur la responsabilité du fait des produits en cas de dommage personnel ou de mort, approuvé en septembre 1976 par le comité des Ministres du conseil de l'Europe.

— et de la proposition de directive de la commission des communautés européennes relative au rapprochement des législations des Etats membres concernant la responsabilité du fait des produits défectueux et dont le dernier état de projet est du 1er octobre 1979.

Il est à noter que ces législations européennes viendront s'ajouter et non pas remplacer, les droits contractuels et non contractuels, qui existent actuellement au plan des droits internes.

Je rappelle, que ces 2 projets établissent une responsabilité stricte du fabricant. Pour autant cette responsabilité est limitée car le fabricant n'est tenu responsable que des dommages résultant d'un défaut du produit. Mais quand on sait que dans les 2 textes est considéré comme défectueux «tout produit qui n'offre pas la sécurité qu'on peut légitimement en attendre», on peut affirmer qu'une véritable obligation d'innocuité du produit est imposée au fabricant.

De surcroît, la charge de la preuve est renversée, et, c'est au fabricant de prouver que le défaut d'insécurité n'existait pas au moment de la mise en circulation du produit. Mais comment le pourra-t-il ?

Quant aux dommages qui se réalisent pendant la vie du produit après sa mise en circulation mais qui résultent de vices absolument indétectables à l'époque de lancement du produit, ils n'en demeurent pas moins, selon ces 2 projets, des dommages d'insécurité.

Ainsi la proposition de directive précise clairement, tant dans ses considérants qu'en son article 1er, que le producteur est sans aucun doute tenu pour responsable des défauts de développement.

Le texte de la convention est moins net mais le rapport explicatif de cette convention affirme le même principe considérant que si des défauts de developpement n'apparaissent qu'à la lumière de connaissances scientifiques acquises souvent après la commercialisation du produit défectueux, il n'en reste pas moins que le produit était défectueux dès l'origine quoique de manière cachée.

CONCLUSION

En conclusion, comme dans bien d'autres domaines, on se trouve face à une attitude qui consiste à faire primer sur les principes juridiques traditionnels, des techniques destinées à répondre à des objectifs de caractère social et politique.

C'est pourquoi la protection qui s'attache aux principes juridiques classiques a tendance à devenir de moins en moins efficace au profit, encore une fois, de cette volonté politique de placer la charge du risque sur le producteur plutôt que le consommateur.

En somme tout fabricant qui produit est par nature un responsable en puissance.

Sécurité et médicaments (1982), pp. 177-182

The Physician's Labeling — An American Point of View

L.G. MILLSTEIN

Food & Drug Administration, (HFD-107) 5600 Fishers Lane, Rockville, Maryland 20857, USA

Abstract — The Food & Drug Administration (FDA) published, on June 26, 1979, a regulation, "Labeling for Prescription Drugs Used in Man". This rule for the package insert or professional labeling describes in detail the information required in the insert and even suggests how it may be said. The changes corect the tendency on the part of some manufacturers to describe to practitioners the merits of the drug without giving information regarding its hazards and special precautions necessary for maximum safety and effectiveness. The regulation directs the use of explicit information on indications and the replacement of generalities with specifics. In effect, all labeling will be brought to a uniform level — that of the best product monographs written. The section on Clinical Pharmacology will now include specific biopharmaceutics data on the drug(s), specific pharmacokinetics and any other information which is pertinent to the drug's clinical use. The section on Precautions is now made up of nine subsections — one section, pregnancy, will identify a category (A, B, C, D or X) that applies to the drug. The categories will tell the practitioner the potential risk for the fetus and a progressive degree of caution that should be exercised accordingly in the various categories. For Adverse Reactions, incidence and severity data will be provided for the practitioner. Other information about the drug product is provided in separate sections to inform the prescriber on the safest and most effective use of the drug.

When Dr. Burke asked if I would present a paper on the product monograph, he suggested that I feel free to take off my regulatory and medico-legal cap and address the subject from the point of view of "how can the prescriber be best informed on the use of a drug so that the patient can be given the most effective treatment with the least possible chance of harmful effects." After spending many years in the pharmaceutical industry prior to joining the Food and Drug Administration (FDA), with much of it spent preparing the necessary labeling documents for review by the Agency, it is not so easy to remove the caps Dr. Burke mentioned. Rather, let me pass on to you what I have learned about the kinds of communications that can best inform the prescriber, and how it is best presented so that it may be utilized as the most complete resource document about the drug not summarized elsewhere.

Labeling starts out in the drug approval process as a summary expression of experimental data in the New Drug Application (NDA). It is a unique form of communication serving a selected audience. It uses relatively few words to summarize large amounts of data with broad implications. Because of this, it deserves to have specific guidelines for the audiences it is to be used for[1]

Much time is spent in developing a package insert that has the most up-to-date information and presented in such a manner that it can serve serveral publics at one time — the physician and other health professionals, the drug manufacturer and the government agency responsible for the drug approval process ; however, because of this we are immediately faced with an inconsistency in our thinking. Many hours are invested to provide just the right word and the proper nuance and yet we are fuly aware that the therapeutic usage of drugs is hardly influenced by these subtle distinctions of language. In spite of this apparent peculiarity, the drug labeling has become increasingly recognized as a document of significance.

It was not until 1962 when amendments were added to the Food, Drug & Cosmetic Act[2] that the scientific quality of the package insert began to show improvement. With these amendments, drugs were not only to be shown they were safe, but also that efficacy be proven by adequate and well-controlled studies appropriate to the indications to be used in the labeling. In 1974, the FDA initiated the Prescription Drug Labeling Project specifically to assure that marketed prescription drugs are labeled with current information for safe and effective use and that such labeling is presented and distributed in the best way possible. To prepare for the writing of a more detailed regulation that would make the practitioner's package insert a more useful instrument and increase its value as an informational resource to prescribers, a few questions would have to be asked. First, what is the goal of the document, and second, how should it be reformatted and what new areas should be included ?

It has been generally agreed that the goal of this document is to inform the prescriber of current relevant knowledge — a condensate of periodically up-dated material and technical information that permits the safe and intelligent use of drugs [3].

As for the question of format, this was addressed specifically in a proposal in 1975 when the FDA published the notice indicating the new format and content for professional labeling[4]. This publication gave the medical community an opportunity to re-examine the basic concepts and purposes of labeling and to express our plans for improving scientific communication. Prior to this period, in 1961 the FDA had promulgated a regulation to remedy the situation whereby a physician was not always made aware by the drug manufacturer of a drug's side effects, contraindications and precautions. This has come to known as the "full disclosure" rule. The regulation required that a package insert be on or within all bulk prescription drug packages and bear adequate information for its use. This includes indications, effects, dosages, routes, methods and frequency and duration of administration, as well as any relevant hazards, contraindications, side effects and precautions under which practitioners can use the drug safely and for the purpose intended. This includes all purposes for which it is advertised or represented. Certain other information was not conveyed by the package insert, for example, that relating to the diagnosis and treatment of disease. In effect, only the drug's dosage, safety and efficacy are included in the insert[5, 6, 7]. The listing of an indication requires proof that the drug meets the necessary requirements for safety and efficacy for the designated purpose. This proof is sustained only by adequate and well-controlled clinical evaluations.

Now, we come upon another problem area. Once a product and its labeling are approved, the manufacturer may begin other clinical trials to obtain additional indications for his drug product. Since approval of any data submitted to the FDA is necessary before the firm may add it to the labeling, it is evident that a time-lag occurs between the publication of studies, approval of the claim and its appearance in the package labeling[8]. Often a claim for a new use of a drug is made in the literature, but no further studies are forthcoming to substantiate the investigation and, occasionally, additional studies do not substantiate the initial claim and no further effort is made. As a result, the practicing physician is often left in a quandary as to how and whether to use the medication beyond the approved claims. The quandary has its basis in the medico-legal significance of the package insert. Clearly, the labeling is increasingly being used to determine negligence in medical malpractice suits against physicians and hospitals and to that end there is little alternative to the proposition that package inserts must be solid, authoritative documents based on substantial evidence[5, 8]. The FDA has stated often enough that it does not regulate the practice of medicine. The practitioner must be free to use a drug for an indication not in the package insert when such usage is part of the pratice of medicine and for the benefit of the patient. However, when a physicians prescribes a drug for a use not in the approved labeling, he or she invokes two responsibilities. The first is to be well-informed about the drug and to base the non-approved use of it on firm scientific and medical contributions, and the second is to be ready and able to cite the information (text, journal article, public presentation) upon which the decision was made, or show that the use is reasonable and consistent with the sound pratice of medicine[9]. This should not be a difficult task, and it has been well-established that many unapproved indications are widely accepted long before the FDA approves the use. However, the physician cannot and should not ignore the approved information in the package insert.

Although physicians may hear of or discover the many innovative ways in which drugs are used in patient care, some of which are not in the approved labeling, another official document detailing these newer uses is not yet needed nor warranted. The package insert's most important educational value derive from the fact that it is a well-reviewed, authoritative document[8]. Should a phyician wish to extend the claim structure to new, innovative areas and act as sponsor for the new use of a drug solely as a research tool or for early clinical investigation of a drug of therapeutic or diagnostic potential, the FDA requires a «Notice of Claimed Investigational Exemption for a New Drug» (IND), be submitted for review before the use of the drug may begin. This enables the FDA to accumulate data on the safety and efficacy of the drug for that kind of treatment and to share the information with other physicians. Physician-sponsored INDs make up approximately 55 % of the workload at the FDA in this particular area, which is a good indication of the pursuit of new areas where drug firms have either no particular interest because of minimal commercial appeal or the company has decided to fund research of new drug entities and not re-examine already approved drugs. Drug firms must encourage physician-sponsored INDs by providing the required background information on animal studies and manufacturing controls when they themselves have no interest, since this area offers the broad opportunity of gathering, correlating and evaluating the facts that are collected. The IND system can function as a central point in the development of a drug's new usage. The physician's experience will not be lost and may be added to the total available information if he files an IND in these circumstances.

Of greatest importance is that a physician should be aware of the information in the package insert prior to investigating new, unapproved uses. The Congress of the United States intended that the courts, not the FDA, judge whether a physician has met his obligations in the event of patient harm from a marketed drug. Thus, it is important that the physician have the most complete, up-to-date information available and a compelling reason for the development of more detailed labeling regulations to provide this information.

To this end, in June of 1979, the FDA published the regulation entitled "Content and Format for Labeling of Human Prescription Drugs"[10]. The FDA's accumulated experience with labeling, the cognizance of the purposes labeling serves and the responsibilities to provide clear criteria to meet scientific and regulatory requirements are embodied in the new regulation. When the regulation was prepared, the suggestion was made for the elimination of interesting, but nonessential sections, including animal pharmacology (unless related to human pharmacology), clinical studies (although their conclusions will be included) and literature references[11]. These three section headings may be included, if appropriate, and meet the criteria explained in the regulation.

The section previously called "Actions" is replaced with "Clinical Pharmacology" which is expanded to include specific biopharmaceutic or pharmacokinetic data (absorption, distribution, metabolism, elimination and binding) to assist the phyician in utilizing his own background in pharmacology. The "Precautions" section is now made up of nine sub-sections — including information on interactions, use in pregnancy, labor and delivery, nursing mothers and use in children. Any required printed patient information (Patient Package Insert or PPI) to be distributed to the patient is referenced in the "Precautions" section and the full text reprinted at the end of the labeling. This will help the physician to be responsive to the patient's questions following receipt of the information from the pharmacist.

The "Pregnancy" sub-section appears in the labeling if a drug is absorbed systemically or if a drug has a potential for indirect harm to the fetus. These drugs are identified with a category (A, B, C, D or X) and the statement required under the category. The categories communicate to the practitioner the potential risk for the fetus and a progressive degree of caution that should be exercised accordingly in the various categories. The categories are based on animal studies and human clinical experience with the drug or drugs of the class. The D and X categories represent the drugs with the greatest risk to the fetus. Information in these categories is referenced to the "Warnings" and "Contraindications" sections. These D and X categories are for drugs with known human fetal risks and, therefore, demand stronger statements than merely labeling for caution[10, 12].

The sections on "Warnings" and "Adverse Reactions" will now provide estimates of the frequency of undesirable reactions so that the endless, and often uninterpretable, string of such reactions that were previously only listed, will now give way to information of real clinical relevance[1]. Thus, a statement that stomach upset may occur in 1 to 6 patients and peptic ulcer in about 1 in 100 patients from clinical trial experience is more meaningful and helpful than a "laundry-list" of side effects.

For the first time, specific sections on "Drug Abuse and Dependence" for controlled drug substances and "Overdosage" are to be included where this information is available and appropriate. The "Dosage and Administration" section will include the usual dosage range, dosage intervals, the optimal method of titrating dosage and modifications needed for special patient groups — children, the elderly or in patients with renal or hepatic disease.

The principles behind these labeling changes developed gradually out of past experience, and were part of the natural evolution of the need for more and better information about the drugs in the marketplace. It is most important that a prescribing physician be able to pick-up a drug compendium and turn to the drug of his choice and have available detailed, practical information taken from the approved package labeling. Although textbooks are extremely important, they are, by necessity, behind current events at publication and cannot serve as a comprehensive alternative source of therapeutic information. It is also necessary that there be a systematic up-dating and revision of drug labeling so that the labeling does not decline in usefulness with age. The FDA has attempted to do this by way of a labeling format revision program started in November 1980 in accord with the regulation published in June 1979[13]. By November 1982, the revised labeling for all prescription drug products approved by the FDA for marketing in the United States will have been submitted for review under the required new format and content. Our plans call for regular reviews of this type. By this method, we hope to achieve consistency of terminology, elimination of promotional and extraneous information and the use of explicit information on indications, and the replacement of generalities with specifics. Clearly, a major undertaking, but one long needed in the United States.

It is important to recognize what the physician's labeling is, and also to recognize what it is not. The most important feature, and the one that distinguishes it form other sources of information and makes possible its use as an authoritative reference source, is that its content must be based on substantial evidence[1]. Because of this, we are faced with the anomaly of meeting this requirement and being fully up-to-date. However, one can expect some lag between the discovery of reasonable new uses of the drug, and their inclusion in the approved labeling, until the required substantial evidence has been submitted to the FDA.

In summary, we at the FDA believe that the major purposes of the package labeling can be divided into three categories — these are : 1. to provide adequate information to the physician for safe and effective use of the drug for its intended use, 2. to act as an educational instrument regarding a specific drug and 3. to provide the factual basis and limitations for the promotion of the drug to the medical community.

I am certain that with the new format and guidelines to be used by the American drug industry, the labeling to be used by physicians and other health professionals will increase in accuracy and usefulness. They will be welcomed by physicians as a valuable reference to what is well-established, rather than as a bureacratic impediment to their practice of medicine[1].

REFERENCES

1. Gagliardi V.J. and M.J. Finkel, Labeling Plans of the Food and Drug Administration, presented as part of a symposium on "Regulation of Therapeutics: Package Inserts and Their Significance to Physician, Patient and Pharmacists", AMA Annual Convention, June 17, 1975.

2. Federal Food, Drug and Cosmetic Act, As Amended, October 10, 1962, 21 USC 301.

3. Holland A.H. Jr, Drugs, Doctors and Directives, *J. Amer. Geriat. Soc.* **7**, 19 (1965).

4. Proposed Regulation on "Labeling for Prescription Drugs Used in Man", Federal Register **40**, 15392, April 7, 1975

5. Hirsh H.L., The Medico-legal Significance of the Package Insert, *J. Faily Pratice* **4**, 1141 (1977).

6. Curran W.J. and E.D. Shapiro, *Law, Medicine and Forensic Science*, Boston, Little, Brown, 1970, pp. 728-38.

7. Reinstein P.H., Drug Labeling as a Standard for Medical Care, *J. Leg. Med.* **4**, 22 (1976).

8. Crout J.R., In Praise of the Lowly Package Insert, presented at the Food and Drug Law Institute, Washington, DC, Decembre 11, 1973.

9. Use of Drugs for Unapprovet Indications : Your Legal Responsibility, *FDA Drug Bulletin*, October 1972

10. Content and Format for Labeling of Human Prescription Drugs, *Federal Register* **44**, 37434, June 26, 1979.

11. Temple R., Legal Implications of the Package Insert, *Medical Clinics of North America* **55**, 1151 (September 1974).

12. Perez T.H., L.G. Millstein and B.P. Lewis Jr, New Look to Prescription Drug Labelling, *American Pharmacy* **NS21**, 39 (February 1981).

13. Content and Format for Labeling for HUMAN Prescription Drugs, Clarification of Effective Date, *Federal Register* **45**, 32550, May 16, 1980.

Sécurité et médicaments (1982), p. 183

Drug Safety — Information Systems

J. CROOKS

University Department of Pharmacology and Therapeutics, Ninewells Hospital & Medical School, Dundee, DD1 9SY, Scotland, United Kingdom

Abstract — The explosive increase in both the number of drugs available and the amount of information which has to be known about them to be able to use them effectively and safely constitutes a major problem in modern therapeutics. The problem is exacerbated by the recognition of the difficulties of ensuring that prescribing instructions are accurately carried out. This paper describes studies which have revealed drug hazards both in hospital and community practice. It also describes a variety of methods of communicating information about drugs to those prescribe, administer and dispense them, which may increase both their efficacy and safety.

Sécurité et médicaments (1982), p. 185

Future Systems in Providing the Prescriber with Drug Information

H. Ducrot

Groupe Hospitalier Necker Enfants Malades, Consultation de Médecine, 149, rue de Sèvres, 75730 Paris Cedex 15, France

Abstract — Up to now, the main way of recording and transmitting medical information was printed matter (books, journals...). We think that, in the near future, this function will be, at least partially, played by computer technics, and mainly by data banks. These have certain advantages : apparent data volume independent of the real volume, possibility of searches using multiple criteria, possibility of specific processings (for instance, search for interactions between several drugs) and mainly fast updating, as frequent as requested. However, before we fully succeed in using these methods in a really operational way, some progress has to be made. Some concerning logic or software : better standardization and analysis of medical vocabulary, design of "cordial" query languages different of complex languages presently used in automatic documentation. Other areas involve hardware : cheap and efficient public information media such as viewdata, increase of microcomputer capacity by the use of very compact peripheral memories (video disc...).

Methods for the recording and spread of medical knowledge have varied little since the era of Gütenberg. Printing has played a virtualy exclusive role. The place occupied by audio-visual methods has remained marginal, and they are used above all in teaching. In the quite near future, within the next few years, it is possible to predict marked changes related to the development of Informatics. Part of the role played by printed matter will be taken over by a special category of data bank, knowledge banks (or factual data banks). May I remind you that a data bank consists of two parts : a data base, i.e. one or more structured collections of data, and secondly, programs used for retrieval, updating and the exploitation of data. The word "structure" is particulary important in this definition. It signifies that information must be organized in chapters, subchapters, headings, etc., in an identical manner for all the "objects" described in the bank. For example, in setting up a data bank on drugs, all drugs must be described in the same form. This limitation must be respected if it is to be really possible to treat the data and not only reproduce them in their original form.

What are the advantages of a data bank over traditionel written records ?

1. The volume occupied by the information is *transparent* for the user. When seeking to set up a collection of immediately useable information by means of books or journals, the amout of space available rapidly becomes a limiting factor. To have a great deal of information available implies the need for a whole library in close proximity to the user's office. By contrast, when using a data bank, it is sufficient to have access to a terminal taking up no more space than a typewritter. The space necessary for the

terminal will be the same, whether the data bank is empty or full of data. It can also provide access to an undefined number of different and complementary data banks.

2. It is possible to use multiple *search criteria*. Traditional systems are in general suitable for the easy use of a search criterion (alphabetical index). However it is most often impossible to use several, in particular when dealing with criteria of a different nature linked by "logical operators" such as AND, OR, EXCEPT. By contrast, informatic techniques make possible the simultaneous use of an undefined number of criteria, at least in theory. In practice, the number of criteria is limited to two or three by the complexity of boolean logic for non-professional users.

3. The *time* required to seek a piece of information is independent of the total volume of information. This also contrasts with the situation applicable in a library. In reality, the time is not totally independent of volume but the differences are too slight to be noticed by the user.

4. Informatic methodes may be used for *data treatment*. In the field of therapeutic information, this applies above all to the search for interactions between several drugs. Once again, alphabetical indexes can provide the answer but are time consuming. Simultaneous prescription of five drugs, which is not encommon, at least in France, results in ten drug combinations taken two by two. In addition, physicians prescribe drugs individually and using their proprietary names, whilst the scientific litterature often mentions only groups (chemical or pharmacological) or generic names. A computer is rapidely able to establish the necessary correspondences.

5. Finally, and perhaps most important, the *permanent updating* of data is possible. The updating of printed texts, manual or treated, is very slow. For technical and economic reasons, at least one year elapses and often far longer between two successive éditions of a book.

Medical data and in particular information concerning drugs evolve rapidly : new drugs and above all new information concerning old drugs. All modern data bank systems offer the possibility of immediate updating, often via several working stations simultaneously. The collection of information represents a heavy task for the producer of the data bank but the exploitation of new data is possible immediately at such a price.

Despite the advantages described above, the implementation of automated drug information systems still poses a certain number of problems. We shall limit ourselves here to a description of the principle ones only.

1. The optimal function of a data bank requires *standardization of the vocabulary* used. This is far from a spontaneous occurrence in the field of medicine. In particular, information concerning drugs uses a very extensive vocabulary. The terms used to describe therapeutic indications or contraindications and side effects cover almost all medical specialities. The usual vocabulary of physicians, whatever their mother tongue, is completely anarchic. The normalization of medical vocabulary being utopian, it is necessary to create a sub-set of this vocabulary, specific to the data bank. In order to question the latter the use of a printed thesaurus (a hierarchical list of terms used in a documentary system) is necessary, but this is often time consuming. There remains a need for further research efforts to make it possible for such a thesaurus to be manipulated automatically by the computer at the same time as the question is asked.

2. Physicians or pharmacists using drug data banks will always remain "*casual*" *usuers.* Questioning the system only from time to time (even if this means several times a day) they will have neither the time nor the training to use effective but complex query languages, such as those used in on-line bibliographical documentation systems (Medline, Pascaline, etc). The development of "cordial" languages is essential but this requires true cooperation on the part of future users.

3. Technical problems must also be resolved, chiefly with regard to the mode of *access to data.* It must be borne in mind that in countries like France the number of potential users exceeds 100,000. It is out of question that all could be linked directly to a central computer. Several solutions may be invisioned. The most simple consists of the creation of several "information bureaus" equipped with a terminal linked to a distant computer. Users pose their questions by telephone to individuals working in the bureau who then question the computer directly. This solution, which can be quickly set up, is costly since it requires a human interface. A second solution consists of distribution of the data base between a certain number of computers to which users are linked directly by terminals and telephone lines. However the updating of such decentralized data bases is far from easy. A final possibility lies in individual use of micro-computers. The latter has begun to spread in the medical profession. At the present time, they are unable to treat data bases as large as those containing necessary information concerning drugs. Whithin a few years the capacity of micro-computers will certainly be greatly increased, in particular by the use of large capacity peripheral memories (video-discs).

4. A final problem is that of *finance.* The great majority of physicians and pharmacists work alone and have limited budgets. What are the most economical means to offer them access to a data base ? In solutions involving access to a distant computer, it is necessary to separate the price of terminals and those of transmissions. The price of terminals may be considerably reduced in the cases of generalized use of standard television screens (viewdata, video-tex). However, the addition of a small printout facility will remain necessary in view of the complexity of the information and problems of legal responsability. The price of transmissions will certainly become negligeable with the availability of public data transmission networks (Transpac in France). The other solution (individual micro-computer) remains relatively costly. But is must be borne in mind that such micro-computers could be used by physicians or pharmacists for multiple tasks (office or shop administration, accounting, appointments, medical records...). In addition, they could be used themselves to provide access to distant computers.

In conclusion, it would seem to be reasonable to predict that whithin 3 to 5 years, information concernint drugs for "peripheral" physician and pharmacist users could quite extensively benefit from informatic methods.

REFERENCES

Several articles describing drug data banks may be found in the following book .

Ducrot H., M. Goldberg, R. Hoigne and P. Middleton eds, *Computer Aid to Drug Therapy and to Drug Monitoring*, Amsterdam, North Holland, 1978.

Sécurité et médicaments (1982), pp. 189-192

Rôle du prescripteur dans l'information du patient sur les effets du médicament

P. GUILLET

21, rue Cujas, 75005 PARIS, France

Abstract — L'action du prescripteur se situe à l'intersection du territoire scientifique médical et du territoire culturel du patient. Il doit non seulement expliquer, mais traduire son information dans un langage accessible.

Les drogues actives étant plus nombreuses, la rédaction de l'ordonnance devient complexe. Pour être fiable, elle doit comporter deux faces : l'une concerne plus particulièrement la relation médecin-pharmacien, c'est la prescription contrôlée par la Sécurité Sociale ; l'autre concerne la relation médecin-malade et l'administration des médicaments. De présentation claire et affichable, elle permet de restituer les contraintes des médicaments et leurs interactions, qui s'ajoutent souvent à une auto-médication.

Le rôle du médicament ne se limite pas toujours à une simple action métabolique : il va souvent beaucoup plus loin. L'information sur les effets des médicaments ne saurait ignorer le moment de la maladie et la personnalité du patient. L'intolérance peut être autant due à la drogue qu'à un refus de dépendance ou un rejet du médecin. En médecine, la façon de prescrire est aussi importante que la prescription.

L'efficacité d'un médicament est étroitement liée à la participation du patient à son traitement. Ce qui suppose : un praticien bien formé en thérapeutique ; un praticien impliqué dans la conception du médicament ; des formes nouvelles de rencontre entre praticiens et usagers.

LA PRESCRIPTION PAR LE MEDECIN

Après avoir été conçu et expérimenté en laboratoire, le médicament est, en bout de chaîne, prescrit par le médecin à la fin de sa consultation.

La prescription du médicament est enseignée aux praticiens de ville par des médecins hospitaliers, à partir de connaissances scientifiques liées à la nature de la drogue et à son métabolisme. Or, en milieu hospitalier, l'administration du médicament est très particulière : le comprimé, souvent anonyme, est donné par un infirmier, le soluté est injecté dans la tubulure d'une perfusion, ce qui escamote totalement la phase d'explication par le médecin des effets du médicament sur son malade.

Or, en ville, le mode de prescription est tout différent : ce que le patient va emporter chez lui, ce n'est pas un médicament, c'est surtout un "message" écrit sur son ordonnance. Sommes-nous toujours bien sûrs que ce message sera bien reçu ?

Le patient a son idée sur l'action (bénéfique ou maléfique) du médicament, et il faut souvent traduire l'information médicale dans son langage ; autrement dit, s'exprimer dans le même "patois" que lui. Avant d'expliquer, il faut souvent savoir ce que l'autre attend du médicament.

Par exemple : «Cet antibiotique va me fatiguer, docteur, est-ce bien nécessaire?» Ou bien : «On donnait ce calmant à mon père pour son cancer, donc c'est grave ?» Ou encore : «Ce médicament pour mes hémorroïdes, c'est curieux, c'est le même que ma femme prend pour ses règles douloureuses !»

On nous demande souvent de relier l'action d'un médicament à un symptôme, et les craintes que font naître d'autres médicaments ont parfois des origines bien mystérieuses.

LA REDACTION DE L'ORDONNANCE

Pour que le savoir du médecin et sa culture scientifique ne se heurtent pas au savoir de son malade et à sa culture familiale ou populaire sur le médicament, il faut plus écouter que parler, plus répondre qu'"ordonner".

La clé de voûte de la relation médecin-malade, en thérapeutique, c'est l'ordonnance. Il faut donc que cette ordonnance, par sa forme et son style, s'approche le plus près possible de la prise réelle du médicament. Assez souvent peu lisible, elle est en fait surtout destinée au pharmacien, qui va bien se débrouiller pour la traduire, et transformer les signes en boîtes ou flacons pulvérisateurs de toutes formes et de toutes couleurs. Elle est aussi, cette ordonnance, objet de contrôle pour les services de la Sécurité sociale : surchargée de tampons et de vignettes, elle témoigne de l'importance de la maladie (et du malade !).

LA GRILLE THERAPEUTIQUE

Aujourd'hui, les drogues actives sont de plus en plus nombreuses et, pour être efficace, l'ordonnance devrait se perfectionner. Nous suggérons par exemple de la rédiger en deux temps, sur deux feuilles distinctes :

— La première — ordonnance classique — comporterait l'énumération des médicaments : doses, rythme de prise, durée... Cette ordonnance concerne surtout le pharmacien et la Sécurité sociale. Elle est suffisante lorsque le malade sait la lire.

— Sur la deuxième, on ferait figurer une *grille* comportant, en abscisses, les différents moments de la journée (matin, midi, soir) et, en ordonnées, la liste des médicaments à prendre à ces différents moments. Le patient pourrait afficher cette grille dans sa cuisine, intégrant la prise de ses médicaments à sa vie quotidienne.

A l'usage, cette nouvelle façon de transcrire l'ordonnance se révèle plus riche qu'il ne paraît : le médecin est étonné de voir que son ordonnance comporte un si grand nombre de comprimés ; les interactions médicamenteuses apparaissent clairement quand, par exemple, dans la colonne "matin au petit déjeuner", s'ajoutent plusieurs médicaments, dont il faudra bien préciser la prise en fonction des aliments.

Les avantages de cette grille sont évidents :

— Grâce à elle, le malade pénètre dans l'ordonnance, en prend possession.

— Elle est plus claire à lire pour une personne de l'entourage du malade qui contrôle le traitement.

— Chez la personne âgée, elle est indispensable.

— Elle permet de recueillir des informations sur la tolérance des médicaments : par exemple, l'intéressé peut expliquer l'effet de tel médicament sur son appétit ; le malaise provoqué par tel autre avant le repas, et supprimé si la prise est déplacée ; pourquoi il a supprimé celui-là, qui lui paraissait sans effet.
— A votre propre liste — qui peut paraître parfois déjà longue —, viennent encore s'ajouter tout naturellement les prescriptions des autres médecins (ophtalmo, gastro-entérologue, rhumatologue...).
— Enfin, apparaît également sur cette grille l'auto-médication, qui ne figure jamais sur l'ordonnance classique. Cette auto-médication — qui peut être exceptionnelle ou systématique chez de nombreux patients — peut éclairer le médecin sur l'origine d'un trouble secondaire inexpliqué.

Autrement dit, la prescription sous forme de "grille thérapeutique" approche de plus près l'information sur le médicament, mais surtout permet de mieux recueillir les nuances des effets principaux et secondaires.

Table 1. Exemple de grille thérapeutique

	Matin	Midi	Soir
Médicament A	1	1	1
Médicament B	1		
Médicament C			1
Autres prescriptions	**	*	*
Auto-médication	*	**	*

PARTICIPATION DU PATIENT

La sécurité de la prescription est ainsi plus grande. On est pourtant loin de l'absence de tout trouble secondaire. Dans la mystérieuse "cuisine" que chaque individu fait à partir de sa maladie, de son médecin, de sa famille, de ses craintes d'aggravation de son état ou de la mort, qui peut dire ce qui déclenche le rejet ? La potion peut devenir poison ou, au contraire, un trouble secondaire peut être accepté comme "prix à payer pour guérir". C'est la part"divine" du médicament, qui échappe à notre pharmacologie. Et comment en serait-il autrement, avec des drogues qui détournent la mort ou changent le cours de la vie ?

L'intolérance peut être autant due à la drogue qu'à un refus de dépendance ou à un rejet du médecin. L'efficacité d'un médicament, sa sécurité aussi, sont étroitement liées à la participation du patient à son traitement. Elles dépendent aussi de la formation des médecins en thérapeutique.

FORMATION DU MEDECIN

Nous sommes de plus en plus nombreux à penser que la réflexion sur la prescription est la base de la formation médicale continue du praticien. Un médecin ne peut pas prescrire avec sécurité s'il n'est pas suffisamment informé sur toute la dynamique du médicament, ses actions multiples et ses interactions avec d'autres. Cette connaissance implique, à notre avis, que le praticien participe très tôt à la conception du médicament et à son expérimentation.

La formation thérapeutique doit mieux tenir compte des réalités de la vie quotidienne du praticien.

Des formes nouvelles sont à concevoir dans l'information sur le médicament et la formation à prescrire.

Sécurité et médicaments (1982), pp. 193-198

Pharmacist Contribution to Patient Information and Drug Safety

J.R. WUEST

College of Pharmacy, Cincinnati OH 45267, USA

Abstract — Health care providers are morally and legally obligated to provide patients with adequate and understandable information on the drugs they are taking in order to maximize therapy and prevent adverse effects. Prescribing physicians have traditionally been responsible for this function but there is a growing belief among health professionals, governmental policy makers and patients themselves that the amount and quality of this information must be improved. This paper reviews the contributions that pharmacists can provide towards meeting this goal. Examples of patient information sources and how they are used by pharmacists will be presented.

It undoubtedly is strange for a presentation on this topic, i.e. pharmacist contribution to patient education and drug safety, to begin with a statement — "not anywhere at the level that it could be" — but I will nonetheless. There is no doubt that pharmacists should, because there is a long standing principle in American Law that health care providers are obliged to render adequate and relevant patient education.

Two major potentiel problems, as they relate to patient safety, that can and reportedly do occur when proper patient education is lacking are noncompliance and adverse reactions.

Noncompliance can involve too much drug being taken leading to toxicity, or, inadequate self-dosing resulting in therapeutic failure. Both of these are certainly harmful to the patient.

Adverse reactions, although inherent in the overdosing expressed above, also occur in normal doses as well as the result of interactions between concurrently administered prescription drugs, OTC's taken in self medication by patients, previously undiagnosed but underlying disease states and the like.

Several studies have pointed out that the above occur much more often than we care to think. In reviewing them preparing this paper it appears that an estimated 30 % of patients in the U.S. do not comply with their therapeutic instructions and one-third of the studies report noncompliance of 50 % or higher.

In the instance of adverse reactions (and I am including drug interactions in this) several sources have estimated that around 10 % of all hospital admissions are due to drug-associated conditions.

A major reason for this occurring is what I like to call the "problems of multiples", situation, which may be unique to the U.S. In America, health care has evolved in such a manner that today we have multiple drug therapy prescribed by multiple physicians being dispensed by multiple pharmacists. When one throws in the non-prescription drugs (which by the way are highly advertised in all media, especially television) the situation becomes mind-boggling.

While this paper is not meant to be a discussion of social values in America certain items should be pointed out to those of you unfamiliar with our system so that you may better understand why we stand where we are today.

Firstly, let me relate that in general, the U.S. certainly has one of the best health care delivery systems in the world today for crisis intervention. Quality care is available to all who will avail themselves of it. I will skip over everything else and get to drug therapy so that we can zero in on how the "problems of multiples" has occurred. The two basic premises of medicine in the U.S. are that potentially dangerous drugs requiring medical diagnosis and supervision of therapy are available only from a physician or on his prescription to be dispensed by a pharmacist. Additionaly there are those which are considered to be safe for self-medication and are available without a prescription. We will call them OTC drugs. They are sold not only in pharmacies but also in supermarkets, department stores, gas stations, toilet facilities other establishments with similar potential for patient counseling.

Looking at the latter first, it is my observation that there is a significant portion of our society that believes there are "pills for all ills". The OTC drug industry, under very few restrictions until recently, has, in too many instances promoted its products in much the same manner as automobiles, food, clothing or any other commodity.

Individuals watching television are told from morning till night how to relieve their upset stomach, "cure" their cold, alleviate their itch, and, my favorite, overcome a disease that doesn't even exist i.e. irregularity. The list goes on and on but the point I want to make is that there is a lot of evidence that a lot of people over-medicate themselves and have somewhat of a disrespect for drugs. There is a great potential for OTC-Rx drug interactions.

On the prescription side we have gone throught a period during which it was considered unethical for pharmacists to discuss the patient's disease state and its therapy. For example, when I went to pharmacy school we were told that such activity was "counter-prescribing" and therefore damnable.

It is also unfortunate that during this same periode, let's call it the first two decades after WW II, pharmacists were evolving from being preparers of concoctions from herbs and roots to merchandisers of convenience items and what we euphemistically call "health and beauty aids". Alas, pharmacists became more merchant than professional.

Also, merchandising and advertising have been a major determinant in the direction of prescription medication evolution.

It is my observation that the lay public has been bombarded with information that generics are cheaper, and, which pharmacy has the lowest prices, rather than the importance of compliance and selecting health providers that give a better value through enhanced professional services even though it costs more. Pharmacists have not helped themselves by traditionally charging for prescriptions based on percentage mark up on the drug rather than services rendered.

Two truly unfortunate contributory factors have been the unwillingness of many pharmacists to accept the responsability of patient counseling, and, the efforts of individual physicians and organized medicine to prevent intrusion into what they believe to be their domain.

A case in point is my own state of Ohio where I am on the Board of Pharmacy. Since I have held this position I have striven to have our, in my opinion, antiquated practice of pharmacy law changed. For several years I have tried, with the board, to promulgate rules to elaborate on the current wording of the law which stipulates that to practice pharmacy means to compound and dispense. We have attempted to extend to include that pharmacists may, among other things, advise patients of the therapeutic values, hazards and use of the drugs they take. This effort culminated recently in representatives of the state Medical Association being able to stop the promulgation of the rules by means of a threat (which it is powerful enough to carry out) of introducing a bill into our Legislature that would prevent the board from making rules.

Since I didn't come here to wash out our laundry, and, obviously we all have our own problems regardless of where we practice, let me say that we have hopes of correcting ours if for no other reason, society will demand (and according to the FDA and Consumer Advocate groups) is already demanding more information on the drugs it takes.

There are four concepts which appear to be implicit in their desires and in the obligations the American Courts have imposed on physicians regarding patient education, namely :

— disclosure of the pertinent facts about the patient's relative health or disease state.

— forewarning them of the hazards and risks of prescribed therapy.

— counseling them on alternative therapies.

— instructing them on the skills and knowledge needed for informed self care.

Functions one and three above are definitely in the realm of the physician alone but certainly others can assist in warning of the hazards and instructing in self-care.

Since the bulk of self-care involves taking drugs, it is only natural that pharmacists share these responsibilities with the physician.

I must add that much of the current patient education that is being offered is uncoordinated. To a great extent this is due to the problems of multiples stated earlier. Before addressing the concept of how pharmacists should contribute to patient education and drug safety I feel I must mention that patients have some responsibility, also. Unless they are willing to choose health care providers with whom they can communicate, tell them every appropriate piece of information about their condition, not shop around for doctors that agree with their desires and for pharmacies that have the lowest prices but no professional services, and, until they are not afraid to admit they don't understand their instructions, patient safety will never be maximized.

Now with that little bit of background out of the way let me bring to you the news of all the neat things that are going on and how pharmacists are contributing to patient information and drug safety. This leads to a few questions that must be answered :

Firstly, what does the patient need to know ? This has been stated over and over by persons far more qualified than I, but, I do believe that the basic information that should be presented to them includes :

— Why was the drug prescribed.

— How should it be correctly administered.

— When are the correct times to take it.

— What signs should they look for to warn of impending adverse reactions.

— What potential drug interactions should be avoided most specifically in relation to OTC medications.

I don't think we need to elaborate extensively on these since it should be obvious that a patient is more likely to be motivated to comply if he understand why the medicine was prescribed, the basics of what it does and how to avoid problems during its use.

A second important question is why should the pharmacist be involved in patient education — especially in a health care system in which he has long been uninvolved ?

The reason why pharmacists should assist physicians that come to my mind are myriad, but to mention a few, — he would serve as a reinforcement to what the physician said and this certainly is helpful.

Additionally, the setting and format in which patient counseling is given is extremely important. As a general rule, when the patient sees the physician he is sick or he wouldn't be in the office in the first place, he has had to wait for some period of time to see the physician, he will have some amount of anticipation, even fear, while waiting, and he will often see instruments and machinery that he does not understand and may associate with unpleasant thoughts. After his examination there is usually a great deal of relief, or unfortunately, some bad news. The question remains, is this setting as conducive to paying attention to instructions as the neighborhood pharmacy which in our country has been designed to be pleasant, and, is full of all the wonderful things that the "tele" has told them are helpful ? The answer seems obvious.

Another and very important factor is that the pharmacist is the last health care person to see and talk to the patient before he will independently take the drug without direct medical supervision.

Add to this the fact that only the pharmacist can show the medicine to the patient while explaining the appropriate instructions. These are mighty convincing reasons.

The third question is what kind of media should be used to relate the information to the patient ? I should think that the answer to this is more opinion than proven truth. So, I will give you mine, which I believe is pretty well documented by what I have read and seen.

It seems as though currently used label instuctions are not enough. Several studies have reported this view. One that comes to mind is the study that asked 67 or so patients to interpret 10 prescription labels. Not one was interpreted the same way in all instances. Experience verifies this in my own mind. Verbal instructions are not adequate either. They are non-standard and easily forgotten.

Perhaps the answer is straightforward label instructions followed by verbal discussion which is reinforced with simple, meaningful and unencumbered printed material.

Care must be taken with the latter, however, in that even though printed material is standardized and retainable for later reference, it must be interesting and understandable or the patient will not save it and refer to it. It must be written in a style that can be comprehended by the majority of its readers and must be an open and frank discussion of the medication without scaring the patient into non-compliance on the low side. Several studies have reported that the highest level of recall of knowledge regarding drugs and therapy is achieved in those partients receiving both verbal and written instructions.

I have brought several examples of the type of patient information materials that are available. They represent the effort of our national professional association — APhA ; our Medicine/Pharmacy compendial organization — USPC and private enterprise.

One of the major endeavors APhA has undertaken and produced is the NMAT — National Medical Awareness Test — a slide presentation designed to be made by pharmacists to community organizations. Its purpose is to help consumers become aware of and understand how to correctly take their medications.

The program reviews the purposes of medications, the concept of administration techniques, dosage regimens, side effect, drug interactions, and understanding directions. This is followed by a question and answer discussion period that reviews key points and assures that the audience understands the concepts presented.

APhA also publishes what is called the personal Drug Information Checklist which is meant to assist pharmacists in explaining drug therapy to patients when dispensing drugs.

The USPC, which as stated earlier, is a joint undertaking by medicine and pharmacy, has recently shifted its emphasis of 150 years from being an organization responsible for compendial standards to playing a much more active, actually a major role in providing health care practitioners and patients with information about medications and how to take them correctly.

Within the last two years USPC has begun making several extremely important informational publications available. The USPC Dispensing information is for practitioners and provides an excellent reference for the uses, doses, side effects, precautions, drug interactions, patient advise and storage requirements for most drugs on the American market.

USPC has several publication available for patients, the most extensive of which is a complete set of monographs called Advice for Patients, abridged edition called About Your Medicines is also available for sale to consumers. It contains selected monographs and covers the most frequently prescribed medications.

USPC publishes a newsletter for consumers on a bimonthly schedule. It covers new and contemporary concepts of medications and their use. It plans to publish separate sheets that can be dispensed with the appropriate medications. They represent the individual monograph for each respective drug. These monographs provide information on things to consider before taking the drug, its proper use, precautions to keep in mind while using it, its side effects and whatever other information that is appropriate.

Several private companies also have patient information materials available. The simplest and most used variety is what are called auxiliary or cautionary labels. It is my understanding that more than 1/2 of the pharmacies in the U.S. use these or similar labels. Their intent is to increase patient compliance, maximize therapy and reduce the potential for interactions with OTC drugs.

The systems available range all the way from a simple chart with suggestions of what labels to use for what drugs up to more in depth programs that have companion hardcopy or microfiche drug monographs that explain the background of why the labels are suggested, what drug interactions may occur and other appropriate patient information.

More advanced patient counseling systems involved advisery leaflets. They are available from local and state pharmacy association, and, from private enterprise. One particular brand contains information on the purpose of the medicine, its correct method of administration, or, when appropriate, how to assemble the administration apparatus, side effects, specific activities to avoid, I/A involving OTC drugs, storage requirements and other helpful information. It is available for purchase and dispensing with the prescription as a complete set, in a binder placed in the pharmacy for patient reference, or, in book form for sale to consumers.

Many, many other counselling systems are available including the traditional, and often must effective, person to person discussion between the pharmacist and patient.

The point I would like to leave you with is that the pharmacist can serve a significant contributary role in patient education and drug safety. The strides made in pharmacists increasing their patient counseling in the past few years has been tremendous. More and more materials are becoming available. Patients seem to accept and appreciate the counsel. It is my hope that physicians will accept and appreciate the services as well.

Working together, the net result will certainly benefit the patient, increase patient compliance and maximize drug safety.

Sécurité et médicaments (1982), pp. 199-205

The Patient Package Insert
The FDA Concept and Plans

L.G. MILLSTEIN

Food & Drug Administration, (HFD-107) 5600 Fishers Lane, Rockville, Maryland 20857, USA

Abstract — The programs of the Food & Drug Administration (FDA) are designed to achieve a single over-all objective — consumer protection. Originally, the labeling or product monograph for prescription drugs was intended as prescribing information for the physician. More recently, written information for the patient beyond the instructions given on the container label is in demand as an increasingly important part of the communications between physicians, pharmacists and the patient. This results from two movements — the "Right-to-Know" and the interest of consumers in participating in decision-making regarding their own treatments. Moreover, in today's world, both the visual and written media serve to augment and reinforce our thinking and concepts of the impact of verbal communications. The taking of drugs requires clear, precise information regarding their desired benefits, possible side effects and instructions for proper use. Studies have shown that patient knowledge of warnings, precautions and side effects is consistently improved by written information. On September 12, 1980, the FDA adopted the final regulation establishing the requirements and procedures for the preparation and distribution of patient labeling for prescription drugs. The patient package inserts (PPIs) are intended to promote the safe and effective use of drugs and ensure that patients have the opportunity to be informed of the benefits and risks involved. The regulation will be applied initially to 10 drugs or drug classes. Evaluation over a 3-year period of the costs and benefits will guide the FDA in deciding whether to extend, revise or defer these requirements with respect to the majority of prescription drug.

The programs of the United States Food and Drug Administration (FDA) are designed to achieve a single over-all objective — consumer protection. This year will mark 75 years that this agency has sought to carry out this goal. As part of the FDA's mission to ensure safe and effective drugs that are honestly labeled, the Prescription Drug Labeling Program was developed in support of this objective.

The original concept of providing labeling or a package insert for prescription drugs was to provide the necessary prescribing information, including any cautionary statements, for the physician. More recently, written information for the patient beyond the instructions given on the container label of prescription drugs is in demand as an increasingly important part of the communications between physicians, pharmacists and the patient. This results from two movements — the "Right-to-Know" and the interest of consumers to participate in decision-making regarding their own treatments. Moreover, in today's world, both the visual and written media serve to augment and reinforce our thinking and concepts of the impact of verbal communications. Clearly, the taking of drugs requires clear, precise information regarding their desired benefits and possible side effects, and instructions for proper use.

Several studies have shown that patient knowledge of contraindications, warnings, precautions and side effects is consistently improved by written information[1].

Patient Package Inserts (PPIs) are not a new phenomenon. In fact, in a review of the European experience, T. Douglas Whittet in 1977, discussed the legislation in several countries and the collective action by the Council of Europe and by the European Economic Community on the interest in and the type of information given to patients about medicines[2]. Several countries have been providing leaflets about their products for distribution to patients for some time. In some countries it is compulsory, in others usual but not obligatory, and this applies to both prescription and over-the-counter products. It is interesting to note that of the 19 countries surveyed, 15 use original package dispensing with one of the 15 not using the original pack only in special circumstances.

The FDA has required PPIs for drugs only where proper ingestion or use was found to be critical because of the potential for serious adverse effects. The beginning of providing mandatory written information to patients in the United States was prompted by an epidemic of deaths following drug therapy of asthma in the early 1960's. Accumulating reports in Australia and Great Britain of young patients dying suddenly after using aerosol bronchodilators containing isoproterenol for the relief of asthma led to a thorough investigation of the causes, since Canada and the United States reported no increase in mortality despite large sales volumes of the aerosol nebulizers[3, 4].

An epidemiological study revealed evidence which suggested that the preparations used overseas were more highly concentrated than the preparations used in North America and might have contributed to the severity of the epidemic of asthma mortality[4]. Patients responded favorably when the inhalation preparation was discontinued. Based on this finding, the FDA concluded that the labeling for such drugs must bear adequate information for their safe use. It was also concluded that in view of the manner in which these preparations are self-administered, it is necessary for the protection of users that warning information to patients be included as part of the label and as part of any instructions to patients included in the package dispensed to the patient[5]. Accordingly, on June 18, 1968, the order was signed by the Commissioner of the Food and Drug Administration establishing the language and procedures to be followed regarding the warning for isoproterenol inhalation preparations for human use, which states essentially that the dose prescribed by the physician was not te be exceeded.

Patient labeling requirements for oral contraceptives had its beginning during the 1970's. PPIs for these products were followed by patient information for progestational drug products, intrauterine devices and estrogens. These products were considered appropriate for an official PPI because of the potential health risks associated with these substances and the possibly elective nature of their use in healthy women.

Following the development of the PPI for oral contraceptives, the FDA began an evaluation of the usefulness of this form of patient information by examining whether the PPIs should be required generally, and what would be the best way to present the information to patients. In 1974, the Patient Prescription Drug Labeling Project was created to investigate these issues and whether to expand the effort. Since the project began, the FDA has — 1. reviewed the scientific literature about patients' needs and desires about the prescription drugs they take, 2. reviewed the existing methods for communicating drug information to consumers and patients, 3. held open discussions on the PPI issues with interested groups and potentially affected persons:consumers, physicians, pharmacists and drug companies, and 4. conducted research projects to evaluate existing and model patient labelling.

In 1975, a consortium of consumer groups petitioned the FDA to require written warning information on labels of some prescription drug products and to require separate and detached information leaflets to be given to patients when the prescription drug products are dispensed[6]. Singled out were those drugs most likely to cause side effects, to interact adversely with other drugs and, specifically, those used in pregnant or breast-feeding women (hypnotics, tranquilizers, amphetamines and chloramphenicol). The petitioners felt these drugs have been overprescribed and can have serious adverse reactions.

In 1976, nearly 700 health professionals and consumer representatives attended a symposium on patient labeling co-sponsored by the FDA, Drug Information Association (DIA), American Medical Association (AMA) and the Pharmaceutical Manufacturers Association (PMA). A great majority of viewpoints and presentations were heard on the kinds of information that should be contained in patient labeling. Potential distribution problems and the effects on patients were also discussed[7]. As a result of this symposium, efforts were focused on necessary additional research and information required before a regulatory policy could be developed.

In 1978, the FDA sponsored a two-day conference on the content and format of PPIs[8]. Approximately 300 health professionals, drug industry, marketing and advertising representatives and consumers participated to resolve problem areas, provide direction and suggest methodology to provide the best possible communication for patients.

Also in 1978, a survey of over 2000 adults showed that they believed that it was important that printed patient labeling be included with prescription drugs[9]. Over 60 percent felt the labeling should be provided compared with approximately 30 percent who felt that current practices were adequate. This 2 to 1 percentage for patient labeling was consistent across all age, sex and educational sub-groupings. Thus, in 1978, approximately 64 percent of the United States population was in favor of patient labeling, an increase of 16 percent over those in the population in favor of patient labeling five years earlier. Neither of these surveys showed, however, that consumers wanted patient labeling to replace verbal communication.

On July 6, 1979, the FDA published the proposed regulation for patient labeling of prescription drug products[10]. The proposal not only set forth requirements for the leaflets, but also contained an analysis of the need for PPIs and the process by which the Administration had decided to require PPIs.

The response to the proposed regulation consisted of over 1 300 comments and came from a diversity of interests. Public hearings were also held in three major U.S. cities to give an opportunity to anyone to comment on the proposal. Individual consumers provided the majority or feedback and were nearly unanimous in their support of patient labeling. Many personal incidents were related where information about the drug they were taking might have prevented discomfort or harm. They acknowledged that written information was not generally available and was needed. On the other hand, the health community, pharmaceutical industry and professional and trade organizations voiced an almost unanimous opposition to the proposal on the basis that the PPIs were not needed, were unproven and would be too costly.

At the time the proposed regulation was published, the FDA contracted with the Institute of Medicine of the National Academy of Sciences to assemble experts to review the state-of-the-art of patient information about prescription drugs and recommend a research agenda for the evaluation of the effects of PPIs. The Institute study committee examined the existing literature, held a public hearing and discussed research needs and evaluation approaches at several meetings before reaching conclusions that they stated in their report in August 1979[11]). Significantly, the Institute supported the concept of PPIs, noting that patients' evaluations of package inserts have been positive and that little evidence of negative effects has been shown. Among their conclusions was that the PPI consumer use patterns should be studied by FDA supported pilot tests in different types of medical and pharmacy settings. They urged that studies be conducted on how the PPIs are used and the extent to which they stimulate communication between the medical community and the patient, or whether the PPI causes qualitative changes in the physician relationships and decision-making. In effect, the studies should determine how PPIs are distributed and used in natural, rather than controlled settings and what the impact is on patients behavior and knowledge of drug therapy.

After extensive review of the comments submitted in response to the proposed PPI regulation, on September 12, 1980, the FDA published the final regulation for patient labeling requirements, as well as draft guideline labeling for ten drugs or drug classes[12]. These are — Ampicillin, Benzodiazepines, Cimetidine, Clofibrate, Digoxin, Methoxsalen, Phenytoin, Propoxyphene, Thiazide diuretics and Doxylamine with Vitamin B6 (more commonly known as Bendectin or Debendox). Many changes were made in the final rule based on the comments submitted and the FDA's re-examination of the entire concept. First, a 3-year test program would be implemented to closely examine costs and benefits. Second, the program would be limited to ten drugs or drug classes during the pilot test program. Third, PPIs would be required only for new prescriptions and not refills, unless the patient specifically requested the information. Fourth, greater flexibility would be allowed in the distribution of PPIs to enable some costs and time savings to occur in the marketplace. Fifth, manufacturers will provide Spanish language PPIs upon request of the distributor or dispenser, and sixth, pharmacists would be reimbursed for Medicaid prescriptions through the Federal Government Health Care Financing Administration.

As part of the Final regulation, a budget analysis indicated that during the first three years, the PPI regulation will have a total annual cost of $21 million. This includes manufacturer, distributor, retail pharmacy and hospital and nursing home costs. Assuming that these costs pass through in their entirety to the consumer, they would result in a price increase for the drugs subject to the regulation to about 0.18 per prescription if applied only to new prescriptions.

The FDA believes that increased patient understanding and awareness of the need for observing precautions and following directions in taking drugs will produce health benefits by reducing the incidence or minimizing the effects of — excessive or inappropriate use, adverse drug reactions and adverse drug-drug and drug-food interactions and therapeutic failures due to poor compliance with drug regimens. Calculated in dollars for certain events associated with non-compliance as workday losses, hospital stays, revisits to physicians and refilled prescriptions, gross benefits of $20 to $80 million per year might be realized.

What about the studies and surveys that have been conducted over the past few years by both the United States government and non-government sources ? Some of these surveys show that a high proportion of Americans taking prescription drugs either do not understand or do not follow the instructions on the container label. Further, the surveys show that patients often cannot retain physician information because of their attention span and preoccupation with diagnosis information. Does this indicate the need for written information ? The studies also show that patients often cannot understand physician information. Does this indicate a need for understandable information ? Studies have shown also that patients often do not clearly understand the benefits and risks of taking certain drugs. In a large study of women who were taking oral contraceptives and had received patient labelling, many of their responses were that they thought that the information was important to their decision to use certain contraceptives and to their health protection[13]. This survey and another done by non-FDA sources indicated that the oral contraceptive package insert was generally well received, read, understood and positively evaluated[14].

What about the future of patient drug use information ? Three basic issues have emerged over the years — What does the patient need to know ? What is the best way to communicate this information ? What are the effects of patient labeling ?

The FDA is not in a leadership role with the PPI. There are many textbooks and drug counseling guides commercially available and several firms, in addition to pharmaceutical companies, have a large number of drug brochures now available for physicians and pharmacists to dispense to their patients and customers. The patient needs to be educated about prescribed drugs, but great sensitivity and insight must be exhibited by those undertaking patient counseling. We view PPIs as a method for making drug therapy and more successful through patient education, and we believe that the manufacturers who voluntarily prepare PPIs for some of their prescription drug products share that view.

In a recent publication on patient counseling and health education, the authors presented some principles relating to the transfer of drug use information not unlike that which has been shown both in FDA and non-FDA sponsored research[15]. These are — present only the minimum essential information for the patient needs — 1. how to use the drug, when it should not be used, potential safety hazards, precautionary statements, risks of developing dependence or tolerance, overdose or missed dose and possible side effects, 2. write the instructions in the sequence they are to be performed with emphasis on the most important point or concept, 3. use illustrations that show the patients' point of view, 4. use common (non-technical) words — "doctor" rather than "physician", "use" rather than "utilize", and short sentences, 5. emphasize the desired patient action or behavior rather than underlying theory or principles — "limit your intake of alcohol", "if you miss a dose, do not take twice as much the next time" and "do not stop taking without first checking with your doctor" and 6.

pre-test the instructions while they are still in a preliminary form. In addition, I would add that the information should not be promotional in tone or content, it should be consistent with the professional labeling and the presentation should be in an adequate print size.

We have made every effort to utilize the above principles in preparing the PPI guidelines ; however, until these leaflets are placed into commerce in the United States for a variety of drugs with a variety of messages to be tested in real world situations, we cannot be sure of the ultimate benefit to everyone's satisfaction.

As I speak now, the PPI regulation and the ten PPIs that were to enter the marketplace beginning in May of this year are being stayed by the FDA until further notice. This was requested to give the new administration an opportunity to review the regulation and further assess its economic impact. However, the research will continue with a national survey to measure changes in patient knowledge and attitudes about drugs and diseases resulting from PPIs in a pre- and post-PPI evaluation, and a study to determine the effects of PPIs on the quantity and nature of patient interaction with physicians and pharmacists in a pre- and post-PPI evaluation. Research will also continue on patient understanding and the kinds of knowledge consumers need if they are to properly use drugs. PPIs, by emphasizing and reinforcing the advice and encouragement of health professionals, should also help patients become more active participants in their own health care. Most of the research effort will be devoted to evaluating the effects to be expected from PPIs.

As there is no perfect world, life does not provide us with perfect choices. To ignore reality is to compound the problem. Providing and promoting education and information about drugs to the patient will not make them become physicians or pharmacists, as I am sure has been shown in Europe, but it just might help during a trying and, on occasion, crucial time of their lives.

REFERENCES

1. Morris L.A. and J.A. Halperin, Effects of written drug information on patient knowledge and compliance : A literature review, *American Journal of Public Health* **69** (1979), 47-52.

2. Whittet T.D., The Viewpoint of the European Experience, *Drug Information Journal* **26S** (1977).

3. Doll R. and P. Fraser, An Epidemic pf Asthma Deaths and its Relation to Drug Therapy, *in* : *Proceedings of the European Society for the Study of Drug Toxicity*, Baker S.B., Dec. ed., Vol. 12, I. C. S. 220, Amsterdam, *Excerpta Medica* **133**, 1971.

4. Stolley P.D., Why the United States was Spared an Epidemic of Deaths Due to Asthma, *American Review of Respiratory Disease* **105** (1972), 883.

5. Code of Federal Regulations §201. 305, revised as of April 1, 1978, p. 34.

6. "Petition to the FDA to Require More Adequate Patient Labelling of Prescription Drugs." Center for Law and Social Policy, March 31, 1975.

7. Various authors : Joint Symposium on Drug Information for Patients — The Patient Package Insert, *Drug Information Journal* **11** (January 1977), 15-82.

8. *Patient Package Inserts : Content and Format*, Washington, D.C., HEW Publication (FDA) 79-3089, 1979.

9. Roper Report, 7803, 1, 1978.

10. *Federal Register* **44**, 40016, July 6, 1979.

11. *Evaluation Patient Package Inserts,* National Academy of Sciences, Publication 79-05, Washington, D.C., August 1979.

12. *Federal Register* **45**, 60754, Septembrer 12, 1980.

13. Morris L.A., M. Mazis and E. Gordon, A Survey of Oral Contraception Patient Information, *Journal of the American Medical Association* **238** (1977), 2504.

14. Fleckenstein L., P. Joubert, R. Lawrence, B. Pastner, J. Mazzullo and L. Lasagna, Oral contraceptive patient information, a questionnaire study of attitudes, knowledge and preferred information sources, *Journal of the American Medical Association* **235** (1976), 1331-36.

15. Doak L.G. and C.C. Doak, Patient Comprehension Profiles : Recent Findings and Strategies, *Patient Counseling and Health Education* **2** (Third Quarter 1980), 101.

Sécurité et médicaments (1982), pp. 207-211

Evaluation de l'observance

E. WEBER

Abteilung Klinische Pharmakologie der Medizinischen Universitätsklinik, Heidelberg Bergheimer Straße 58, D-6900 Heidelberg, West Germany

Résumé — Savoir dans quelle mesure les patients suivent les recommandations qui leur sont faites par leur médecin, est une notion importante lorsqu'il s'agit de juger de l'observance du malade pour le médicament qui lui est prescrit. Nous ne traiterons ici que de l'appréciation des résultats d'une étude clinique, de l'efficacité d'un traitement chez un malade particulier ou du taux d'apparition d'effets indésirables. Nous avons donc besoin de méthodes simples, précises, sensibles, exactes et en même temps faciles à mettre en œuvre pour évaluer l'observance des malades. Nous sommes loin d'en être là. Les quelques méthodes objectives que nous connaissons n'ont qu'une valeur limitée. Elles consistent dans la détermination du médicament lui-même et/ou de ses métabolites dans le sang ou dans les urines. Souvent des méthodes analytiques valables ne donnent qu'une information qualitative, ne permettant pas de juger de la quantité du médicamant que le patient a pris. En plus il y a de nombreuses difficultés pour obtenir des échantillons de sang ou d'urine de manière répétée et randomizée et sans que le patient en soit averti d'avance. En outre les résultats de certaines méthodes peuvent être faussés par le patient. Par exemple lorsque des interrogatoires oral ou écrit sont utilisés ou de la comparaison du nombre d'unités pharmaceutiques prescrites pendant une période donnée avec le nombre que l'on trouve au domicile du patient ou qu'il apporte à la consultation.

Depuis qu'il est possible de traiter les patients ambulants avec psychose ou tuberculose par pharmathérapie on commence à étudier d'une manière scientifique en quelle proportion les ordonnances médicales sont réellement suivies. Il est universellement reconnu que sur tous les terrains de pharmacothérapie la quantité des médicaments pris est nettement inférieure que celle ordonnée. La non-observance varie de 0 à 100 % des médicaments prescrits et peut aussi être dépassée. L'insuffisante consommation des médicaments conduit à quelques conséquences fâcheuses, dont deux importantes sont indiquées ci-après :

1. L'ignorance de l'ampleur de non-observance empêche le docteur de juger l'effet d'un médicament. Il ne peut se prononcer sur la part que la non-coopération du malade ou le choix peu approprié de remède a sur la non-réussite du traitement.
2. Les résultats des examens cliniques sont inemployables s'ils n'ont pas été obtenus en observation stricte des règles du protocole, spécialement ce qui concerne les doses des médicaments prescrits. Ni l'efficacité thérapeutique ni les effets secondaires — favorables ou nocifs — peuvent être jugés en qualité et quantité.

Ces difficultés ne peuvent être contournées que par un nombre suffisant de tests, renseignants sur le comportement du patient quant à la consommation des médicaments. Pour valoriser ces témoignages, deux conditions sont nécessaires :

1. Il doit être défini ce qui est entendu par observance et un écart de celle-ci.

2. Il faut disposer d'une méthode appropriée pour évaluer l'observance.

Ces deux conditions semblent évidentes et simples. Cependant elles offrent de sérieuses difficultés. Pour chaque examen il faut à nouveau définir sur quoi le témoignage doit s'étendre.

Le tableau 1 indique un choix de paramètres qui viennent en ligne de compte. Seule la dose non appliquée doit-elle être repérée ou également d'autres fautes dans le régime des médicaments ? Les tests doivent-ils être répétés en permanence, si oui à des temps choisis par randome ? A partir de quelle mesure une coopération est constatée, et à partir de quand une non-observance ? Les différentes possibilités de définition d'une observance imparfaite font que — mis à part les nombreux facteurs qui interviennent — il est si difficile de nommer une non-compliance moyenne.

Entre les méthodes qui peuvent être employées pour mesurer l'observance distinguons trois groupes :

1. Dosage des substances à appliquer et/ou leur(s) métabolite(s) dans le sang ou l'urine.
2. Détermination de l'observance par un effet pharmaco-dynamique.
3. Détermination basée sur des informations données par le patient.

Il faudrait que les méthodes soient chacune simple à réaliser et — en analogie aux procédés analytiques en chimie clinique spécifiques, exactes, précises et sensibles.

DETERMINATION DE L'OBSERVANCE PAR METHODES DIRECTES

Le jugement basé sur la détermination du médicament lui-même ou de ses métabolites, peut sembler être de prime abord le meilleur. Mais même cette méthode pour différentes raisons est chargée de sérieuses difficultés. Les progrès de la chimie analytique nous permettent aujourd'hui il est vrai de résoudre presque chaque problème même s'il s'agit d'analyse de spécimen de source biologique. Cependant bien souvent le dosage des médicaments les plus modernes et les plus efficaces, prescrits en petites

Table 1. No complaisance in use of medications[10]

1. Incorrect dosage per intake and/or per 24 hours
2. Drug taken though unnecessary
3. Drug no taken though necessary
4. Schedule incorrect
5. Incorrect schedule with reference to the meals
6. Incorrect route of application
7. Drug not appropriated for the purpose
8. Drug expired
9. Drug not stopped against presciption
10. Drug stopped against prescription
11. Drug not procured
12. Forget to take the drug

doses, nécessitent un personnel hautement qualifié et des appareillages coûteux. Nous en possédons que peu de méthodes qualitatives simples comme la détection dans l'urine d'une fluorescence provoquée par les rayons ultra-violets, par exemple après l'ingestion de la riboflavine.

Le principal désavantage est que, endéans un certain laps de temps qui vacille avec le temps de demi-vie de la substance l'on peut prouver l'ingestion, mais l'on se trouve dans l'impossibilité de juger d'une manière certaine de la quantité ingérée. Une valeur basse de taux sanguin n'indique pas si cela est dû par la prise d'une haute dose longuement antérieure ou d'une petite dose récente. Il en est de même pour l'analyse d'urine. Pour le cas d'une substance à temps de demi-vie longue l'on peut plus aisément conclure à une prise de dose plus ou moins régulière si le steady state dans le sang est élevé, quoique les informations restent limitées à cause de l'interaction de différents facteurs.

Un exemple typique correspondant est le dosage de la digitale. Chez les patients âgés avec une masse musculaire réduite et souffrants d'une insuffisance rénale non reconnue le taux de digoxine peut très bien faire croire à une plus haute adhérence au traitement qu'elle n'est en réalité. D'autre part, dans une population depuis longuement digitalisée, l'on repère aisément le patient qui n'a pas ou rarement pris les tablettes de digoxine. Dans une clientèle de banlieue nous avons repéré 16 patients sur 33 qui appartenaient à cette catégorie[1].

Des difficultés se présentent aussi pour le groupe de substances à temps de demi-vie courte, car la prise d'échantillons de sang ou d'urine doit se faire tôt après l'ingestion de la substance. D'ailleurs la récupération des échantillons de sang et d'urine posent des grands problèmes d'ordre pratique, ce qui fait que lors d'un examen clinique le test de l'observance ne se fait en général qu'une seule fois. Des prises renouvelées, par exemple d'urine, pourraient influencer spécialement le comportement de malades ambulants, dont l'adhérence à la pharmacothérapie prête un intérêt particulier. Cette influence serait souhaitable si la question à résoudre porte sur la pharmacodynamie de la substance mais est à éviter, si l'acceptance du médicament est le problème qui se pose.

Nous aurions beaucoup d'avantage à connaître des substances "marker", qui — de leur côté chimiquement et physiologiquement inertes — peuvent être ajoutées aux préparations galéniques sans déranger celles-ci et dont le dosage pourrait se faire aisément selon les critères établis ci-haut. Même si telles substances étaient à nôtre disposition nous aurions hélas en principe la plupart des difficultés que nous venons de décrire. En plus pour toutes études cliniques il faudrait spécialement confectionner des préparations galéniques contenant la substance marker. La biodisponibilité de ce nouveau produit ne peut pas être jugé d'avance inchangé comparé avec la préparation standard.

Peu de substances marker appropriées nous sont connues, dont la riboflavine, le rouge de phénol, des sels de bromure, la quinine et — sous réserves importantes bien entendu — des radioisotopes.

Nous donnons un exemple avec le bromure de sodium auquel nous avons fait mélanger 40 mg à la dose journalière de la sito-stérine en poudre. Au contraire des patients coopératifs ceux n'obéissant pas aux prescriptions de leur médecin se lais-

Table 2. [4]

Jour	Heure			
1	7.00	12.00	17.00	
2	8.00	21.00		
3	5.00	11.00	21.00	
4	6.00			
5	5.00	11.00	17.00	19.00

saient identifier par le manque d'augmentation du taux sanguin en bromure. L'étude clinique avait à répondre à la question, si la sitostérine est en mesure d'abaisser d'une façon certaine le taux plasmatique du cholestérol. Un résultat positif n'était obtenu que si les données de tous les patients ne montrant pas une augmentation adéquate du taux plasmatique en bromure étaient éliminées avant l'examen statistique[2].

Si une préparation galénique supplémentaire à celles qui sont indiquées par l'état de santé du patient, est prescrite, portant une substance marker, une mesure indirecte de l'observance peut être effectuée. Certains problèmes se posent dès que le patient exige des explications sur la raison de la prescription de cette préparation.

Une substance convenant bien pour une étude de ce genre est la riboflavine par la détection facile de fluorescence dans l'urine. Chez 306 patients en clinique, auxquels en outre de leur médication journalière une capsule contenant 15 mg de riboflavine leur a été portée au lit journalièrement pendant dix jours de suite, nous avons trouvé que 204 — soit 34 % — ont pris chacune de ces capsules, 25 % les ont prises à 1 — 2 jours des dix journées, le reste correspondant à 40 % l'ont négligé trois ou plusieurs jours[3].

Une méthode originale pour juger le comportement des patients vis-à-vis d'un médicament ophthalmologique ordonné montre Kass[4]. Il donnait à 38 patients avec glaucome à chacun un flacon de gouttes pour les yeux, qui adapté à un système électronique, enregistrait chaque fois qu'une goutte de solution de pilocarpine était enlevée du flacon, date et moment. L'exemple d'un patient montre tableau 2. Non seulement

Table 3. Comparaison of compliance in children on penicillin prophylasis[7]

	By interview	By pill count
	n = 113	109
Good	73 %	55 %
Questionable	19 %	35 %
Poor	8 %	10 %

la dose journalière de 4 gouttes par œil et jour n'est pas atteinte, mais l'intervalle entre les applications est des plus fantaisistes. L'entièreté des 38 patients n'appliquaient en moyenne que 2,6 gouttes par œil et jour au lieu des 4 gouttes prescrites.

DETERMINATION PAR EFFETS PHARMACODYNAMIQUES

De par la grande variabilité les effets pharmacodynamiques ne conviennent en général pas pour le contrôle de la compliance. Vu que l'atténuation de l'aggrégation plaquettaire par l'acide acétosalicylique par exemple peut être détectée pendant 5 à 7 jours après l'ingestion d'une dose unique, cet effet est également utilisable comme indice de l'observance que sous réserve.

DETERMINATION PAR METHODE INDIRECTE

Un dernier groupe de procédés souvent employés sont ceux dans lesquels les patients sont plus ou moins directement engagés. En premier lieu ce sont les connaissances basées sur les réponses des patients concernant leur comportement vis-à-vis de leurs médicaments. Les interrogatoires peuvent être oraux, par écrit, francs ou dissimulé. Il n'est pas étonnant, comme il a été démontré, qu'en faisant la preuve des réponses obtenues par l'examen objectif on obtient souvent des discordances dans les résultats. Des exemples sont démontrés aux tableaux 3 et 4.

Dans la clientèle de banlieue citée antérieurement nous avons demandé à 67 patients combien des médicaments prescrits ont été pris régulièrement. D'après leurs données nous comptons 30,7 % en moyenne, malgré qu'il ne s'agissait que de l'ordre de 2,4 médicaments avec 3,7 tablettes, dragées etc. en moyenne par jour[1]. Egalement dans l'étude citée sur la consommation de la digoxine les patients ont été interrogés. Leurs réponses correspondaient avec les taux sanguins en digoxine[1].

Si la valeur des dépositions des patients peut être mise en question, elles peuvent quand même être une base non négligeable à condition d'employer une méthode adéquate.

Une dernière méthode à citer est le décompte des médicaments utilisés lors d'une consultation chez le médecin ou le contrôle des médicaments trouvés en possession du

Table 4. Compliance in ambulatory tuberculosis patients[9]

	COMPLIANCE	
	n	%
By own statement	24	96
By physician assessment	20	80
By urine test	18	72

Table 5. Comparison of compliance in children prescribed ten days of penicillin[6]

	Percent complying by	
on day	urine test	pill count
3	46	44
6	31	29
9	8	18

malade en son domicile. Nous connaissons maintes expériences de ce genre[5]. Ces méthodes peuvent conduire à une solution valable. Un exemple est cité au tableau 5. Elles portent cependant un caractère d'intervention plus prononcé que les méthodes citées antérieurement.

Il est hors de doute que les résultats des méthodes de ce genre peuvent être manipulés par le patient. Certes il serait souhaitable d'ajouter des techniques pour évaluer le degré de cette manipulation.

REFERENCES

1. Gundert-Remy U., C. Remy and E. Weber, Serum digoxin levels in patients of a general practice in Germany, *Europ. J. Clin. Pharmacol.* **10** (1976), 97-100.

2. Oster P., G. Schlierf, C. Heuck, H. Greten, U. Gundert-Remy, W. Haase, G. Klose, A. Nothelfer, H. Raetzer and B. Schellenberg, "Sitosterol in type II-Hyperlipoproteinemia"*in : Lipoprotein metabolism*, Gretten H. ed., Berlin, Heidelberg, New York, Springer, 1976.

3. Gundert-Remy U., U. Möntmann and E. Weber, Studien zur Regelmässigkeit der Einnahme der Verordneten Medikamente bei stationären Patienten. I. Methodik und Basisdaten. II. Erläuternde Feststellungen zu sozialen und krankheitsbedingten Fakten sowie zur Selbsteinschätzung der Erkrankung durch den Patienten, *Inn. Med.* **5** (1978), 27-33 & 78-83.

4. Kass M.A., *in : Noncompliance with Miotic Therapy : The Views of Four Leading Clinicians*, interview organized and conducted on behalf of Alza Pharmaceuticals, Paolo Alto, California by KFR Infor/media Corp., New York, N.Y., 1978.

5. Gordis L., "Conceptual and methodologic problems in measuring patient compliance" *in : Compliance in Health Care*, R.B. Haynes, D.W. Taylor and D.L. Sackett eds, Baltimore and London, John Hopkins University Press, 1979, pp. 23-45.

6. Bergman A.B. and R.J. Werner, Failure of children to receive penicillin by mouth, *New Engl. J. Med.* **268** (1963), 1134-38.

7. Feinstein A.R., H.F. Wood, J.A. Epstein, A. Taranta, R. Simpson and E. Tursky, A controlled study of three methods of prophylaxis against streptococcal infection in a population of rheumatic children. Results of the first three years of the study, including methods for evaluating the maintenance of oral prophylaxis, *New Engl. J. Med.* **260** (1959), 697-702.

8. Gundert-Remy U., C. Remy and E. Weber, Eine Untersuchung zur Langzeitmedikation in einer Allgemeinmaxis, *Verh. Dtsch. Ges. Inn. Med.* **83** (1977), 1624.

9. Preston D.F. and F.L. Miller, The tuberculosis outpatient's defection from therapy, *Am. J. Med. Science* **247** (1964), 21-25.

10. Schicke R.K., *Sozialphprmakologie : Eine Einführung*, Stuttgart, Berlin, Köln, Mainz, Verlag W. Kohlhammer, 1976.

Sécurité et médicaments (1982), pp. 213-220

Cross Cultural Problems with Regard to Product Information and Drug Safety

L.A. SALAKO

Department of Pharmacology & Therapeutics, University of Ibadan, Ibadan, Nigeria

Abstract — The safety of any given drug can be influenced by a number of factors including idiosyncrasy of subjects using it, genetic differences in different populations, different environmental factors, adequacy of the information about the drug to consumers and compliance with such information. Informing patients about drugs in developing countries is beset with problems which stem from a number of factors prominent among which are multiplicity of languages, low literacy level, living habits which majority of the health personnel are unfamiliar with and conflict between the traditional and the modern concepts of the nature, causation and treatment of disease. These problems are compounded by high population-doctor and population-pharmacist ratios. The result is that a relitively higd percentage of the population have no information at all on the drugs they take or obtain whatever information they have from unconventional sources. The problems of drug information in developing countries thus differ in many respects from those of developed countries and different solutions, which take into consideration the peculiar social, cultural and economic circumstances of developing countries, have to be adopted.

There are two broad aspects of drug information :

1. information directed to the health profession and
2. information directed to the public in general and to patients in particular.

In many developing countries, particularly those in Africa, it is important that information be directed to the health profession as a whole rather than to the classical prescribers (doctors) or the dispensers (pharmacists) alone. This is because in many localities, nurses, midwives and medical auxilliaries have about as much role to play as doctors, dentists and pharmacists in the subsequent dissemination of information to patients. In many developing countries, these paramedical groups play a central role in the health care delivery programmes. This central role arises as a result of severe shortage of doctors and pharmacists and the concentration of the few available ones in the major towns and cities so that health care in the rural areas is largely in the hands of paramedical personnel like nurses, midwives and medical auxilliaries. An idea of the size of the problem can be gained from the following figures for Nigeria which is the largest country in Africa with an estimated population in 1976 of 80 million, and one of the more technologically developed countries in the continent. In 1976, the number of doctors was 4000, pharmacists 2000, dentists 250 and nurses 34,000. There was therefore a doctor: population ratio of 1 : 20,000 and a pharmacist population ratio of 1 : 40,000. (These figures contrast sharply with a population per doctor ratio of less than 1000 for European countries). Since the large majority of these few doctors are based in the major towns and cities, it is not difficult to see why many of the population of the rural areas will not have the benefit of being treated by a Western-style doctor from cradle to grave. On the other hand, the much larger number of nurses and their more even distribution in the rural areas where they administer the primary health care system ensure the contact of the rural population with this cadre of health personnel and their prominent role in the dissemination of drug information can therefore not be overemphasised.

SOURCES AND TARGETS OF DRUG INFORMATION

The sources of information on drugs in developing countries do not differ to any great extent from those in the developed world. The most important source of information is, of course, the pharmaceutical industry.

Most drugs marketed in developing countries emanate from the major multinational pharmaceutical industrial complexes and they have to provide information on their products to the consuming countries. Such information varies from product to product and it is especially important to know whether the product is a new drug being introduced into the country for the first time for use in man, whether it is an old drug for a new indication or whether it is just a 'me too' product. Ordinarily, information emanating from the manufacturers could be directed to :

1. The drug regulatory authorities for the purpose of registration of the product for distribution in the target country.
2. The health professions but subject to approval by the drug regulatory authorities.
3. The health professions but not subject to approval by the drug regulatory authorities.
4. The health professions and the public alike as with package inserts for prescription and non-prescription drugs.

The technical complexity of any given information varies with the target. It is not often realised by developing countries that data on pre-clinical testing and initial clinical evaluation of drugs often demanded by their national regulatory authorities are highly technical scientific data the evaluation of which may be beyond the technical expertise of these authorities. A certification scheme on the quality of pharmaceutical products moving in international commerce, like the one introduced by the World Health Organization in 1975 and now participated in by about 58 member states of the organization offers the best protection at present for developing countries for ensuring the quality of drugs entering their countries. When this scheme is combined with a rigid application of the World Health Organization requirements for 'good practices in the manufacture and quality control of drugs', then the quality and safety of drugs in developing countries will be assured even when such countries are not in a position to evaluate complex pre-clinical and initial clinical evaluation data on their own.

DRUG INFORMATION FOR THE HEALTH PROFESSIONS

Information directed to the health professions in developing countries has to take cognizance of the fact 1. that the number of doctors is small in relation to the population served, 2. that these doctors are usually overworked and so have little time to devote to complicated reading especially on what, to their practice, may well be obscrure drugs, 3. that only a few drugs are essential to their practice — thus, 90 % of their patients may be served by not more than 100 drugs and 4. that the information is directed not only to doctors and pharmacists but also to nurses, midwives and medical auxilliaries.

The aims of drug information directed to the health worker in developing countries should be :

1. To familiarize him with the relevant pharmacological properties and clinical uses of the drugs to enable him pick the right drugs for any particular disease requiring drug treatment.
2. To familiarize him with the side effect profile of the drugs to enable him make his choice of drugs with full knowledge of the benefits and risks.
3. In situations in which scanty financial resources are available, there is always a financial constraint on the health worker's freedom in selecting drugs. Although it is conceded to him that financial considerations should not compromise that the largest possible number of people benefit from the available resources or he will lose the confidence of the health authorities. Information on drugs to the health worker should therefore include cost to enable him consider the cost : benefit ratio in making his selection.
4. To increase his ability to detect and therefore monitor adverse reactions to the drugs he uses.
5. To inform patients accurately on various aspects of the drugs he administers.

The health professions in developing countries obtain their information on drugs from the manufacturers in the form of package inserts and promotional literature, from the ministries of health in the form of local formularies and from drug compendia prepared and distributed by interested pharmacists and physicians. It is, however, widely recognized that this information falls far short of the minimum required to achieve the aims enumerated above.

Herxheimer and Lionel[1] proposed a set of minimum information for prescribers. Their proposals can be adapted to meet the needs of different countries. For example, for most developing countries, apart from citing a drug by its generic name, the names of all the brands available in the country should be given, with the manufacturers' names and countries of origin. Fixed dosage brand drugs containing the active generic compound should be similarly recorded. It should be stated whether the country of origin or the manufacturer participates in the World Health Organization certification scheme for the quality of pharmaceutical products moving in international commerce. This information is necessary because many developing countries do not possess the capability to undertake quality control of drugs on their own and this scheme may be the only way of ensuring the quality of the various products. To be attractive to the majority of non-specialist potential users the information should preferably be in a pocket-book size and should contain only the essential drugs as determined by individual countries[2]. Compilation in loose-leaf form allows revised information to be inserted in place of old ones at intervals without the need to reissue new editions of the book. Although the need for such a book is widely recognized, the problems of the logistics of writing it — who, how, when and where to write it — have generally proved unsurmountable.

DRUG INFORMATION FOR THE PATIENT

The first problem about giving drug information to patients in developing countries is that of who to give the information. Experience has shown that to achieve the optimum result all those who have a role to play in the delivery of health care should be actively involved in the activity.

The question of why inform the patient has been ably answered by Hermann, Herxheimer and Lionel[3]. The patient needs to know how to take the drug, when to take it and for how long, what the drug is being taken for and what it is expected to do, the precautions to take whilst using the drug, what problems could arise whilst using the drug and what to do when they arise, and how to store the drug. Adequate information on these points will increase the patient's co-operation and enhance compliance.

Two situations need to be considered with respect to where to give the information. One is with a patient seen in hospital and the other is with a patient who presents at a pharmacy with or without a prescription.

With Patients seen in hospital initial information has to be given by the doctor or his assistant. As many of the patients will not be literate in the official language of communication, effort must be made to find someone who can communicate with the patient in his own language and ensure that information is not distorted during interpretation. Another problem is that of reducing the clinical information to what can be readily understood by patients. This requires patience and experience both of which may be lacking in a busy clinic manned by relatively junior staff. In a study of patients' understanding of the prescriber's information, patients attending the medical outpatients department of the University College Hospital, Ibadan, Nigeria, were questioned about the prescription information given by the doctor within ten minutes of receiving the information. Thirty-five per cent repeated the information wrongly[4, 5]. This high percentage of misunderstanding of information emphasises the problem of drug information to a largely illiterate patient community.

When patients procure their drugs at licensed pharmacies, it is not enough for the pharmacist to direct the patient's attention to the package inserts. It is equally important for him to go through the information in the package inserts step by step with the patient, carefully explaining all the information there. This is necessary whether the patient is literate or not. Experience has shown that literate patients do not care to read package inserts even when they have been directed to do so but will listen carefully to information from their medical attendants, and, as much as possible, follow instructions given by them.

The problem becomes more difficult when patients procure over-the-counter drugs from unlicensed pharmacies or 'patent medicine' stores where the attendants themselves may not know much about the drugs and have poor understanding of the information in the inserts. To solve this kind of problem, a number of governments in Africa have instituted public enlightenment programmes with regards to drugs. In these programmes, the more common over-the-counter drugs like aspirin, paracetamol, fixed dosage combinations of analgesics, amongst everal others, are made the subjects of discussion and information in mass media like newspapers, radio and television and also in schools and hospitals. As a result of all this, most households would have some members who possess reasonable information on the drugs commonly bought without prescription and can therefore advise their less informed kins and neighbours on their use.

Explaining what the patient must know to him is, however, not so easy. The problems are those of education, language and socio-cultural habits and these vary enormously from one community to another and even in the same community. If one takes the example of how to take the drug, there would be patients who might be able to understand and follow such relatively complex instruction as 'take 500 mg morning and night and 250 mg in the afternoon 1-2 hours after food or ' 10 mg/kg body weight per day in 3 equal divided doses 8 hourly', and there would be those who might misunderstand a simple instruction like 'take 2 tablets once daily'. As a rule dosage schedule should be as simple as is compatible with efficacy and safety. Thus, if 3 times daily administration of a drug will do the same thing as 4 times daily, the former should be preferred ; 2 times daily is better still whilst once daily is ideal. Prescription for children given by the weight is almost certain to be misunderstood. The prescriber or supplier should ideally weigh the patient and the quantity of drug to be administered should then be stated in tablet number or in volume in the case of a mixture. When prescriptions are made in volume, the measuring spoon should be supplied with the medicine since many people have different ideas as to what a teaspoonful, a dessertspoonful or a tablespoonful is. Some even do not use spoons at all and therefore do not have them. As much as possible drugs of the same generic compound but of different brands should have the same strength. It will then be possible to prescribe them in tablet numbers without running the risk that overdosage or underdosage will be taken. For example, all brands of aspirin could be of 300 mg strength, tetracycline 250 mg, metronidazole 200 mg or chloroquine 150 mg. There is little advantage in having the same dosage form of a drug in different strengths.

Social habits and culture also affect drug use and this should be borne in mind. For example, flexibility in the timing and manner of drug administration should be exploited so as not to clash with the patients habits, as such a clash would be certain to lead to non-compliance. A patient who normally has one or two meals a day who is requested to take a drug 3 times a day after food has a dilemma. He probably will not change his eating habit because of the drug. The chances are that he will take the drug only two times daily. The responsibility of the prescriber when drug administration is related to meals is to find out how frequently the patient eats and harmonise that with drug administration.

Information should be as flexible as possible to take care of varying levels of education, social class and intellectual ability. For example, asking patients to take drugs at precise hours of the day or at definite time intervals would be meaningless to peasants who keep no clock. Duration of treatment needs to be particularly emphasised since many patients stop their drugs as soon as symptoms disappear. They will only continue to take the drugs if it is emphasised to them that disappearance of symptoms does not mean cure. In chronic, sometimes symptomless conditions like hypertension, patients' co-operation can only be obtained if the result of failure to persist with treatment can be conveyed to them in dramatic terms like the risk of sudden death or what is generally considered to be worse, the risk of paralysis. Even this approach will not often succeed since the idea that sudden death, paralysis and such catastrophes are due to supernatural forces and can therefore not be staved off by conventional treatment, is deep-rooted in many cultures.

Storing of drugs is always a problem in the tropics where, because of high environmental temperature and humidity, chemicals deteriorate very rapidly. Drugs that have to be kept in refrigerators are of little use in mass treatment since refrigerators are commodities to be found in a few homes and even those cannot guarantee continuity of electricity supply to keep the drugs at the required temperature. It would be enough to inform patients to keep drugs in a cool dry place but the ultimate solution is with formulations that can withstand heat and moisture for long periods. In any case, it is not very helpful to supply drugs for periods of over one month at any one given time. Tablets and capsules becoming matted together or changing colour are features well known to patients as signifying deterioration in the drugs. When changes in smell are described it is important to use smells that are familiar. Thus the smell of vinegar may not be familiar whereas that of local wines or spices can be readily recognized.

In order to obtain maximum co-operation from a patient during treatment it is necessary to let him know as much as possible of the action of the drug in relation to the disease being treated. For example, in treating an infection it would be useful to let the patient know that his blood, liver, kidney, bladder, lungs or any other tissue or organ is infected with some worms and other parasites. The roles of worms and other parasites in causing disease is well recognized in many African cultures.

Indeed they constitute the second commonest cause of disease after supernatural forces invoked by illwilling persons. Other types of disease processes and the effects of drugs on them should be explained in a similar way.

It is customary in traditional medical practice that when a medicine is prescribed, the patient is given a number of precautions he has to take whilst on the treatment in order to ensure efficacy and prevent untoward effects. Such precautions usually have to do with life tyle and the avoidance of certain foods. With this kind of cultural background patients always expect a checklist of precautions to take and these should be carefully explained.

Another common feature of traditional medicines is that it is not uncommon for changes in urine or stool colour to follow their administration. Patients may therefore not worry when darkening of urine or stool occurs whilst they are on a drug. This could be put down simply to a sign of efficacy of the drug. The fact that the patient becomes weaker in association with such signs may still not alarm him as there is a widespread belief that the more potent the remedy the greater is the disturbance to body function.

We, of course, know that this is not necessarily so. Certain drugs, including sulphonamides, can produce intravascular haemolysis leading to haemoglobinuria in patients with glucose-6-phosphate dehydrogenase deficiency whilst aspirin and other non-steroidal anti-inflamatory drugs can produce gastric bleeding leading to melaena. It is therefore important to warn patients to report any unusual manifestations to the prescriber or supplier immediately.

Patients expect to be told about situations in which it will be inadvisable to take the drug. There is a surprisingly widespread awareness of the danger of indiscriminate use of drugs during pregnancy and to a less extent during lactation. Many pregnant women will not even take aspirin preferring instead to bear their headaches and mild musculoskeletal pains with stoical resignation. The possibility of pregnancy occurring in the course of chronic medication in women of child-bearing age should be borne in mind and information given should include what the patient should do in that event.

The most important source of information to the patient is the manufacturer's package insert supplemented by verbal information by doctors, pharmacists and other health workers and government sponsored health education programmes. In their present form, most package education inserts fall short of the minimum information required by patients and the information they contain is expressed in language too technical for the understanding of the vast majority of drug users. Although in general information on any product should be the same irrespective of the community being served, certain basic sets of information have to be adapted as described in the preceeding paragraphs to meet the socio-cultural differences which may affect the use of drugs in different communities.

In summary, the problems with regards to product information and drug safety in the developing countries of Africa stem from 1. wide differences in social expectation and cultural background, 2. conflict between the Western (modern) and the African's traditional concepts of disease causation and their treatment, 3. difficulties in communication between medical workers and patients due to multiplicity of languages and illiteracy of a large percentage of the people in the language used for official communication and 4. a depressingly low number of doctors and pharmacists necessitating the use of lower level cadres of health workers in prescribing drugs, dispensing them and informing patients on their use. Nevertheless, experience has shown that provided these problems are borne in mind when compiling product information for health workers and transmitting information to patients, it should be possible to obtain maximum benefit and minimum trouble from drugs used in these countries.

REFERENCES

1. Herxheimer A. and N.D.W. Lionel, Minimum information needed by prescribers, *Br. Med. J.* **2** (1978), 1129-32.

2. World Health Organization, The selection of essential drugs, second report of the W.H.O. expert Committee, Techn. Rep. Ser. 641, W.H.O., Geneva, 1979.

3. Hermann F., A. Herxheimer and N.D.W. Lionel, Package inserts for prescribed medicines : what minimum information do patients need ?, *Br. Med. J.* **2** (1978), 1132-35.

4. Salako L.A. and B.K. Adadevoh, Patients attitudes, understanding and consumption of prescribed drugs, *W. Afr. Med. J.* **21** (1972), 140-43.
5. Salako L.A. and B.K. Adadevoh, Patients attitudes, understanding and consumption of prescribed drugs II. Procurment practices, attitudes and facilities for drug dispensing at the hospital pharmacy, *Nig. Med. J.* **2** (1972), 143-47.

Sécurité et médicaments (1982), pp. 221-224

Product Information : Proposal for a Coherent Action Program

A. HERXHEIMER

Department of Pharmacology, Charing Cross Hospital Medical School, Fulham Palace Road, Hammersmith, London W 6 8 RF, United Kingdom

Abstract — The patient needs both spoken and written information about his medicine. The responsibility for informing him is shared primarily between the prescriber and the pharmacist; the manufacturer provides full supporting material. The first two, and often the nurse, need a clear summary of what it is that the patient should know. They can then go through it with the patient and explain it where necessary. The written information for patients could be distributed to prescribers and pharmacists by printing a copy next to, or as part of, the data sheet for the particular product.

Since the minimum written information needed for closely related medicines should be correspondingly similar, it makes no sense for every individual manufacturer to preduce his own separate product information set. Collaboration beween manufacturers and others will be needed to develop effective and congruent information sets.

The preceding speakers have discussed the various ways in which the patient gets or could get information about his treatment, and who should or could provide the information. What I want to talk about is how we can put all this together in a coherent way, so that everyone concerned — the patient and those near to him, the prescriber, the nurse or receptionist, the pharmacist and the manufacturer — can know what is expected of him or her, and how his or her role fits in with those of the others. All that I shall say will apply primarily to a developed Western country, but I hope that with suitable modifications it could be applied elsewhere too.

Let us start by considering what the patient wants or needs to know about his medication. These needs have been well summarised by Freya Hermann[1]. They fall into three categories, according to the time when the information is relevant (Table 1). First, at the time of the consultation with the doctor the patient wants to know why he is to take the drug, and the benefits, risks and possible inconveniences of doing so. Ideally that information should enable him to participate in the treatment decision. Second, when the decision has been made and the prescription written, the patient goes to the pharmacist to get the medicine. From the time that he takes charge of the medicine he needs to know how to store it appropriately, and when and how to take it. The patient must understand the dosage regimen from the very first dose, so that he can fit it into his daily routine. The doctor is of course likely to have discussed or mentioned the dosage regimen during the consultation, but at that point the patient could not make any use of this information.

Table 1. When the patient needs different items of information

A. During consultation:	benefits, risks, inconveniences
	the treatment plan in outline
B. When the pharmacist dispenses the medicine:	dosage regimen manner of taking the medicine
	how to store it
C. After starting to take the medicine:	what effects to expect and when
	possible side effects and interactions
	what to do if specified events occur

Thirdly, only after the patient has started taking the medication will he actually *need* to know about its effects and possible side effects. He may *want* to know about these during the consultation with the doctor, but he will not have to act on this information until later. For example if the therapeutic effect does not occur when it should have occured, or if something untowards happens, then the patient must decide whether to go on taking the medication, to alter the dose, to inform the doctor urgently or less urgently, and so on. As this time the patient is not with the doctor or pharmacist — he is on his own, and therefore the package insert becomes of paramount importance.

It is clear that the patient pakage insert cannot be an effective substitute for what the doctor tells the patient or for what the pharmacist says or puts on the label — if only the patient will either not be in possession of the insert or not be able to read it at the right time.

We also have to look at the information the patient needs in another way, and consider from whom he can best get each item — the doctor, the pharmacist or the manufacturer. In Table 2, I have underlined what is probably the best source for the various items of information, but note that many of them can also be obtained from one or more other sources. Inevitably the patient will receive a patchwork of information, and it follows that the messages he gets from the doctor, the pharmacist and the PPI have to be congruent and to complement one another harmoniously. This will not be easy to achieve.

We can now begin to see how the manufacturer (or anyone else) who produces a data sheet for the prescriber and a package insert for the patient, can best make his contribution. Since he can communicate only in print, his contribution cannot be tailored to individual patients. The PPI must be applicable to all the patients who will be prescribed the drug. It is the doctor and to some extent the pharmacist who have to tell the patient about the particular points that apply specifically to him. However, the manufacturer can use his data sheet to provide support for the doctor and pharmacist, by drawing their attention to the points on which the patient may want or need information, and perhaps even by suggesting simple words or phrases that can help to get the information across.

What I envisage is that the data sheet for a product would be accompanied by 1.

Table 2a. The best sources for different items of information (1)

Benefits ("how will this medicine help me?")	doctor
Risks, inconvenience	doctor
Name of medicine	doctor, pharmacist, label
"How important is it for me to take it? "What may happen if I don't take it?"	doctor
"Can I tell if it works?"	doctor, pharmacist

an aide-mémoire for the prescriber which reminds him of the points that may need discussion with the patient, and 2. a copy of the patient package insert. The aide-mémoire and the PPI could be printed side by side, as outlined in Table 3. At the end of the consultation the prescriber can briefly go through the important points with the patient, and explain that the patient will get a copy of the PPI to keep.

Table 2b. The best sources for different items of information (2)

Dosage regimen manner of taking	doctor, *pharmacist*
Side effects, interactions and what to do about them	doctor, pharmacist, *PPI*
How to store it	pharmacist, *label*, PPI
What to do with tablets no longer needed	doctor, pharmacist, label, PPI

Table 3.

Aide-memoire headings	PPI headings (from F. Hermann *et al.*, BMJ 1978, 2, 1152)
1A how it will help	
1B what may happen if you don't take it	1 What the medicine does
1C effects to expect	
1D what to do if they don't occur	
2 How *you* should take the medicine	2 Taking the medicine, important details
	3 Storing the medicine
4 Problems to watch for — refer patient to PPI	4 Possible problems
— note particularly relevant items	

Many doctors will object that they don't have time to do this, but I think that is a blinkered reaction which raises some fundamental questions about prescribing. On occasions it will take the doctor less time to explain why he is not giving the patient a prescription than it takes to tell the patient what he needs to know about a prescribed medicine. We know that prescriptions which are inadequately explained often do little good, and not infrequently do harm. The number of prescriptions written will have to be brought into balance with the time needed to explain them adequately to the patients.

So far I have talked about methods for harmoniously pouring out for the patient relevant information from different sources. But if we pour it out for the patient, that does not mean that it will go into him in a way in which he can use it. Effective transmission of information depends as much on the recipient as on the transmitter. The message can get in only if the receiver is switched on and tuned in to the transmission. In our context, "switched on" means paying attention, "tuned in" means understanding the specific purpose of the message and the underlying concepts. The physician, the pharmacist and the manufacturer can all make it easier for patients to switch on and tune in. Patients will pay attention if they are convinced that the information is important to them and if they are not swamped by its bulk and complexity.

Ley[2,3], who has done much work on this subject, suggests that one can lend importance to a statement by mentioning it as the first of a number of statements, giving it primacy, by repeating it, and by expressing it with great specificity. Enabling the patient to tune in is a different matter : he needs to grasp a few very basic general concepts relating to medicines. The patient will understand the physician, the pharmacist and the PPI much better if he understands the notion of a benefit/risk relationship, and that it is influenced by the nature and seriousness of an illness ; that the body gets rid of drugs, and that the speed with which this happens affects the frequency of doses ; that a drug can have effects on the body that are not intended ; that medicines do not keep for ever. We have to find ways of teaching patients these elementary ideas, but have hardly begun to do so. It should not be difficult to devise posters, leaflets, tape-slide programmes, etc. for waiting rooms in surgeries, clinics and pharmacies. We should also aim at school teachers, so that future citizens can learn all this as children at school. They will then be able to teach their parents as well !

Having tried our best to make the patient switch on and tune in, we still need to find out whether our message has been received and correctly understood. The doctor, the pharmacist, or whoever has been giving the patient information, can of course ask him to repeat it or explain it to check whether he has understood it. But is probably better to get the patient to ask questions. Ideally he should know what he needs to get from the message, so that he can ask the right questions if he does not get it. Patients are often reluctant to question professionals, partly because they feel a bit overawed and inhibited and partly from a fear that their questions will seem silly. It is therefore a good idea for doctors and other professionals to encourage patients to ask important and sensible questions. A simply way of doing this is to give them examples of questions to which they may reasonably expect to be given answers. I made up a list of such questions some years ago[4] ; they concern the points already discussed (Table 2). A list like this[5] could be distributed by doctors' receptionists, pharmacists, community health councils and many others. The questions could also be included in patient package inserts ; they occupy little space. However there is one major obstacle that must be overcome. Before most doctors and pharmacists will accept the distribution of questions and take part in it, they have to feel confident and comfortable about answering the questions. At present many of them do not.

So it is clear that all of us who are primarily concerned with medicines — medical

Table 4. Elementary concepts wich patients need to tune in to the message

* The benefit/risk relationship, and that it varies with the seriousness of an illness.
* The body gets rid of drugs. The speed with which this happens determines the interval between doses.
* A drug can have effects on the body which are not intended.
* The bigger the dose, the greater the effect.
* The bigger the dose, the greater the variety of different effects.
* Medicines don't keep for ever.
* Doctors (or scientists) don't know everything about medicines, even commonly used ones.

V

FREE COMMUNICATIONS AND POSTERS

COMMUNICATIONS LIBRES ET POSTERS

Sécurité et médicaments (1982), p. 229

A Diploma Course in Pharmaceutical Medicine

B.T. MARSH and D.K. LUSCOMBE

Leo Laboratories Ltd., Aylesbury & Division of Applied Pharmacology, UWIST, Cardiff, United Kingdom

Abstract — A postgraduate course in Pharmaceutical Medicine is held in Cardiff under the auspices of the Association of Medical Advisers in the Pharmaceutical Industry, the Association of the British Pharmaceutical Industry and the University of Wales. This two year part-time training programme prepares candidates for the Diploma in Pharmaceutical Medicine of the Royal Colleges of Physicians of the United Kingdom. The course consists of 20 days of teaching each year, comprising lectures, workshops and seminars, divided into five residential sessions each of four days. The course is now in its fifth year and between 15 and 20 candidates sit the examination each year. Approximately 20 % of those attending the course represent pharmaceutical companies outside the United Kingdom, particularly in France, Switzerland, Holland and Germany.

Sécurité et médicaments (1982), p. 231

Diploma in Pharmaceutical Medicine (D.P.M.): A survey of Attitudes of A.M.A.P.I. members.

R.P. BAX and D. MCCULLEY*

*Roussel Lab. Ltd., Roussel House, Wembley Park, Middlessex HA 9 ONF, United Kingdom

Abstract — 400 AMAPI members were invited by post to complete a questionnaire on their personal history and attitudes to the D.P.M. and the JAC course. 142 replies on personal history, 40 on the exam and 39 on the course were received. 60 % of Pharmaceutical Physicians (P.P.) came directly from hospital medicine, the remainder from general practice. 5 % of the total have higher qualifications other than D.P.M.: 28 % hold the D.P.M. but 57 % of the rest do not intend to sit the exam. The majority of companies appear unimpressed by D.P.M. and exert little pressure on P.P. to take it.

72 % found the course relevant to the exam and the out of hours activities, i.e. meeting other medical advisers, useful.

Of the subjects offered on the course 53 % considered coverage adequate, 28 % poor and only 19 % good. The exam pass rate approaches 100 %. The best covered subject was Statistics with 94 % of replies stating that the course was well or adequately covered. The worst was Principles of Pharmacy with 50 % of respondents stating that the course was badly covered. The remaining found the subject was covered adequately.

Further data analysis and comment will be presented.

Sécurité et médicaments (1982), p. 233

Test of Small Airways Function in Monitoring Respiratory Effects of Medicinals

B.M. COHEN

546 Irvington Avenue, Elizabeth, New Jersey 07 208, USA

Abstract — Toxic and therapeutic respiratory drug effects are commonly monitored by FEV1.0 or PEFR tests which may be less sensitive than derivatives of flow/volume loops. Even the latter may not be as reliable as newer tests of the small airways in detecting the impact of bronchoacdtive substances, functional abnormalities and their degree of reversibility. We tested assumptions by comparing older spirometric indices with derivatives of MEFV curves on air and He/02 breathing, single breath N2 data and the volume of isoflow in two randomized trials. In the first, guaifenesin, or matched placebo, was given in divided oral doses for 7 days to 20 subjects with chronic bronchitis after a 1 week placebo washout. The second trial, also incorporating resistance measurements, compared the acute effects of inhalation of a mixture of aromatic vapors with water in 24 adults with acute coryzal rhinitis; gas chromatographic analysis of air samples provided the concentration of aromatics. Our data show 1. the methodology is feasible for monitoring ambulatory subjects; 2. treatment differences may be inapparent unless small airways functions are tested (trial 1); 3. when changes occur in both large and small airways, deviations in indices of the latter be of greater statistical import (trial 2); 4. changes in the phase III slope of the alveolar plateau (delta N2 %) may be the small airways test most sensitive to treatment differences (both trials).

Sécurité et médicaments (1982), p. 235

Algorithms and the Science of Systematic Drug Development

F.W. WOLFF

Institute for Drug Development, 800 Notley Road, Silver Spring, Maryland 20904, USA

Abstract — Advances in the basic and clinical sciences and growing demands of regulatory burocracies are complicating and prolonging the development of promising new molecules. The twenty years it took to develop minoxidil, the evidence for indifferent planning, poor collation of data, slow and tedious reviews, and clinical problems in drugs such as amiloride, nifedipine, verapamil, bumetanide, oxprenolol, timolol, ticrynafen suggest the need for a Science of Drug Developpment. In this the various stages necessary for logical drug work-up are planned to interdigitate, a chronology is etablished, time limits are setand a series of algorithms portray the necessary effort.

Constant and open contact before and during each stage with the appropriate regulatory group, without slavish adherence to preset quidelines, emphasis on innovative concepts and technology, shortcuts as long as they are logical and rational should lead to economy of effort, saving of precious time, and a marked improvement in the too frequently poor relationship between scientists and regulators working for private industry, government or academia. Enthusiasm for therapeutic advances and technological excellence may in time replace the current censorious and carping attitude of the regulatory authority. Industrial laboratories and research organisations will benefit from interaction with free standing, independant consultative groups with a background of the positive and negative aspects of the participants, termining a creative and timely approach, laying the groundwork of a strategy and tactics which each participant group by itself might not embrace.

The five cardinal sins in drug development with pertinent examples in this presentation, will lead to the description of an outline of suitable corrective solutions.

Sécurité et médicaments (1982), pp. 237-245

Management of Clinical Trials in Developing Countries

E.W.J. DE MAAR

W.H.O., avenue Appia, 1211 Geneve, Switzerland

Abstract — Clinical research is an important bottleneck in attempts to improve health in developing countries. When in developing countries novel measures to improve poor health require assessment, clinical research is complex, because of specific needs and constraints in patients, in diseases and in trial circumstances.

Experience have been drawn from clinical research in developing countries in evaluating new regimes for leprosy, schistosomiasis, malaria, tuberculosis, filariasis, and contraception. Locations are in geneal more or less confined to hot and often humid climates.

The main objectives should be to reveal new information. For instance, when there are different genetic, nutritional or climatic conditions, differences in drug metabolism or obvious lower body weight may make different dosage recommendations necessary. Therapies for specific diseases endemic in developing countries can be evaluated properly only in those countries. But when trial conditions are very much the same, plain repetition aimed at confirming existing information in developing countries is neither ethically nor logistically desirable.

To proceed smoothly and to obtain reliable and innovative results, broad guidelines are suggested which are not, however, intended as a rigid prescription. Specifics will be considered for protocol, location, staff patients, ethical clearance, operations and data.

Clinical trials on better agents and methods for health are a major bottleneck in improving health in developing countries. When novel measures to improve health require assessment in those countries, clinical trials are complicated because of specific needs and constraints in diseases, in patients and in trial circumstances[1]. Experiences have been drawn from evaluating new regimes for filariasis, leprosy, malaria, schistosomiasis, tuberculosis and contraception and from locations which are in general more or less confined to hot and often humid climates. They include, Brazil, Ghana, Indonesia, India, Mali and Zambia.

Predictions on safety and efficacy under local conditions which derive from trials on affected populations in another region, cannot always be accepted as reliable indicators of future regional performance. It is highly desirable that the study be carried out where the disease is endemic. The main objectives should be to reveal new information. For instance, when there are different genetic, nutritional or climatic conditions, differences in drug metabolism obvious lower body weight may make different dosage recommendations necessary. Therapies for specific endemic diseases can be evaluated extensively and properly only in those developing countries. But when trial conditions are very much the same, plain repetition, aimed at confirming existing information in those countries is neither ethically nor logistically desirable.

To proceed smoothly and to obtain reliable and, hopefully, innovative results, broad guidelines and minimum requirements are suggested which are not, however, intended as a rigid prescription, nor need they oblige every international activity to comply with them. It is not intended in this paper to expand on the general management of clinical trials[2] or to duplicate existing check lists for the planning of clinical trial protocols[3], or to assess reports of therapeutic trials[4], or even to examine reports of adverse drug reactions[5].

It is mainly intended to consider certain additional or different specifics ; if these are observed, clinical studies can proceed as smoothly as trials carried out in more developed, temperate climates. The results obtained will be just as reliable. Needless to say that with so much to cover, there will be both generalization and lack of details. For each of the following subjects, others may wish to provide more definitive and up-to-date papers :

ON THE PROTOCOL, ITS STANDARDIZATION AND PROJECT WORKSHOPS

A planning group with the broadest possible representation draws up a protocol stating objectives and procedures at an initial workshop. Held preferably at the testing location and with all future participants thus involved, the protocol is never imposed, but developed through extensive consultation and coordination.

Its initial aim, particularly for cooperative clinical trials is to determine whether a specific study is feasible. Initially, research ovjectives, taking into account the stage of development of the new method or agent, should be restricted to answering a few simple but meaningful questions. Answers on future regional application as well as feedback to continuing research on improvements are both important. A strict correlation of the requirements of the protocol with the real "field" conditions of the treatment of the target disease should exist.

Sophisticated therapeutic regimens, which cannot be applied in field conditions, where supervision is lacking and where the patient's compliance is a major limiting factor, require that one should anticipate environmental conditions, It assures the opportunities for the execution of a standardized protocol. such a standardized protocol is repeated in a comparative fashion as a necessary condition of the scientific method. However, to define regimens suitable for a large "field" application, the "absconders-"rate, the regularity of drug intake, the possibility of re-infection, and all other possible sources of variability due to a peculiar environment should be taken into account.

The information in the protocol includes :

— the aims and objectives of the trial ;

— a very clear definition of clinical parameters, both for inclusion and exclusion as well as assessment. Even seemingly obvious ones, such as, for instance, sudden death, if not exactly defined, can cause ambiguities during analysis of the data ;

— a detailed description of clinical procedures, laboratory tests, biopsies, etc. plus frequency-timing of these observations and follow-up ;
— a precise definition of parameters which depend on individual investigator evaluation (so-called "soft parameters") to assist in uniformity of measurement between investigators ;
— case report forms, kept as simple as possible and which can be made part of the patients' records ;
— consent forms and warning notices written in the local language ;
— the treatment allocation procedure and individual treatment charts, particularly when regimens are reallocated or changed ;
— the labelling code and emergency code-breaking and referral procedures. Precise guidelines for evaluation and management of known adverse reactions (mild, moderate, severe) to assist in uniformity, and work manuals for the pharmacist or drug supervisor.
— the investigational drug data brochure.

Many tropical diseases remain ill-understood and consequently there may be a large amount of guesswork involved in the designing of the protocol. If the protocol is too rigid, the trial runs into difficulties later. A protocol planning group may be unable to project the rate at which suitable patients can be obtained to enter a trial. In a schistosomiasis endemic area of 30 % overall prevalence, it was found that serial analyses of urine samples of up to a week in any one individual increased the yield of patients beyond the most optimistic expectation.

In case of doubt about the logistical feasibility of a particular trial, consider starting with a trial run of the test procedures, using an established drug, to detect potential problems concerning availability of scientific and technical expertise, equipment or reagents. The pilot study may reveal an unexpected situation like the need to feed patients before the administration of a drug, even a potentially innocuous one. For example, during a trial of the metrifonate in Mutenda, Zambia, several of the school children "collapsed" after the administration of the first dose, only 7 mg/kg. It was found out that they had their last meal at about 6 p.m. the previous evening and some of them had walked up to 6 kilometres to school. The drug was administered at 11 a.m. These children took the tablets not on an empty stomach but in a fasting state. Since then, it has been necessary to feed all the patients before any drugs could be administered. By the way, the children alluded to above had no side effects after the administration of further doses of metrifonate on a full stomach.

Local capability will vary and, in some places, change continuously. Problems may exist only in certain neglected areas of clinical research. A second standardization workshop for the core items of the protocol contributes to the precision of clinical and Laboratory results with respect both to the assessment of patients and of responses. Byproducts of the worshop are a great sense of fellowship in addition to training and motivation. For multi-centre studies, a workshop is essential. In cooperative studies, a third workshop of principal investigators to review progress is also highly desirable. It can help to overcome flagging interest.

ON STAFF AND SUPERVISION

It is essential to select a competent, dependable and enthusiastic principal investigator, available for the full duration of the study. The principal investigator should ideally be a member of the local medical profession and, where possible, fully paid by the project. He/she should be knowledgeable about clinical trials or willing to learn, and should have been a member of the protocol working group. The principal investigator should keep to the protocol, except in case of danger for the safety of patients, in which he alone should be allowed to make the decision to discontinue one or more affected cases.

It would be useful to appoint drug supervisors who observe intake of the prescribed drugs and social workers who should be motivated to follow up poor attenders and absentees. The latter should know each patient, usually having interviewed them during their selection for a study and having on record one or all addresses where they can be contacted, as well as, if possible, a polaroid photograph of their faces.

Other medical and supporting personnel, such as physicians, nurses, secretaries, a pharmacist or drug supervisor, a financial or administrative officer, a statistician, and a clinical pathologist, are organized and prepared to substitute for each other in case of sudden unforeseen absences. Even the best motivated groups may experience the full range of causes of absences, from accidents to unexpected departures. National counterparts should be appointed for any non-local, temporary staff.

In addition, a coordinator, familiar to the trial groups and not alien to their culture, who adheres to high scientific standards and can appreciate local problems, is very useful for the necessary liaison with other trial groups in different locations, and with the sponsor of the trial. For sponsored trials it might be necessary to state that a sponsor-appointed monitor will have unrestricted access to patients, the laboratory and all data.

Consultant services should be arranged from the local hospital, and the night and weekend services should be checked in case research patients have problems outside research clinic hours. Also, consult such local health dignitaries as the traditional medicine man and the dispenser or pharmacist ; their cooperation and understanding of the clinical trial should be sought. Their displeasure may jeopardize the whole study. Finally, the opportunity for advice from a national body in charge of the scientific evaluation of the project could be considered.

Permanent national or international advisory committees to guide the research can be helpful by giving broad support, but they are expensive when their travel and other expenses have to be covered.

Training of staff

In order to improve the standards of clinical research, motivation by training plays an important role with staff who are attending to the running of the trial, in particular items such as :

— identifying eligible patients
— comprehension of protocol and its demands

— how to fill out a case record form and especially how to later include laboratory data accorately
— and a general review of concomitant challenges to the success of a piece of research, e.g., medication misuse, problems of compliance, seriousness of any concomitant unprescribed medication.

ON LOGISTICS AND LOCATIONS

Make a project contract with local and national authorities, including national research councils, so that any agreement will extend throughout the administration from the Ministry of Health to the local authorities. The project is designated as national or local with no emphasis on internationality.

Even though the target problems or diseases are widespread, suitable trial sites may be difficult to identify. These should be carefully chosen to avoid conditions that might prevent application of adequate scientific standards, whether a permanent base or a temporary arrangement is foreseen. Determine what cooperative arrangements can be made. Make full use of all local, available experience in relevant medical research. An integrated effort with local scientists builds into a project a continuity by the local commitment to clinical research. For difficult procedures, explore whether cooperative arrangements can be made in the form of an inter-institutional twining arrangement with a group with proven experience, particularly, for instance, for clinical pharmacology or pharmacokinetics.

In reference to diseases and patients, check the will to investigate a disease problem of local importance and preferably with global consequences, and the prevalence and incidence of the target disorder and of relevant endemic or other concomitant diseases, and the adequacy of any mechanism in existence for case detection. For infectious diseases, what are the possibilities of reinfection during the trial or follow-up period ? Can the tests discriminate between suppression with relapse and cure with reinfection ? Are there local variabilities in patient tolerance or disease susceptibility likely to affect safety or efficacy ?

Is the medical and paramedical infrastructure capable and willing to support the project according to protocol and to manage any unforeseen complications, besides the provision of ordinary medical care requested by patients. If not, what is the need for strengthening the infrastructure through training or with equipment. Does the Laboratory have the proper specific expertise in endemic infections, particularly in scanty mixed infections ? Do rooms need to be air conditioned for coulter counters or multianalyzers. Serious consideration should be given to the possibility of carrying out a series of small studies rather than one large one. Success at a small study which has been quickly carried out tends to breed enthusiasm and interest for further studies. Local medical capability and infrastructure areas which require strengthening can be easily assessed. This really shows the importance of a pilot study.

Check your staff and patients' need for transportation. Are there adequate vehicles, is there a steady supply of gasoline or petrol and are the vehicle permits in orde ? Is there ready access to study areas with reliable, adequate transportation in season of study ? Could adding satellite field centres reduce transportation time, promote recruitment of patients and encourage participation by all interested persons in the trial area, if they offer medical care for conditions other than the one of interest to the study ? The problem of ready access to study areas throughout the year is not to be taken lightly. Rural roads described as not likely to be flooded may in practice turn out to be impassable for months because the health worker cannot afford to spend hours stuck in mud. A follow-up planned for six months later may fall in the rainy season and become impossible.

Responsibility must be assigned for each laboratory test. If assays are performed locally, prestandardization by running control samples is necessary. If laboratory assays are to be run elsewhere, preserved samples should be shipped on a regular schedule. A specimen identification form and a laboratory report form links each patient and his laboratory data. The local and international regulations on export and transport of biological materials should be carefully checked. It is "medical colonialism" to take samples out of a country, leaving no further trace of that export than a publication many years later from a laboratory in another part of the world. Availability of maintenance services for all laboratory equipment should be checked. Power cuts can destroy frozen samples. A back-up generator in working condition is highly desirable. For local conditions, check attitudes regarding tendencies to please, security (be wary of drug leakage for alternative uses of the drug), attitudes towards trials of new agents, investigational invasion of privacy (e.g., blood tests, stool collection and post mortems) ? What is the order of case holding in regular clinics and absences for such occasions as religious holidays, harvest, sickness in the family, funerals ? Special taboos exist in some places for women frequently visiting public places, even hospitals.

Make a realistic estimate of the duration of the study from start to completion. A financial officer should determine the total funds required, preferably on a monthly basis. Consider the financial consequences of delays, inflation and exchange fluctuations, and the time needed for the preparation of the initial coherent research proposal or interim reports to financial sponsors. A flow diagramme of the whole project is useful.

ON DRUGS AND COMPLIANCE

Try to obtain all needed drug supplies at once. Include recommendations about storage conditions of test drugs, as studies may fail because of drug spoilage. The regimen for post-trial follow-up treatment supplies when waiting for the final assessment of the trial results should be decided in advance and supplies obtained it possible. Test medications should never be smuggled into any country ; a worthy scientific purpose is no excuse. Research drugs are new chemicals which cannot be classified by customs. A full formula should be placed on the tear-off label and the problem of unrealistic value assessments should be discussed with the manufacturer. Check the necessary national clearances for investigating new agents ; permits may be needed from review body, a manufacturer, or from an authority.

An independent measure of patient compliance must be agreed upon. This will avoid branding as ineffectual a compound that the patients have not actually taken, or having the design of the study blamed for results that are difficult to explain. A patient eating only one meal a day cannot take medication three times a day with meals. Concomitant unauthorized medications are a very serious problem. Native remedies supplied by traditional healers continue to be taken, as can be the case with anything patients buy from street vendors that may unknowingly contain active drugs.

Care should be taken during selection of a study population to avoid groups that have easy access to conventional medical treatment, for they might obtain treatment which could interfere with the clinical trial. For example, in selection of school children for a clinical trial of a schistosomicide, urban schools or rural schools located near a clinic are to be avoided. A longer pretreatment period than usual, with careful clinical histories, might be required.

Care must also be taken not to confuse the symptoms of a co-existent illness and the side effects of the trial drug. For example, during a trial of a new schistosomicide it was found that a significant number of patient volunteers complained of nausea, dizziness and abdominal discomfort after the administration of the drug. Some of these complaints were later found to be due to malaria in an area endemic for P. falciparum infections.

ETHICS

Projects should be reviewed and approved by an independent local group, practising the highest standards of protection of the rights of the individual. If such a group does not exist, is should be created. In cross-cultural research, review should take place at both ends. A well-tried way to obtain ethical clearance for clinical trials in developing countries is to ask the Ministry of Health to form the local Ethical Committee. The Principle Investigator could then be a non-voting secretary of such a group. Verbal or written informed and meaningful consent must be obtained from each patient. But the manner in which it is obtained may vary from practices in developed countries. Sometimes, due to the very limited education of the patients, some of the necessary information for consent might be difficult to explain such as :

— aims and expected duration of the project and the monitoring and follow-up of the projects ;
— alternative methods of treatment of the target disease and the procedures which are experimental ;
— any known immediate or long-term risk or possible discomfort to which subjects are liable ;
— benefits anticipated for subjects or others ;
— any incentives, like out-of-pocket expenses or treatment services to be given to subjects in exchange for their participation ;
— the degree of freedom of each subject to withdraw from the study at any time ;
— confidentiality of any information relating to patients obtained during the course of the study.

The manner (oral or written) in which this information will be conveyed should be included, as well as the names and status of those who transmit this information to potential subjects and who ascertain that it has been understood and that consent is freely given. Handing out consent forms to people who may at best be semi-literate does not suffice. In some areas, the act of signing any paper is considered an act of self-incrimination and is therefore not feasible as a method of indicating consent. One may have to seek additional consent from the traditional "head" of the unit, from parents as well as from the head teacher for school children. The consent of a husband for participation of his wife may need to be obtained in some areas. Withdrawal of subjects after several weeks or months is the penalty for neglect.

Any invasive procedure, especially repeated venepuncture, should be clearly explained and repeatedly demonstrated to the patient volunteers. It is no easy to explain to many patients that 300 mls of blood taken by venepuncture over a period of two months has no untoward effects in an adult with a Hb of 100 %. Nevertheless, frequent informal talks to the patient volunteers as a group in the presence of some other health workers has been found to be very helpful.

Recently, some patients refused further venepuncture. One of them complained that about two litres of blood had been taken from him (10 c.c. at a time !) The situation was explained to the group and the patient concerned was asked to demonstrate how two litres of blood could have been taken with a 10 c.c. syringe over the period in question. Immediately he started his demonstration his erroneous ideas were highlighted. The other patients then laughed and the clinical trial progressed satisfactorily.

DATA COLLECTION AND ANALYSIS

Data collection starts with defining the population from which the trial subjects will be drawn. For identification of subjects, photographs, in addition to careful records of name, household, domicile and occupation, may be useful. A calendar for clinic visits be agreed upon and special clinic hours arranged. A low degree of patient intake into a study, or a high drop-out rate, can result from many with acute illness phases or a high incidence of other disease conditions incompatible with the particular phase of the trial. Too rapid early intake, or too slow or unsteady intake can lead to incomplete data collection, missed visits and general disappointment of staff in projects with logistic complexity. If a long-term follow-up is needed of people in scattered villages one should try to assess mobility as nearly as possible before work is started. If underestimated, too many subjects may not be traceable due to migration. Obtain cooperation also from all inhabitants of the area under study. When the community understands what is going on, work is facilitated. Neighbours may even see to it that patients turn up on days of study.

The handling of data should not be compromised because of the state of development at the selected location, particularly as multi-centre, short-term trials rapidly produce large amounts of data suitable for tabulation. Mechanized methods for data collection using precoded forms for storage, and analysis are particularly desirable in developing countries to promote accuracy and thus ensure acceptability of the information to others. It promotes close surveillance with quality checks as data are generated.

But guard against collecting masses of information which cannot be easily analysed. Many clinical trialists will give examples of materials they collected several years ago and have been unable to find time to analyze. In short, do not collect information that may be impossible to "digest". Continuous tabulation may be useful to detect trends for studies of longer duration, or those involving many patients. Whether, at the risk of engendering biases these results should be supplied to all concerned, should be carefully considered.

The final goal is a scientific publication. There should be agreement on confidentiality and ownership of data. Who is to analyze interim and final results and where ? What about publication policy (e.g. acknowledgements) and public announcements ? Investigators in developing countries may prefer that results be published in local journals, which do not have international distribution. The possibility of simultanous publication of articles in local and international journals should be pursued.

REFERENCES

1. Maar E. de and J.M. Kofi Edue, Facilitation of Clinical Trials in Developing Countries. Proceedings, Conference on Pharmaceuticals for Develloping Countries. Division of International Health, Institute of Medicine, Nationale Academy of Sciences, Washington, D.C., U.S.A., 1979, pp. 359-66.
2. Ledermann H. and M. Glocke, *Principles of the Clinical Trial of Medicines and Medical Statistics*, Baden-Baden, Cologne, New York, Verlag Gerhard Witztrock, 1980.
3. Chaput de Saintonge D.M., Aide-mémoire for preparing clinical trial protocols, *Brit. Med. J.* **1** (1977), 1323-24.
4. Lionel N.D.W. and A. Herxheimer, Assessing Reports of Therapeutic Trials, *Brit. Med. J.* **3** (1970), 637-40.
5. Herxheimer A., "Check List for Assessing Reports of Adverse Effects of a Drug, Chemotherapy Vol. 4 : Pharmacology of Antibiotics", *Proc. 9th Int. Congr. of Chemotherapy*, London, New York, Plenum Press, 1976, 287-91.

Sécurité et médicaments (1982), p. 247

The Pathologist's Role in the Interpretation of Carcinogenicity Studies on Laboratory Animals

J.M. FACCINI

Centre de Recherches, Laboratoires Pfizer, 37400 Amboise, France

Abstract — The burden of the interpretation of the results of a long-term carcino-genicity study in rodents falls squarely on the shoulders of the pathologist : his findings have ultimate legal, economic and political connotations.

There are three critical decision points — diagnosis, interpretation and evaluation.

The diagnosis, as in man, depends on a full clinical history being correllated with the pathological findings.

The most difficult task is to distinguish inflammation from hyperplasia, hyperplasia from neoplasia and the benign from the malignant form of the latter.

Interpretation is deciding, with all the information available, chether the substance is carcinogenic in the rodent species employed and evaluation is deciding whether the substance should, therefore, be considered to be carcinogenic for man.

Sécurité et médicaments (1982), p. 249

Methodological Problems in the Detection and Evaluation of Adverse Events during the Phases I, II and III of the Drug Development

L. Bossi, J. F. Henry, M. Vadrot

L.E.R.S. 58, rue de la Glacière, 75013 Paris, France

Abstract — The importance of a correct methodology for the detection and the evaluation of adverse events during the various phases of the development of a new drug is obvious. However, a literature search (1970-1980) showed that the published contributions on this topic will be presented with a critical analysis of the following points :

1. *Advantages* and *disavantages* of *check-lists* as compared to spontaneous reporting. The use of check-lists increases the incidence of symptoms both in "normal" untreated populations and in patients or treated subjects ; spontaneous reporting may lead to underreporting of symptoms but it is more likely to detect relevant side-effects and unexpected side-effects (Greenblatt, Huskinsson and Wojtulewski, Ciccolunghi *et al.*).
2. Problems in the establishing of a *cause-effect relationship* between treatment and adverse events. Several algorythms are proposed in the literature (Lasagna *et al.* ; Kramer *et al.* ; Blanc *et al.*) ; however, they are seldom used in clinical trials, as documented by a literature search in the areas of epilepsy, depression, and schizophrenia. The possible reasons are discussed.
3. The practice of regular *monitoring of drug plasma concentrations* during phases I, II and III clinical studies is very limited, despite the evident usefulness of this tool in the evaluation of drug effects (Morselli *et al.*).
4. Evaluation of the *severity of adverse events* in the context of the severity of the treated pathology (Tallarida *et al.*).

Sécurité et médicaments (1982), pp. 251-256
Pergamon Press France

Post-marketing Surveillance in Italy : A Comparison between Firm-sponsored and Independent Trials with Prazosin

V. FORTE and M. CIAMPINI*

*c/o Medical Department, Pfizer Italiana, Via del Fornetto 85, 00149 Rome, Italy

Abstract — According to Wardell ("Postmarkeing Surveillance : Case-study Approach" *in : Drug Monitoring*, F.H. Gross & W.H.W. Inman eds, Academic Press, 1977, pp. 241-54), uncontrolled postmarketing surveillance (PMS) studies should be reevaluated due to the results obtained in some of them. It is true that they contain — as do many other studies — bias and errors, but these points must not be emphasized more for the socalled "uncontrolled" thant for the other studies.

Prazosin, still according to Wardell (l.c.), would be an interesting example for PMS. We compared the results obtained in three different PMS studies conducted in Italy on prazosin since. 1978, the year the product was put on the market in our country. One of these studies (V. Forte *et al., in : Problemi e prospettive dell'ipertensione arteriosa*, C. Bartorelli *et al.*[1] eds , ESAM, 1978, pp. 325-36) was sponsored by the manufacturers of the drug and involved 1606 hypertensive kpatients. The orthe two were sponsored by independent national medical associations (ANCE and ANMCO) and involved 453 (C. Fernandez *et al.*, in press, *in : Biologia e Medicina*, 1980) and 201 patients (unpublished data). The résults obtained in these three studies were compared in terms of efficacy and safety of the drug during its pratical use by GPs and/or cardiologists. No important difference was observed between the results of the three studies.

The aim of this paper is to compare, in a retrospective manner, three different trials carried out in Italy "in the field" which were designed to study the antihypertensive activity of prazosin, a selective postsynaptic α -blocking drug[1]. Some general considerations may also be drawn, in our opinion, from this very simple comparison.

During 1978, i.e. the time when prazosin (Minipress, Pfizer) was put on the Italian market, 292 Italian general practitioners conducted a multicenter trial on 1606 hypertensive patients[2]. The following year, the Ministry of Health issued a decree[3] on the basis of which postmarketing surveillance of drugs registered in Italy became compulsory for the pharmaceutical firms. Even though prazosin is not included in the list of products subject to this law, we thought it would be a very good trial run — for future uses — to have independent groups repeat the study already performed in the field.

Two different medical associations were therefore asked to organize and monitor the new trials : the Italian association of cardiologists working outside hospitals (a medical figure quite common in Italy but perhaps less so in other European countries) and the Italian association of hospital cardiologists. These two groups agreed to directly organize two different trials on hypertensive patients on the basis of two protocols not really different from the one we used in 1978. The Company's participation in these two trials was limited to sending the samples and handling the administrative aspects of the publications. The two trials are now finished and published [4] or in press [5].

Table 1. Initial blood pressure (B.P.) value in mmHg (average).

	Trial 1	Trial 2	Trial 3
Supine systolic B.P.	191	186	179
Standing systolic B.P.	188	184	177
Supine diastolic B.P.	107	104	109
Standing diastolice B.P.	106	104	111

Table 2. Percentage values of the systolic and diastolic blood pressure in supine position, compared with the baseline measurement (made conventionally equal to 100), for the three trials at the various assessments.

	Supine systolic B.P			Supine diastolic B.P.		
Assessment	Trial 1	Trial 2	Trial 3	Trial 1	Trial 2	Trial 3
I	95.28	97.45	95.94	95.72	97.47	96.09
II	92.67	92.25	---	93.45	92.71	---
III	90.05	89.65	93.06	89.71	90.14	90.56
IV	87.95	---	88.97	88.78	---	88.88
V	85.86	86.70	---	85.98	87.42	---
V	84.81	85.25	87.20	84.11	86.11	86.71

Table 3. Percentage values of the systolic and diastolic blood pressure in supine position, compared with the baseline measurement (made conventionally equal to 100), for the three trials at the various assessments.

	Standing systolic B.P.			Standing diastolic B.P.		
Assessment	Trial 1	Trial 2	Trial 3	Trial 1	Trial 2	Trial 3
	95.74	97.53	93.82	94.33	96.31	94.38
II	93.08	91.62	---	92.45	90.58	---
III	90.42	89.62	89.01	90.56	85.80	92.03
IV	88.29	---	86.12	87.73	---	87.49
V	86.17	86.86	---	85.84	86.00	---
VI	85.63	85.07	86.84	84.90	84.44	84.33

RESULTS

The Pfizer Italiana trial (trial 1)[2] considered 1606 hypertensive patients treated for more than 30 days, with 6 assessments (plus the baseline measurement) during this period. The nonhospital cardiologists trial (trial 2)[4] studied 453 patients, and the hospital cardiologists trial (trial 3)[5] involved 201 cases ; these last two trials were carried out for 3 months, with respectively 11 and 8 assessments (including the baseline measurement).

The accompanying tables show the baseline blood pressure values (Table 1), the percentage values (calculated on a conventional baseline value of 100) for both systolic and diastolic blood pressure measurements in the supine (Table 2) and standing (Table 3) positions, the heart rate during the trials (Table 4), the doses of prazosin (Table 5) and, for trials 1 and 2 only, the clinical results expressed in percentages (Table 6). Tables 2, 3, 4 and 5 report the data evaluated at the various assessments which took place at the same times, with reference to the beginning of the treatment, in all three trials.

Table 4. Average values of the heart rate (b/min) in the supine position at the various assessments during the three trials.

Assessment	heart rate (b/min)		
	Trial 1	Trial 2	Trial 3
Basseline	80	79.5	77.3
I	80	80.0	78.8
II	79	--	--
III	--	79 7	83.5
IV	79	79.2	78.5
V	77	78.4	--
VI	79	79.4	78.5

Table 5. Average doses of prazosin (b/die) used at the various assessments during the three trials.

Assessment	Doses of prazosin (b/die)		
	Trial 1	Trial 2	Trial 3
I	2.5	1.45	1.78
II	2.8	1.7	--
III	3.0	2.05	2.94
IV	3.0	--	4.14
V	3.1	2.23	--
VI	3.1	2.12	4.5

It is impossible to compare the side effects observed during the three trials because trial 1 specified the frequency of the various side effects reported at each assessment, but trial 2 and trial 3 only refer generically to "side effects". However, without going into detail, the type of side effects reported is the same in trials 2 and 3 as for trial 1[5]. The only important difference on this point concerns severe side effects, like faintness at the first administration or immediately following an increase in the dosage : the frequency of these severe side effects is practically the same in trial 1 (Pfizer-sponsored : 0.72 %) and trial 2 (nonhospital cardiologists : 0.88 %) but is higher in trial 3 (hospital cardiologists : 3 %).

DISCUSSION

We have reported the above data principally in order to stimulate some considerations :

1. The aforesaid decree of the Ministry of Health requires Italian pharmaceutical firms to do postmarketing surveillance studies, without assigning responsabilities or specifying the methods to be followed in order to achieve this goal. The spontaneous reports on drugs which filter down from physicians to detailmen are in our country generally unverifiable, anecdotal, and devoid of critical appraisal and objectivity. The attempts made by the Italian center for drug surveillance (an organization connected with the W.H.O.) have so far resulted in no substantial response from doctors and from the majority of the hospitals. The only way the decree can become actually operative is through the extensive cooperation and involvement of the medical department in each pharmaceutical firm.
2. Medical departments in the pharmaceutical firms are not officially recognized by the Italian Ministry of Health, so many bureaucratic duties that, by their very nature, pertain to the province of medical department responsibilities (such as signing the reports for registration purposes) must be handled by the technical director. No one can reasonably ignore the situation of creating responsibilities without designating the person

Table 6. Overall clinical results (expressed in %) of treatment with prazosin in trials 1 and 2.

Results	Trials 1	Trials 2
A – excellent	41.0	
48.96		
B – good	41.0	36.01
Total A + B	82.0	84.97
C – poor	8.7	7.77
D – unsatisfactory	9.3	7.25
Total C + D	18.0	15.02

responsible for them, which currently burdens the medical departments in our country.
3. The results we have just presented herein testify that in practice no difference can be observed, in postmarketing surveillance, between a trial monitored by a pharmaceutical firm's medical department (trial 1) and a trial organized and monitored by independent medical associations (trials 2 and 3).
4. If the duty of postmarketing surveillance is attributed by law to the pharmaceutical firms, the role of medical departments must be recognized by the government authorities, and an attempt must be made to avoid the doubts and criticism recently directed at post-marketing surveillance trials both by the nonmedical press[6,7] and by parliament. It is very strange, in cour opinion, to assign medical duties to pharmaceutical firms but neglect to legally recognize medical departments and the responsabilities connected with them. We hope the Italian situation will change in the future from this point of view as well.

REFERENCES

1. Bartorelli C., A. Bertelli, A. Giotti and U. Teodori eds, *Problemi e prospettive dell'ipertensione arteriosa*, Rome, ESAM, 1978.
2. Forte V. and M. Ciampini, "L'attività antiipertensiva del prazosin in pazienti ambulatoriali — studio policentrico italiano in medicina generale" *in* : C. Bartorelli, A. Bertelli, A. Giotti and U. Teodori eds, l.c., pp. 325-36.
3. Italy, Ministero della Sanità, Presentazione da parte delle imprese farmaceutiche di rapporti informativi periodici sull'impiego di specialità medicinali registrate a proprio nome, *Gazetta Ufficiale della Repubblica Italiana* **83**, 25 March 1980, p. 2644.
4. Fernandez C., G.F. Cuttitta and P. Santoro, Farmacovigilanza sul territorio — studio de ll'attività antiipertensiva del prazosin, *Biol. Med.* **2** (1980), 351-75.
5. Pessina A.C., M. Hlede and E. Piccolo, *Valutazione policentrica dell'attività antiipertensiva del prazosin — studio coordinato dall'A.N.M.C.O.*, in press.
6. Letter to the Editor : "Farmaci a corso forzoso", *Paese Sera*, 9 April 1980.
7. Letter to the Editor : "Indagini policentriche", *Il Giornale Nuovo*, 10 April 1980.

Sécurité et médicaments (1982), pp. 257-262
Pergamon Press France

Current Concepts for Assessing the Drug Adverse event Relationship and their Problems

J. HASFORD

Institut für Medizinische Informationsverarbeitung, Statistik und Biomathematik der Universität München, Marchioninistr. 15, D. 8000 München 70, West Germany

Abstract — The symptomatology of an Adverse Drug Reaction is in general not pathognomonic for a certain drug. The problem of assessing different degrees of prabability of the drug — event relationship e.g. unlikely, possible, definite, gets even more serious because of the polypragmatic therapy most patients receive. The interobserver variability even of experts is considerable. Irey assessed only 220 of 824 alleged ADR-cases as ADRs according to the WHO definition. Similar poor results presented by Koch-Weser and others emphasize the difficulty and the importance of a valid and reproducible assessment of ADRs[5, 11]. Presently available methods to verify a suspected drug — ADR relationship are :
1. Epidemiological criteria (Bradford-Hill), 2. Decision-algorithms[9, 11, 2, 3]. The structure and the criteria used in these algorithms will be described, compared to each other and critically assessed. Basically the use of algorithms diminishes interobserver variability i.e. increases reproductibility of the assessment. Validity presents still a major problem. Moreover some of the criteria create problems of their own. For all that, research should be continued in this field. Physicians, regulating authorities and scientists urgently need a valid assessment of alleged cases of ADRs. As long as this problem is unsolved, terms like adverse drug event or alleged or suspected ADR should be preferred to "ADR".

The wide-spread use of the term "Adverse Drug Reaction" gives the impression that there is the possibility of an effortless diagnosis of a causal drug — adverse reaction relationship. But the assessment of the degree of probability of a true drug — adverse event relationship still presents a major problem.
The interobserver variability even of experts is considerable. Koch-Weser[13] reported that of 500 suspected ADRs evaluated by three clinical pharmacologists only 21 % were definitely assessed as ADRs and they disagreed about the drug most likely responsible for the ADR in 36 % of the cases. Irey[10], Blanc[2], Karch[11] and Naranjo[17] presented similar poor results. The reasons for this rather unsatisfactory situation are among others : Lack of specifity of the reaction, polymorbid and polypragmatically treated patients, lack of empirical knowledge in medicine and lack of data about the specific ADR-case.

Finally, the doctors evaluate the cases with a 'method' characterized by Hammond[6] : "Known data, but unknown human data processing". That's why Feinstein [5] and Karch and Lasagna[11, 12] stronfly emphasized the necessity and importance of a valid and reliable method for identifying an adverse drug reaction and for assessing the cause-effect relationship between the drug and the reaction.

To tackle this problem decision-algorithms have been developed and published in the last years. In the following, I will talk about five of these :
Irey[8, 9], Karch *et al.*[12], Dangoumau *et al.*[3], Blanc *et al.* [2] and Kramer *et al.*[14]

An algorithm is in this context understood as a formalized procedure to process the information about a single alleged ADR-case in order to identify an ADR as such and to assess the probability of a true drug — ADR relationship.

The criteria for the evaluation of the drug — event relationship used in these algorithms are :

Patient Compliance :
Did the patient take the drug before the event started ?

Temporal Sequence :
Was the interval between drug intake and event appropriate (for example : agranulocytosis one day after therapy with Chloramphenicol is not appropriate) ?

Known Reaction to Drug :
Is the event a well known and accepted reaction to the drug (reports in the literature etc.) ?

Dechallenge :
Was dechallenge attempted and did the event improve ?

Rechallenge :
Was rechallenge attempted and did the event relapse or exacerbate ?

Other Drugs :
Did the patient get any other drugs ?

Alternative Etiologic Candidates :
Is the event reasonably explained by clinical state, underlying or not yet recognized diseases or other non drug therapies or diagnostic interventions ?

Event Pattern :
Is the clinical symptomatology typical of a well known adverse drug reaction ?

Drug Levels :
Were drug levels in body fluids or tissue measured ?

Special Disposition :
Did further special examinations take place such as proof of an enzyme deficiency ?

Table 1 shows in a simplified manner the use of the criteria in the different algorithms. Most criteria are used in all the algorithms, except for : Other drugs, event pattern, drug level and special disposition. For the criterion "known reaction to drug" Blanc *et al.*[2] assessed the literature according to their scientific credibility : proved by clinical trial or large scale monitoring › few reports only › no reports at all.
Dangoumau[3] developed a special rating of the literature, which is done separately and after the evaluation of the clinical case in order to avoid bias. Both the clinical case and the assessment of literature are scored separately.

How to work with an algorithm ? Blanc *et al.*, Dangoumau *et al.* and Karch *et al.* use a decision-table, Kramer a decision-tree respectively a questionnaire. The treating physician or the researcher, who wants to assess a single alleged ADR-case goes through all the criteria and tries to answer these within the requirements of the algorithm. The result is scored and leads to a given set of degrees of probability of a true drug — ADR relationship.

Table 1. Use of the criteria in the different algorithms

	IREY	KARCH	DANGOUMAU	BLANC	KRAMER
PATIENT COMPLIANCE	X	X		X	X
TEMPORAL SEQUENCE	X	X	X	X	X
KNOWN REACTION TO DRUG	X	X	X	X	X
DECHALLENGE	X	X	X	X	X
RECHALLENGE	X	X	X	X	X
OTHER DRUGS	X				
ALTERNATIVE ETIOLOGIC CANDIDATES	(X)	X	X	X	X
EVENT PATTERN	X		X	X	
DRUG LEVELS	X		X	X	X
SPECIAL DISPOSITION			X		

These are : (Table 2)
Negative, doubtful, unlikely
Coincidental
Possible, plausible
Probable
Causative, definite, certain.

Did the patient receive more than one drug, the assessment has to be done for every drug separately. The drug with the highest degree of probability is chosen then as the most probable causative agent.

The extent of differentiation of the criteria varies with the algorithms but can't be demonstrated here.

Due to the time limit I can only present some ideas about the advantages and limitations of these algorithms.

1. The use of algorithms ensures that a minimum set of possibly intervening factors is checked and the factors are weighted in the same way. As Hutchinson *et al.*[7] and Leventhal *et al.*[15] reported, the reliability increases considerably with the use of their[14] algorithm. In addition, it is easier to find out the reason of interobserver variability in a particular case.
2. Most algorithms implicitly try to answer two questions : is there an ADR at all, and is there a specific drug — ADR relationship ? Their application works like a screening for true ADRs according to the particular definition of ADR ; it separates the chaff from the wheat. Karch's, Kramer's and partly Blanc's algorithms look for underlying causes of ADRs like overdosage, poor prescribing or drug interaction.
3. As Mayer *et al.*[16] reported, the use of an algorithm takes less time to assess a single

Table 2. Degrees of probability used in different algorithms

	IREY	KARCH	DANGOUMAU	BLANC	KRAMER
NEGATIVE, DOUBTFUL, UNLIKELY	X	X	X	X	X
COINCIDENTAL	X	X		X	
POSSIBLE, PLAUSIBLE	X	X	X	X	X
PROBABLE	X	X	X	X	X
CAUSATIVE, DEFINITE, CERTAIN	X	X		X	X

ADR-case than an unstructured overall assessment. But when you have a patient, who receives a lot of drugs, using an algorithm may be quite time consuming, because the probability for each drug has to be assessed on its own. This may limit the use by the clinician.

4. The decision rules are not sufficiently differentiated, only in Kramer's algorithm more than "yes" or "no" answers are planned. Mayer *et al.*[16] demonstrated that about 25 % og alleged ADRs couldn't be assessed with Karch's *et al.* algorithm, mainly because reality doesn't fit into the rigid frame of this algorithm. The referred publications do't even mention this point.

5. The criteria "temporal sequence", "known reaction to drug" and "event pattern" are not independent from each other. Additionally the criterion "known reaction to drug" creates problems because of its basing on literature. Dangoumau[3,4] and Karch[12].

6. To ascertain the label "definite" rechallenge with exacerbation or relapse is necessary in all algorithms except for Kramer's and Dangoumau's (cases with overdosage excluded). This is problematic, because : ethical considerations mostly do not allow rechallenge. As Hammond [6] reported, the frequency of rechallenge is less than 5 %. Rechallenge is impossible, if the ADR is irreversible or lethal or has a long latency period or the drug hasn't been dechallenged before. Furthermore the ADR is being treated quite often and tolerance versus the ADR can develop. Logically, this together with the weight of "dechallenge" restricts the label "definite" to non serious, short latency and short time ADRs in patients without grave indications for this particular drug. Moreover, there is little help to assess adverse non drug reactions, previously unknown ADRs, therapeutic failures and rebound phenomenons.

7. Criteria and degrees of probability have partly not yet been defined. What is dechallenge ? Does it include dosage reduction or not ? Accordance among the algorithms must not be expected therefore at present. Begaud *et al.*,[1] report and interalgorithm reliability of only 25 %.

8. The algorithms have not yet been fully operationalized. Personal judgement is necessary for "alternative etiologic candidate" and "event pattern" etc. This impedes reliability.
9. Validity still poses a major problem. Karch *et al.* and Kramer *et al.* validated their algorithms with experts' opinion, the others don't mention, how they did it. But even experts' opinion can be wrong.

Despite these still unsolved problems, decision-algorithms seem to be a useful tool to investigate the probability of a true drug-ADR relationship. In order to act adequately the single physician or the researcher in general does not need the definite knowledge of a causal relationship. But he needs an estimation of the probability of a causative drug — ADR relationship to assess the risk — benefit ratio. Regulatory authorities are in a similar situation[18].

To me, it is quite obvious, that the algorithms in their present state are a first step and not a final solution. The problem is now : How to improve them ?

There are to my opinion at least four possible ways of improvement :

1. To try more sensitive criteria within the algorithms in order to make them fit better to clinical reality.
2. To weight the criteria differently, according to their importance to the assessment of causality.
3. To compare empirically the results of decision-algorithms with each other and with the clinical evidence.
4. To find out if there are optimal algorithms for specific ADRs. It may be that there is no single algorithm, which is optimal for all situations.

REFERENCES

1. Begaud B., A. Boisseau, H. Albin and J. Dangoumau, Assessment of Adverse Drug Reactions — A Comparison of four Methods (abstr.), World Conference on Clinical Pharmacology & Therapeutics, London, 1980.
2. Blanc S., P. Leuenberger, J.P. Berger, E.M. Brooke and J.L. Schelling, Judgements of trained observers on Adverse Drug Reactions, *Clin. Pharmacol. Ther.* **25** (1979), 493.
3. Dangoumau J., J.C. Evreux and J. Jouglard, Méthode d'imputabilité des effets indésirables des médicaments, *Thérapie* **33** (1978), 373.
4. Dangoumau J., B. Begaud, A. Boisseau and H. Albin, Méthodes d'identification et d'imputabilité des effets indésirables des médicaments, *Thérapie* **35** (1980), 287.
5. Feinstein A.R., Clinical biostatistics — XXVIII. The biostatistical Problems of pharmaceutical Surveillance, *Clin. Pharmacol. Ther.* **16** (1974), 110.
6. Hammond K.R. and C.R.B. Joyce, "Psychological Influences on Human Judgement, especially of Adverse Reactions", *in : Drug Monitoring*, F.H. Gross, W.H.W. Inman eds, London, Academic Press, 1977, p. 269.
7. Hutchinson T.A., J.M. Leventhal, M.S. Kramer, F.E. Karch, A.G. Lipman and A.R. Feinstein, An Algorithm for the operational assessment of adverse drug reactions : II. Demonstration of reproducibility and validity, *JAMA* **42** (1979), 633.
8. Irey N.S., "Diagnostic Problems in Drug-induced Diseases", *in : Drug-Induced Diseases*, L. Meyler, H.M. Peck eds, Vol. IV, Amsterdam, Excerpta Medica, 1972, p. 1.
9. Irey N.S., Tissue Reactions to Drugs, *Am. J. Path.* **82** (1976), 617.
10. Irey, N.S., Adverse drug reactions and death. A Review of 827 cases, *JAMA* **236** (1976), 575.

11. Karch F.E., C.L. Smith, B. Kerzner, J.M. Mazullo, M. Weintraub and L. Lasagna, Adverse Drug Reactions – a Matter of Opinion, *Clin. Pharmcol. Ther.* **19** (1976), 489.

12. Karch F.E. and L. Lasagna, Toward the operational Identification of Adverse Drug Reactions, *Clin. Pharmacol. Ther.* **21** (1977), 247.

13. Koch-Weser J., E.M. Sellers and R. Zacest, The Ambiguity of adverse drug reactions, *Europ. J.Clin. Pharmacol.* **11**(1977), 75.

14. Kramer M.S., J.M. Leventhal, T.A. Hutchinson and A.R. Feinstein, An Algorithm for the operational assessment of adverse drug reactions : I. Background, description and instructions for use, *JAMA* **242** (1979), 623.

15. Leventhal J.M., T.A. Hutchinson, M.S. Kramer and A.R. Feinstein, An Algorithm for the operational assessment of adverse drug reactions : III. Results of tests among clinicians, *JAMA* **242** (1979), 1991.

16. Mayer I., M. Meuth and R. Schuhmacher, Intensive Drug Monitoring, Medizinische Dissertation, Universtät Heidelberg, 1979.

17. Naranjo C.A., U. Busto, E.M. Sellers, M. Spino, P. Sandor, I. Ruiz, E.A. Roberts, E. Janacek and D.J. Greenblatt, Improved Reliability using a rating Scale to assess the Probability of Adverse Drug Reactions (Abstr.), World Conference on Clinical Pharmacology & Therapeutics, London, 1980.

18. Überla K.K., Statistische Gesichtspunkte zur Überwachung unerwünschter Nebenwirkungen zugelassener Medikamente, Vortrag am Methformin-Symposium, 7. 3. 1980, Wien.

Sécurité et médicaments (1982), p. 263

Methodological and Statistical Problems in the Evaluation of Data on Adverse Drug Reaction

J. SCHERER and A. STRAUSS*

* Psychiatric Clinic of the University of Munich, Nussbaumstrasse 7, 8 000 München 2, West Germany

Abstract — 7 000 inpatients from four psychiatric hospitals were monitored in one year in the course of monitoring adverse drug reactions. During data acquisition via computer, the plausibility and formal correctness were checked immediatily. The time structure of the data was taken into account when establishing the files. During evaluation, for which a separate program package was developed, details on the patients previous history, the clinical findings and the course of the drug therapy were considered in addition to adverse drug reactions. During evaluation, the frequency, the time of occurence and the intensity of adverse drug reaction were determined for the drugs given. The risk that an adverse drug reaction occurs is assessed. The risk means the relative frequency of the occurence of an adverse drug reaction in the case of a drug. The lower and upper bound for the risk of an adverse drug reaction for specific drugs is determined. A procedure for the optimum assessment of the bounds is stated. The problem of the interaction of drugs with respect to an adverse drug reaction is also investigated with the aid of statistical methods. For certain drugs a plausible estimated value for the risk of the occuence of an adverse drug reaction can be given. This was also possible when the drug is given in conjunction with other drugs.

Sécurité et médicaments (1982) pp. 265-273

Post-marketing Surveillance Methodology as Applied in a Pharmaceutical Medical Department

A. EMANUELI and G. SACCHETTI*

*Funzione Medica, Divisione Farmaceutica Italia, Farmitalia Carlo Erba, Via Imbonati, 24, Milano, Italy

Abstract — Postmarketing surveillance is becoming a relevant part of the medical evaluation of pharmaceutical products because there is a real need of an early warning on the adverse reactions which escape detection in premarketing clinical trials. Practical reasons limit the sensitivity of present methods to events with a frequency around 0.5-1 ‰. For rare and much delayed ADRs only spontaneous or pasive monitoring are the methods on which out of necessity we must rely at present.

The Authors review their experience in the methodology concerning validation of ADRs, planning of postmarketing surveillance trials and use of computers for analysing results.

On the basis of such experience the Authors feel that postmarketing surveillance trials which can be carried out by a medical department of a pharmaceutical company should be planned also to supply information on how the drugs are actually employed by practising physicians so as to orient them on their proper clinical use. This approach could help in reducing the frequency of ADRs due to misuse of drugs which are the most commonly encountered and can be easily prevented.

Postmarketing surveillance carried out by practising physicians with the technical aid of the pharmaceutical companies should be a running program meant to monitor also the efficacy of drugs and to identify new fields for their application.

The very fact that for years the subject of post-marketing surveillance has been discussed worldwide means that there is no easy solution to this problem. So far reasonably good techniques have been developed for the demonstration of the beneficial effects of drugs, now we need to improve the available methods for the evaluation of the risk of untoward reactions, especially the rare ones. In fact, at this writing there is no efficient program which can assure that rare events can always be detected in the early phases of marketing. The current interest in this subject has been stirred up by well known disasters as for example the thalidomide or practolol experience, and everyone now concerned with the safety of new drugs wants assurance that dramatic untoward events will not occur in large populations in the future. Consequently, a lot of emphasis has been put on PMS, a term covering all systems suggested for monitoring beneficial and untoward effects of drugs available on the market and their patterns of use in med ical practice. The present situation in this field and how it could reasonably evolve in the near future is illustrated in figure 1. As it can be seen private and public organiza-

tions are involved and the feeling is that PMS will eventually be conducted along the following main lines :
1. large epidemiological studies carried out by public organizations on data bases of hospitals, health care programs etc., possibly with record linkage and coordinated by a state or private non-profit unit for drug surveillance,
2. passive monitoring carried out by pharmaceutical industries and public organizations,
3. PMS prospective trials carried out by pharmaceutical industries for alerting and training of practising physicians to regularly report their drug experiences. In addition, these trials should supply information on the best use of drugs especially in order to reduce the occurrence of untoward reactions due to overdosage, which are the most frequent and likely to be avoided.

Pharmaceutical industries at present have the "know how" to carry out well designed PMS prospective trials on a few thousand or at the most ten or twenty thousand patients using their international facilities.

These studies in our opinion should include as an important issue the training of physicians to observe rare events, and one way to do this is to familiarize them with the

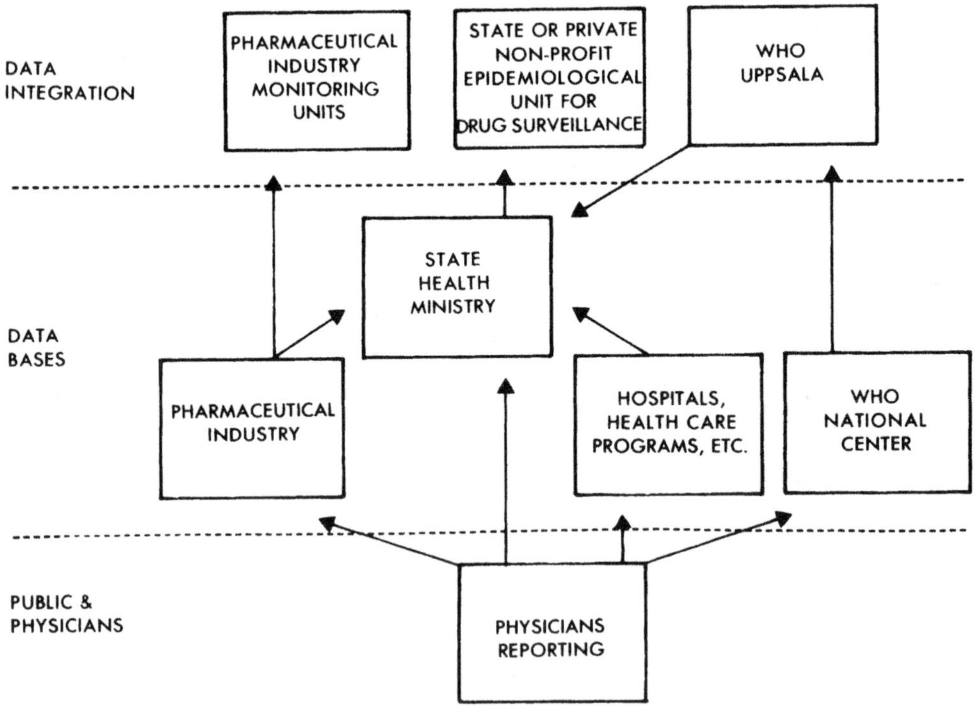

Fig. 1. Scheme of the outflow of information from reporting physicians to data integration organizations including a suggested epidemiological unit for drug surveillance

QUESTIONS

1. Was there an appropriate time relationship between agent and event ?
2. The possibility that clinical state or other therapies may explain the event can be ruled out ?
3. Is the event a known reaction to agent or drugs of the same chemical group ?
4. Did the event cause discontinuation of treatment ?
5. Did the event improve when dosage reduced (or agent withdrawn) or deteriorate when dosage increased ?
6. Did patient experience the event or similar events with similar drugs ?
7. Did the event relapse on rechallenge ?
8. Did patient experience the event or similar events with drugs of the same or closely related chemical groups ?

ANSWERS

1	2	3	4	5	6	7	8	ADVERSE REACTION RELATIONSHIP WITH DRUG
NO	NO	NO						Unrelated
YES	NO	NO						
YES	NO	YES						DOUBTFUL
YES	YES	NO						
YES	YES	NO	NO	NO	NO	YES one or both		Probable
YES	YES	YES	NO	NO	NO	NO	NO	
YES	YES	YES	YES or NO	YES one or both		NO	NO	Almost definite
YES	YES	YES	YES	YES or NO	YES or NO	NO	NO	
YES	YES	YES	YES or NO	YES or NO	YES or NO	YES one or both		Definite

READ QUESTIONS FROM LEFT TO RIGHT. CHECK ANSWERS AND PROCEED TO RIGHT FOR CLASSIFYING ADVERSE REACTION.

Fig. 2. Decision table for the categorization of adverse reactions observed in large scale clinical trials use of an algorithm for the categorization of untoward events. In fact, an efficient algorithm should improve the assessment of the relationship of events with drug therapy and foster critical examination by physicians of all possible information which may be relevant to the early recognition of new adverse drug reactions. In addition, the algorithm approach allows good standardization of judgement and with its aid a new drug adverse reactions profile can be outlined in a more sophisticated manner in comparison with traditional reports[1]. The algorithm which we have suggested is reported in figure 2. It is presented as a decision table based on eight questions. When an event results "unrelated" on the basis of the answers to the first three questions there is no point in proceeding with the other questions. If the event is categorized as "possible" (YES to question 1 and 2), then a positive answer to question 7 or 8 or both turns it into "probable". An event categorized as probable on the basis of the first three questions becomes "almost definite" if also question 4, 5 or 6 have a positive answer. Finally, it is "definite" as far as its relationship with a drug is concerned if question 7 or 8 or both are answered YES. Needless to say, in the individual patient the definition of an event as unrelated to a given drug always leaves the possibility open that it may become suspicious if it is observed in several other patients. In this case specifically de-

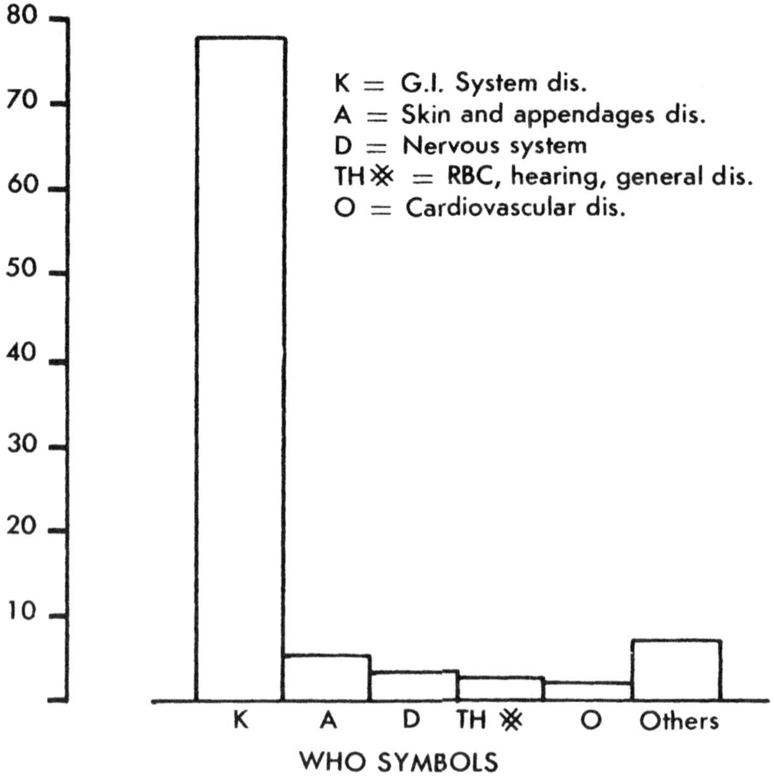

Fig. 3. Breakdown of adverse reactions observed during the Indoprofen PMS prospective trial.

signed studies may be necessary. Algorithms allow only a statement of probability that clinical events may be drug related. They frequently do not tell the truth but are nonetheless invaluable for standardizing judgement between observers. From this angle the proposed algorithm has been validated by a panel examining a list of 30 adverse events obtained from actual cases treated during a PMS prospective trial on Indoprofen, a new non-steroidal antiinflammatory drug [3, 4]. Concordance was obtained in 88.5 % of judgments (Kendall's W = 0.926 HS)[2].

Adverse drug reactions profiles can benefit from categorization of events with an algorithm. For instance the quoted study on Indoprofen gave a pattern of adverse reactions typical of NSAIDs (Fig. 3). How reliable this profile can be assumed to be is shown by the algorithm study of the report ed events (Fig. 4)[4]. This approach represents a clear improvement in the assessment of untoward events, it is of practical use and quite adequate for large scale clinical trials.

As a necessary complement of the proposed algorithm we have prepared a specif-

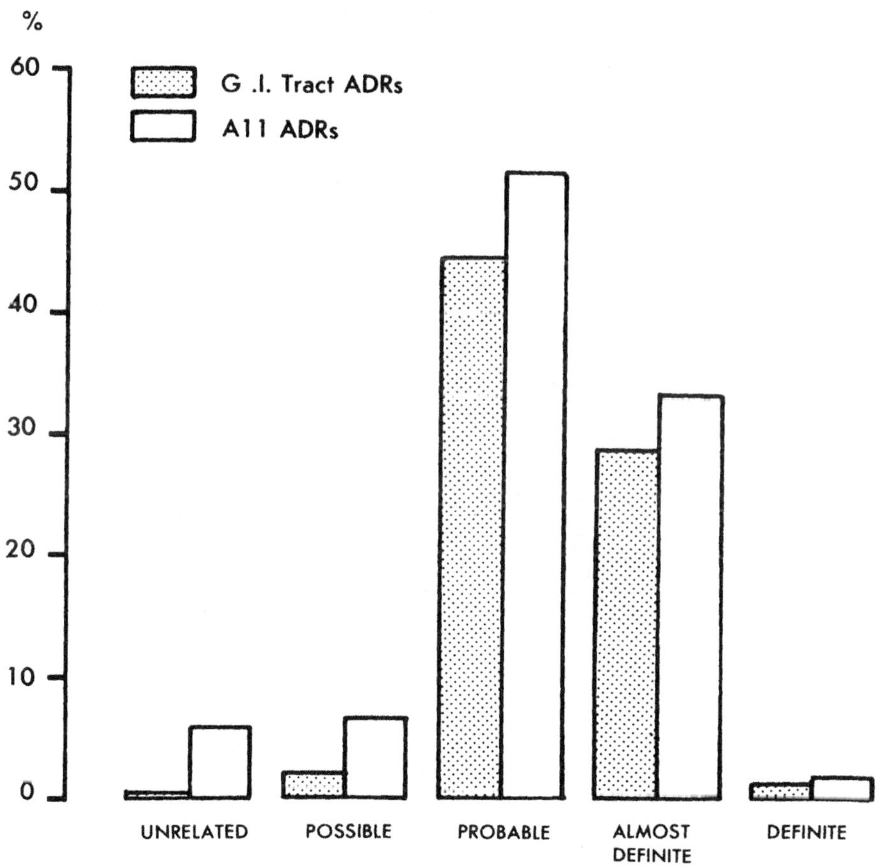

Fig. 4. Adverse reactions reported during the Indoprofen PMS prospective trial and categorized with the decision table shown in fig. 2

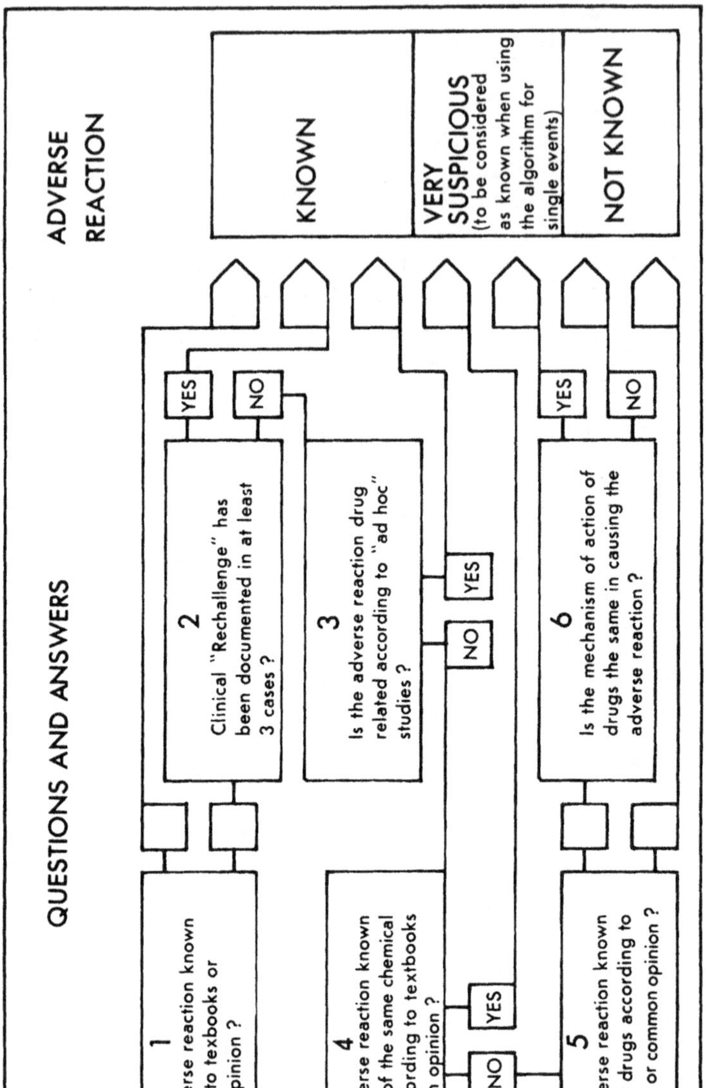

Fig. 5. Algorithm for assessing if an adverse reaction is "known". It should be used when in doubt in answering question 3 of the decision table shown in fig. 2

ic one to define a "known reaction" for a given drug (Fig. 5). This is a crucial point because question 3 of the algorithm for the categorization of adverse reactions if answered YES may shift the decision from "not drug-related" to "drug-related."

Our experience with prospective studies in the area of post-marketing surveillance can be summarized as follows :

1. PMS prospective trials may supply more precise details on the risk of adverse reactions in populations of all ages and with different concomitant diseases and therapies. Better rates of adverse reaction occurrence can be obtained as it is well known that less reactions than expected are reported by investigators in phase 3 studies because mild ones are usually disregarded.
2. Practising physicians usually show interest in PMS studies and are willing to cooperate especially when simple and concise clinical forms are used.
3. No unknown event was detected in PMS prospective trials and the patterns of adverse drug reactions observed correspond to those reported in pre-marketing studies. Also the activity of the drugs was in general confirmed and of the same order of phase 3 trials.
4. Codification of adverse drug reactions for computer analysis is adequate when the WHO list is adopted. In spite of the fact that this list is open ended, nevertheless with some minor adjustement it was shown to be adequate for coding adverse reactions reported in post-marketing surveillance.

The general conclusions that we have reached confirm that PMS prospective trials can be designed so as to duplicate the results of pre-marketing trials both in regard to activity and toleration of drugs with only minor differences. Therefore, they might turn out to be useful to replace some phase 3 studies and allow earlier marketing of new drugs if regulatory authorities are willing to accept them as part of the registration files. PMS prospective trials are most valid for sensitizing large numbers of physicians to the problem of safety studies on new drugs and for making passive or spontaneous monitoring more efficient. It is good that this is done by pharmaceutical companies because doctors are more likely to report adverse reactions to the manufacturer rather than to public organizations. Moreover, only the pharmaceutical industry has the possibility of maintaining frequent and close contacts with practising physicians.

On the basis of our experience we have outlined some proposed guidelines which the industry can adopt for carrying out PMS prospective trials. Most important and critical for the success of these trials is to use them for improving spontaneous monitoring because in past experience it has been frequently contributory and when it failed it was because physicians were not sufficiently stimulated to report their drug experiences.

In conclusion, we expect that each country will set up an epidemiological unit to coordinate adverse reaction reports emerging from data bases containing hundreds of thousands of cases treated with new and old drugs. In this way there might be a definite possibility of an early warning on rare adverse drug reactions. Some years are likely to be necessary before such a program may become operative. Meanwhile, the pharmaceutical industry should concentrate its efforts on stimulating spontaneous monitoring and this can be done with the training provided by well designed and carefully carried out PMS prospective trials.

INDUSTRY ORGANIZED PMS

Proposed guidelines

1. All participants in the PMS should receive the same protocol and forms. Training of physicians to report all clinical events should be firmly emphasized.
2. Adequate selection of physicians should be made, i. e. hospital physicians, general practitioners, etc. In particular, specialists should be enrolled in sufficient numbers on account of their likely experience in observing uncommon signs and symptoms.
3. The number of physicians cooperating in the PMS should be in the order of hundreds so as to ensure an adequate basis for a subsequent efficient passive monitoring.
4. Sampling of patients should be adequate and such as to include special populations as aged persons, children and cases with genetic defects so that interactions may also be revealed between the test drug and other drugs and diseases. Indications for treating patients should be those of the instruction leaflet, because PMS should give a picture of how the drug is actually used when it is available for prescription.
5. The number of patients should be sufficient for detecting events with occurrence of 1 in a thousand, which is the reasonable aim of a prospective trial.
The number of patients should then be over 3.000.
6. Selection of patients should not be biased. For example, if the PMS protocol requires 10 patients to be treated by each physician, then the first 10 patients presenting with diseases included in the prescribing instructions of the product should be treated.
7. All PMS should be planned so as to obtain information on adverse reactions and beneficial effects of the drug as used in ordinary practice so as to allow assessment of the risk/benefit relationship.
8. Adequate validation of adverse reactions should be carried out with an algorithm.
9. The observation of patients should be continued after the end of treatment for as long as possible to provide coverage of at least short-term delayed effects.
10. PMS is to be considered as a program to alert physicians and train them for passive monitoring of untoward events. Physicians, after having reported the data on cases studies for the PMS prospective trial, should also carefully observe all the other patients treated with the test drug, for as long as possible, and report all events observed on special forms for passive monitoring. Physicians should pay particular attention to the study of delayed events, including both therapeutic and adverse effects.

REFERENCES

1. Cuthbert M.F., Adverse reactions to non-steroidal antirheumatic drugs, *Curr. Med. Res. Opin.* **2** (1971), 600-10.

2. Emanueli A. and G. Sacchetti, An algorithm for the classification of untoward events in large scale clinical trials, *Drugs and actions* **7** (1980), 318-22.

3. Emanueli A., V. Mandelli, G. Mascellani and G. Sacchetti, Indoprofen, a new non-steroidal anti-inflammatory drug in the treatment of osteoarthrosis, *Curr. Med. Res. Opin.* **6** (1979), 124-35.

4. Emanueli A. and G. Sacchetti, Extended multiclinical trials and post-marketing surveillance with special reference to the role of the pharmaceutical industry, *Acta Therapeutica* **4** (1978), 313-25.
5. Emanueli A. and G. Sacchetti, Indoprofen in the treatment of osteoarthrosis. Results of a phase 4 multiclinic trial in 1629 patients. IXth European Congress of Rheumatology, Wiesbaden, 2-8th September 1979, abstract n° 4, p. 255.

Sécurité et médicaments (1982), p. 275

Cimetidine as a Model for Post-marketing Safety Assessment

A.C. FLIND and D. ROWLEY-JONES*

*Smith Kline & French Laboratories Ltd, Mundells, Welwyn Garden City, Herts AL 7 1 EY, United Kingdom

Abstract — Tagamet (cimetidine) has provided excellent opportunities for the practical evaluation of both established and new methods of assessing drug safety. The experimental pre-clinical, clinical pharmacological and clinical trial programmes have been extensive and of good scientific quality. Two formal post-marketing surveillance schemes of differing methodology are in progress, one of which described elsewhere in this meeting. Widespread clinical use after marketing in over 100 countries has provided a considerable source of spontaneous reports of adverse events.

Methods of handling, follow-up and evaluation of spontaneous reports to Smith Kline & French U. K. are described. The contribution of data from this source to the solution of specific questions concerning the safety of cimetidine is also described and discussed in relation to that of safety data from other sources. In our experience data from spontaneous reports by themselves have, in rare instances, been conclusive that a problem not detected in pre-marketing clinical trials is associated with cimetidine (e.g. mental confusion in some ill or elderly patients). They can confirm data from other sources (e.g. interaction with anticoagulants), or fail to confirm a theoretical danger (e. g. ulcer perforation on withdrawal of treatment). More often, they add to the large amount of inconclusive information already available. Even so, spontaneous reports of adverse events from vigilant physicians and surgeons have proved so far the most important single source of information on the safety of cimetidine in everyday use since marketing.

Sécurité et médicaments (1982), p. 277

Improving Drug Compliance in a Multi-Cultural Multi-linguistic Society

P.S. TALBOT and L.D. BECKWITH*

*40 Grevillea Way, Blackwood, South Australia 5051, Australia

Abstract — Australia actively promotes the development of an integrated multi-cultural society with retention of ethnic language and English as a second language. Many immigrants have no or poor English ability by virture of their intense cultural ties or lack of language education. Few health professionals have bi-lingual or multi-lingual skills.

This paper studies the cultural and population mix in Adelaide, the South Australian state capital, a city of 933,000 inhabitants and identifies the geographic location of ethnic groups.

Pharmacies are identified which are selected by various ethnic groups for the dispensing of drugs. Pharmacies are geographically pinpointed and the reason for consumer choice differentiated : language, cultural empathy, extended family, peer group referral, ancillary services, locale, and transport. Relevant piospheres are specifically delineated.

Choice bases as perceived by pharmacies are explored in relation to particular ethnic group, also non-choice of pharmacy in equal or better geographic locale, including : available special cultural need or desire, taboos, linguistic ability, ethnicity of staff. Identification is offered of specific measures to ensure patient understanding in the primary language of drug name, type, dose frequency and timing, duration of therapy, common or particular relevant precautions, complications or side-effects.

The study outlines measures for improvement in drug compliance perceived by patient, cultural community and pharmacy.

Conclusion : an outline is presented of existing preferences by non-English-proficient ethnic minorities in obtaining pharmaceutical drugs and outlines measures designed to promote compliance within such sub-cultures.

Sécurité et médicaments (1982), p. 279

1984 and the Committee on Safety of Surgery

D.M. BURLEY

Ciba Geigy, Pharmaceuticals Division Horsham, West Sussex, RH 12 4 AB, United Kingdom

Abstract — The coronary by-pass disaster is described and the events leading to the formation of the Committee on Safety of Surgery in the U.K. Licensing of new surgical techniques has now become mandatory and the consequences of this on the practice of surgery far reaching. New departments of Surgical Techniques have been set up in the major teaching hospitals and a wide range of new surgical journals have come into being.

There is growing concern over the contraction of surgical practice and research, which has led to frustration and a lack of medical students wishing to follow a surgical career.

Sécurité et médicaments (1982), pp. 281-285

Adverse Drug Reaction Monitoring in Psychiatric Hospitals

R. GROHMANN

Psychiatrische Klinik der Universität München, Nußbaumstr. 7,8000 München 2, West Germany

Abstract — In 1979, 4 psychiatric hospitals (with 7650 admissions per year) started an adverse drug reaction monitoring program, designed as a feasibility study for a future establishment of a drug monitoring system in psychiatry in FRG. ADR's were defined as grade I-III according to their seriousness and impact on therapy. Two different approaches were used.
1. Intensiv Drug Monitoring (IDM) : In each of the 4 hospitals 100 patients were randomly assigned to the IDM-procedure. Doctors acting as 'drug monitors' weekly recorded all relevant data of these patients on standardized questionnaires, designed for data processing. 2. Organized Spontaneous Reporting (OSR) : In weekly intervals the drug monitor visited all psychiatric wards including the out-patient department and recorded all ADR of grade III that had occured during the week. An assessment of drug utilisation in the 4 clinics serves as a basis for the calculation of the relative frequency of the observed ADR's. The objective of IDM is an hypothesis-free data collection, the aim of QSR to work as signal-generator and a mediator for continued education of the staff. IDM and QSR are compared in their efficiency in relation to the necessary effort. Preliminary results will be presented. Supported by the Bundesgesundheitsamt Berlin.

Since May 1979 a system of adverse drug reaction monitoring in psychiatric patients has been in operation in the Federal Republic of Germany. Three psychiatric hospitals — those of the universities of Berlin, Göttingen and Munich participate. Together about 3 400 Patients are monitored per year (Berlin = 600, Göttingen = 1 000 and Munich = 1 800 patients) (2).

METHODS

In this system we defined Adverse Drug Reactions (in the following abbreviated as ADRs) according to Seidl *et al.*[1] as 'any adverse response to medication undesired or unintended by the physician'. Inefficacy is not rated as an ADR.

The probability of a causal relationship between drug and unwanted event is rated according to the definition suggested by Seidl *et al.*[1] as 'documented, probable or doubtful'. This rating is done by psychiatrists with extensive experience in psychopharmacology in close contact with the treating doctor.

ADRs are further characterized in our system according to their impact on therapy :

Grade I : The ADR gets registered, but leads to no change in medication.

Grade II : The ADR leads to change in medication which is either a change in dosage or an addition of another drug to counteract the ADR.

Grade III : The ADR leads to discontinuation of the suspected medication, grade III includes as well all new and/or unusual drug reactions.

Our drug monitoring system consists in three elements :
Organized spontaneous monitoring (OSM), intensive drug monitoring (IDM) and the assessment of all drug prescriptions as a basis for the calculation of relative frequencies for the different ADRs.
With the OSM all patients except observed within the IDM are monitored for ADRs grade III exclusively. Weekly the drug monitor — a doctor — visits all wards and asks the doctors whether an alleged ADR grade III has occured.

Then he interviews the doctor for all the necessary data and records these suitably for computer-assisted evaluation. The patient himself is not interviewed by the drug monitor, all the relevant data have to be given by the treating doctor. Anamnestic data, psychopathological and somatic status of the patients at the time of the occurence of the supposed ADR, and details about the ADR like duration, symptomatology etc. are collected. At the time of discharge of the patient a final evaluation of all given drugs, and of the observed ADR is done. This includes an assessment of severity of the ADR too. With the IDM a group of randomly selected psychopharmacologically treated patients — 100 per year and hospital — are monitored intensively from beginning to end of their stay in hospital. ADRs of all grades, psychopathological and somatic status, various laboratory parameters, EEG and ECG data are collected in weekly intervals. Again the main source of information is the treating doctor. The final evaluation is done as it is for the patients within the OSM system.

Assessment of drug prescription is done by taking all information on the prescribed drugs from the patient's records at the end of each year for all in-patients of the year.

RESULTS

Results from the first 18 months of operation of our Drug Monitoring System are presented from the hospitals in Munich and Berlin only. the third participating clinic, Göttingen, started later, so that the results for the first phase of one year of this clinic are not

Table 1. Frequencies of ADRs detected by IDM
Phase I : May 79 - May 80 — Phase II : May 80 - Nov. 80

	Pat.	no ADR	ADR I=II	ADR III
Berlin I	100	29 %	55 %	16 %
Berlin II	30	37 %	43 %	20 %
Munich I	100	41 %	40 %	19 %
Munich II	50	28 %	54 %	18 %

available yet. In both clinics — Munich and Berlin — phase I of one year's duration and phase II of six months' duration have been completed and partly analysed.

The last column (Table 1) demonstrates the frequency of ADRs grade III, that is of ADRs that lead to the discontinuation of the accused medication. In both hospitals and in both phases the frequency was about equal with a rather high rate of 16-20 % ADRs grade III. As for patients who did not experience any ADR at all it seems remarkable that the rate of patients without any observed ADR went down considerably from 41 % to 28 % in Munich in the second phase, mainly due to an increase in ADRs of grad I and II. Perhaps this does not reflect a change in the actual frequency of ADRs but that the doctors begin to look out for ADRs more carefully.

A comparison of the rates of ADRs grade III detected with the IDM versus the OSM system demonstrates the considerable difference of the figures for OSM with 5-6 % in both hospitals in phase I to 16-19 % of the IDM in phase I (Table 2).

Table 2. Frequencies of ADRs grade III detected by IDM and OSM in phase I and II.

Munich I	n=100 19 %	n=1488 6,5 %
Munich II	n= 50 18 %	n= 722 10,4 %
Berlin I	n=100 16 %	n= 440 5,2 %
Berlin II	n= 30 20 %	n= 390 8,2 %

In phase II, the procedure for the OSM has been changed to get a more complete assessment of ADRs grade III. Now the drug monitor on his weekly rounds is 'armed' with a list of all drugs that have been discontinued in the course of the week before. He asks for the reason of discontinuation, so the chance that an event of an ADR grade III is overlooked is lessened. Obviously this led to more complete data, for the rates of ADRs grade III increased in both hospitals to 8 respectively 10 %. Still there remains a striking difference of about 10 % to the discovery rate of ADRs grade III as assessed with the IDM. This difference can't be easily explained but emphasizes the necessity of an intensive drug monitoring system besides the spontaneous reporting, even when this is an organized spontaneous reporting system as ours.

Table 3. Relative frequencies of ADRs grade III connected with neuroleptics, only n $\geqslant$100 patients per drug and only OSM-data included.

Haloperidol	n=743	3,1 %
Perazine	n=419	3,1 %
Laevomeprom.	n=399	1,5 %
Thioridazine	n=186	3,8 %
Penfluridol	n=109	1,8 %

As it is important for the doctor to know the relative risk of ADRs connected with comparable drugs, we calculated the relative frequency of ADRs of grade III for all neuroleptics given to more than 100 patients each in Munich during phase I (Table 3).

The figures include only OSM data. The first column presents the number of patients treated with the drug in the course of phase I. The second column shows the frequency data for ADRs grade III in patients treated with the specific drug in per cent. The rates of ADRs grade III are about 1,5 — 3,8 % and do not differ very much for the five most frequently used neuroleptics with a rate of 3,1 % for Haloperidol, 3,1 % for perazine, 1,5 % for Laevomepromazine, 3,8 % for Thioridazine and 1,8 % for Penfluridol. The corresponding data for antidepressants are slightly higher than those for the neuroleptics and there are greater differences from drug to drug (Table IV).

Table 4. Relative frequencies of ADRs grade III connected with antidepressants, only n = 60 patients per drug and only OSM-data included.

Amitriptyline	n=351	4,0 %
Doxepin	n=104	3,8 %
Clomipramine	n= 98	7,1 %
Dibenzepin	n= 68	4,4 %
Mianserine	n= 67	1,5 %
Tranylcypromine	n= 64	9,3 %

Tranylcypromine shows the highest rate of ADR grade III with 9,3 % and Mianserine — a new tetracyclic antidepressant — shows the lowest rate with 1,5 %. Prior to further conclusions from these data the comparability of the differently treated patients has to be assessed.

Looking for the most frequently observed ADRs grade III in the first 18 months of our system in both hospitals, four ADRs have been observed more than 20 times each (Table V).

These are parkinsonism as the most frequent ADR with 41 cases, akathisia with 40 cases, delirium with 23 and finally depression with 20 cases. Of these data it is most re-

Table 5. Most frequent ADRs grade III observed in phase I and II in Munich and Berlin with IDM and OSM, n = 3300 patients.

Parkinsonism	41 cases
Akathisia	40 cases
Delirium	23 cases
Depression	20 cases

remarkable that drug induced delirium which must be considered a grave drug reaction is among the most frequent ADRs grade III.

Further details about methodology and results which could not be presented here, are to be found elsewhere[2, 3].

In spite of some shortcomings of our methodology we are well aware of, we hope to be on the way of developing, with our drug monitoring system in psychiatry, a useful tool for the assessment of the relative risks of different ADRs connected with the use of different psychotropic drugs.

REFERENCES

1. Seidl L.G., G.F. Thornton and L.E. Cluff, Epidemiological Studies of Adverse Drug Reactions, *Am. J. Publ. Health* **55** (1965), 1170.

2. Rüther E., O. Benkert, F. Eckmann, I. Eckmann, R. Grohmann, H. Helmchen, H. Hippius, B. Müller-Örlinghausen, W. Poser, L. Schmidt, G. Stille, A. Strauß and K. Überla, Drug Monitoring in psychiatrischen Kliniken, Arzneim. — Forsch./*Drug Res.* **30 (II)**, 8 (1980), 1181.

3. Grohmann R., A. Strauss, C. Gehr, E. Rüther and H. Hippius, Zur Praxis der klinischen Therapie mit Psychopharmaka, *Pharmakopsychiat.* **13** (1980), 1.

Sécurité et médicaments (1982), pp. 287-290

A Post-marketing Surveillance Study on Bacampicillin

P. G. PRELLA*, M. CIAMPINI** and E. MICHELETTI***

*Pharmaceutical Division, Pfizer Italiana S. p. A., Roma, Italy
**c/o Medical Department, Pfizer Italiana, Via del Fornetto 85, 00149 Roma, Italy
***Department of Pharmacy, Policlinico Umberto 1, Roma, Italy

Abstract — A decree of the Ministry of Health, issued in March 1980, made post-marketing surveillance (PMS) obligatory by law in Italy. This law requires the manufacturer to send reports to the Ministry of Health twice a year on sales, clinical use and side effects observed during use in the field of recently registered drugs.

PMS data concerning the use by GPs of a new prodrug of ampicillin (bacampicillin) are reported. Bacampicillin was used in more than 3500 patients suffering from infections of the respiratory and urinary tracts as well as skin diseases and needing, in the physician's opinion, antibiotic treatment.

Data were analyzed by a computer on the basis of the age groups, dosage schedule, sites of infection, side effects, and clinical results. All the evaluations were in accordance with the possibilities offered by a normal group of outpatient case histories.

The results are also discussed in relation to the pharmacokinetic properties of bacampicillin.

Drugs registered in Italy after 25 March 1980 must be monitored for the first five years following their introduction on the market[1]. The duty of this monitoring is attributed to the pharmaceutical firms which, every six months (during the first two years ; every twelve months for the remaining three years), must report to the Italian Ministry of Health the number of drug packages sold and the eventual side effects brought to their attention.

In this connection, we report herein on a multicenter trial carried out in Italy by general practitioners using bacampicillin, a relatively new ampicillin prodrug extensively studies in Italy[2, 6], after the introduction on the Italian market of this product at the beginning of 1980. In the first part of our study, 576 patients were evaluated[7], but in this paper we are referring to a different group of 4123 cases. A comprehensive report on the total number of 4699 cases treated in Italy will be published in the future.

A total of 4123 patients were treated, of whom 42.7 % were females and 49.9 % males (sex was not specified in 7.4 %). As regards age, 552 patients (13.4 %) were less than 12 years old ("pediatric age", according to health insurance criteria) ; 493 (12 %) were more than 64 years old.

Table 1 shows the distribution of patients according to the localization of the infections. Fever (meant as body temperature higher than 37° C), one of the most obvious signs of infection, was present before the beginning of bacampicillin treatment in 3391 cases (84,1 % of the cases, considering that in 94 cases no information was given about the presence of fever).

Table 1. Distribution of patients according to diagnostic groups

ENT infections	1713	cases	(41.5 %)
RTI	1205	cases	(29.2 %)
UTI	491	cases	(11.9 %)
Skin and soft tissue infections	361	cases	(8.8 %)
Mouth infections	347	cases	(8.4 %)
Diagnosis not specified	6	cases	(0.1 %)

The patients were treated with 800 mg bacampicillin tablets in 3414 cases (84.3 %) and with 400 mg tablets in 621 cases (15.7 %) (in 88 cases the size of the tablet was not specified). The highest percentage of 800 mg tablet users is found in UTI (91.1 %) and the lowest in ENT infections (78.5 %). Tables 2 and 3 illustrate, for the various localizations of the infections, the number of daily administrations of bacampicillin tablets. It is evident that most of the patients were treated with two or three administrations a day, with a general preference for the twice-daily administration when 800 mg tablets were used.

Table 2. Distribution of cases according to the number of daily administrations of 800 mg bacampicillin tablets.

No. of administrations	UTI	RTI	ENT	Skin	Mouth
1	27	59	74	13	14
2	232 (52.7 %)	558 (52.6 %)	763 (57.6 %)	160 (53.5 %)	160 (55 %)
3	147 (31.1 %)	368 (34.7 %)	385 (29.2 %)	104 (34.8 %)	88 (30.2 %)
4 or more	12	24	19	5	6
Not specified	22	51	79	17	23

Table 3. Distribution of cases according to the number of daily administrations of 400 mg bacampicillin tablets.

No. of administrations	UTI	RTI	ENT	Skin	Mouth
1	7	6	20	3	2
2	11 (25.6 %)	46 (40 %)	184 (51 %)	21 (40.4 %)	21 (42 %)
3	21 (48.8 %)	56 (48.7 %)	134 (37.1 %)	22 (42.3 %)	23 (46 %)
4 or more	2	4	11	1	3
Not specified	2	3	12	5	1

Table 4. Clinical results according to the size of the tablet.

	Excellent	Good	Satisfactory	Poor	Unsatisfactory	Unassessable	* Total
400 mg	309 49.7 %	241 38.8 %	45 7.2 %	3 0.5 %	6 1.0 %	17 2.7 %	621
800 mg	1 732 50.7 %	1 315 38.5 %	234 6.8 %	37 1.1 %	34 1.0 %	62 1.8 %	3 414

* In 88 cases, the size of the tablet used was not specified.

Table 4 shows the clinical results obtained, as evaluated by the physician, in terms of therapy with 400 mg and with 800 mg tablets. In practice, the use of 400 or 800 mg tablets did not yield any observable differences, but the lower dosage was evidently chosen in less severe cases. Table 5 illustrates the clinical results obtained in the various localizations of the infections independently of the dosage used.

Interestingly enough, the number of days of therapy was significantly lower in the group of patients using 800 mg bid than in that using 800 mg tid (5.78 $\pm$ 2.80 vs. 6.02 + 2.58 ; $p < 0.05$), and the same was observed for those subjects using 400 mg tid or bid (5.56 $\pm$ 2.47 vs. 5.08 $\pm$ 2.07 ; $p < 0.01$). It appears that, irrespective of the dosage, the bid schedule is able to significantly reduce the number of treatment days in comparison with the tid schedule. This suggestion is confirmed by the evaluation of the period needed in order to obtain defervescence (2.73 $\pm$ 1.61 with 800 mg bid vs. 3.14 $\pm$ 3.66 tid ; $p < 0.01$; 2,63 $\pm$ 0.95 with 400 mg bid vs. 2.79 $\pm$ 1.05 tid ; $p < 0.05$). These differences are reported in table 6.

As far as side effects are concerned, no side effect was reported in 3708 out of 4123 cases (89.9 %) ; one or more side effects were reported for 346 cases (8.4 %) (no information was given in 69 cases = 1.7 %). In terms of the size of the tablet used, the percentage of side effects was 7.2 % in the cases treated with 400 mg tablets and 8.7 % in those treated with 800 mg tablets. Using 400 mg tablets, no difference was observed between the bid and tid schedule as far as the frequency of side effects is con-

Table 5. Clinical results according to diagnostic groups.

	Excellent	Good	Satisfactory	Poor	Unsatisfactory	Unassessable	Total
UTI	213	209	40	10	12	7	491
RTI	575	497	101	6	11	14	1205
ENT	938	611	93	18	11	42	1713
Skin	163	142	37	5	3	11	361
Mouth	199	124	13	2	4	5	347

Table 6. Average length of treatment and time needed for defervescence according to differentbacampicillin dosage schedules. Statistical comparaison ("Student's" t test).

Number of treatment days	800 mg bid 800 mg tid	5.78 ± 2.80 6.02 ± 2.58	p	0.05	(df 2853)
	400 mg bid 400 mg tid	5.08 ± 2.07 5.56 ± 2.47	p	0.01	(df 516)
Number of days required for defervescence	800 mg bid 800 mg tid	2.73 ± 1.61 3.14 ± 3.66	p	0.01	(df 2242)
	400 mg bid 400 mg tid	2.63 ± 0.95 2.79 ± 1.05	p	0.05	(df 427)

cerned (respectively 7.4 and 7.0 %) ; for 800 mg, the frequency of side effects was higher with the tid schedule (9.7 % as opposed to 8.0 %). Most of the side effects reported were not severe (276 out of 346 = 80 %).

As a summarizing comment, a general practitioners trial confirmed bacampicillin's activity as well as the good tolerance of the drug. The bid regimen seems to be preferred for the better activity it produced (evaluated by using the criteria number of days of treatment and number of days needed in order to obtain defervescence) and for the reduced frequency of side effects. This appears in agreement with other results[8] and may be due to the fact that other pharmacokinetic parameters are possibly more important than the blood levels[9].

REFERENCES

1. Italy, Ministero della Sanità, Presentazione da parte delle imprese farmaceutiche di rapporti informativi periodici sull'impiego di specialità medicinali registrate a proprio nome, *Gazzetta Ufficiale della Repubblica Italiana* **83**, 25 March 1980, p. 2644.

2. Renzini G., G.P. Ravagnan and F.M. Cannistrà, Bacampicillin. Quaderni di Antibiotica, April 1980.

3. Garagnani A., Valutazione clinica dell'efficacia di due diversi schemi terapeutici di un nuovo profarmaco dell'ampicillina (bacampicillina) – nota preliminare, *Cl. Europ.* **19**, 3 (1980), 607-18.

4. Petrucci D., F. Rollo, V. Tini, V. Campanella, D. Pavan and E. Micheletti, Bacampicillina e ampicillina : confronto clinico, *Biol. Med.* **2** (1980), 341-50.

5. Bellentani G., L. Aquino and W. Ingrosso, La bacampicillina in pneumologia, *Riv. Patol. Clin. Tuberc. Pneumol.* **51**, 3 (1980), 209-18.

6. Martelli A., A.M. Martelli and N.G. Melilla, Considerazioni sull'attività clinica di un nuovo profarmaco dell'ampicillina, la bacampicillina, *Cl. Europ.* **19**, 3 (1980), 498-508.

7. De Rosa F., Esperienze cliniche con una nuova aminopenicillina, paper read at the incontro di studio "Nuovi aspetti della terapia con aminopenicilline", Naples, 20 November 1980.

8. Maesen F.P.V. and B.I. Davies, Pulse dosing of bacampicillin in acute exacerbations of chronic bronchitis : a new method of treatment, paper read at the International Symposium "Pulse dosing : theoretical and clinical aspects", Dorado Beach, Puerto Rico, 8-9 May 1980.

9. Bergeron M.G., Continuous or intermittent (pulse) administration of antibiotics : tissue penetration and *in vivo* efficacy, paper read at the International Symposium "Pulse dosing : theoretical and clinical aspects", Dorado Beach, Puerto Rico, 8-9 May 1980.

Sécurité et médicaments (1982), pp. 291-300

Post-marketing Surveillance : Computerized Evaluation of Side Effects

U. QUAST

Behringwerke AG, Postfach 11 40, D. 3550 Marburg/L., West Germany

Abstract — The spontaneous reports of side effects are of great value for the manufacturer and increase largely the safety of a pharmaceutical preparation. However, it is indispensable to completely compile, evaluate and document them. A compilation and evaluation system by means of electronic data processing is described. Documentation is made by a processing machine type HP 1000, the data base system IMAGE 1000, and by self-made programs. About 30 different data are stored for each individual case. The system of coding all symptoms given by the doctors is discussed in details. Description and evaluation of side effects are strictly separated from each other. Also statements which are relevant to biologics are discussed. The documentation should give the possibility to recall, individually or in combination, all storage data, and to use them for control, comparison and statistical purposes. This object has been achieved. Meanwhile the data base in question store 6000 reports of side effects compiled during the last 10 years. It works routinely since January 1st, 1978. So there is an extensive continuously working documentation of side reactions of biological preparations that is available at any time.

Behringwerke have been collecting all adverse reactions (ARs) reported since 1970 in the case of their preparations for human use, regardless of whether a connection of the As with the application of the preparation is probable, improbable or even to be excluded. Precise data on the ARs reported are obtained by the pharma representatives from the physician concerned by means of a comprehensive questionnaire.

The data were originally recorded on margin-punched cards.

In 1977 the increasing volume made it desirable to use an electronic data processing.

The following points had to be borne in mind :

1. The preparations of Behringwerke are "biological" preparations having their own special features. Those preparations are shown in the first table.

Table 1. Biological preparations with different mechanisms of action

1. Killed vaccines
2. Live vaccines
3. Immunoglobulins (from human plasma)
4. Immune sera (from animal sera)
5. Human plasma derivatives as infusion solutions
6. Infusion solutions derived from gelatins
7. Coagulation preparations
8. Fibrinolytic agents
9. In vivo diagnostic aids

2. The original collection of an estimated 150 000 individual data items on about 5 000 individual cases should also be utilized.
3. New accessions of about 600-800 cases annually were to be expected.

Table 2. Individual data stored for each case

1. *Data on preparation and case*
– Name of preparation
– Batch No.
– Documentation number
– Date report received
– Behring branch office
2. *Data on patient*
– Initials
– Domicile
– Age
– Sex
3. *Case history*
– Allergic patient
– Primary diseases (4 inputs possible)
– Indication for application (4 inputs possible)
4. *Data on the adverse reactions described (10 inputs possible)*
– Context
– Causes (2 inputs possible)
– Sequelae
5. *Data on application*
– Date of administration
– Interval before onset of the adverse reaction
– Mode of application
– Prior treatment with the preparation
6. *Number and nature of concomitant drugs (3 inputs possible)*
7. *Physician and reporting date*
8. *Clear text as required*

4. It should be possible to inquire each single input individually or in combination.
5. The print-outs of the computer should be in clear and undestandable text.

The data to be acquired are listed in the next table.

These demand were possible only with coded data.

The ages of the patients, for example, were divided into relevant andreadily aparent age groups ; domicile of patient and physician could be representet with the aide of the postcode used in the Federal Republic of Germany, and modes of application coded with the aid of a numeric code, a.s.o.

Difficulties arose in connection with the following points :

I. *The primary disease*

The intention was to use an already proven code, and after some hesitation we decided on an easily modified form of the 3-digit ICD code (4). In this manner it was possible pass on the already coded primary diseases to the German Medical Commission or the competent superior authorities*, and finally to the WHO, without the risk of input errors during recoding.

II. *The concomitant medication*

Because in biological preparations the concomittant medication is usually irrelevant, we decided to use the only 2-digit number of the "Red List", a German index of manufacturet drugs (6).

III. *The adverse reaction*

We hakd to develop our own code for inputs of the ARs : For this purpose we first analysed our reports. It emerged that over half concerned vaccines. Other reports were expected to centre on gamma-globulins, fibrinolytic agents and infusion solutions.

Table 4. Adverse reactions reported 1970-1979*

Préparation	Number of AR	Percentage
Vaccines	4364	69,4 %
Infusion solutions	1289	20,5 %
Immunoglobulins	326	5,1 %
Heterologous sera	61	1,0 %
Fibrinolytic agents and coagulation preparations	156	2,5 %
Other	93	1,5 %
Total number	6289	100,0 %

*All reports are counted regardless of our judgement concerning the causal connection with thed preparation.

Since in these cases the bulk of te symptoms reported are of the allergic-analylactic form, we had to develop our own code specially attuned to such symptoms.

We decided on what we call a "multiaspect code", in which we separated.

* Federal Public Health Autority or Paul-Ehrlich-Institut

1. *the anatomy*
i. e., the organ in which the AR takes place ; it is stated in hierarchic order. The main groups are reproduced in table 5.

Table 5. Main anatomical groups

Code	anatomy
< 100	not known
100	skin
200	site of application
300	respiratory tract
400	cardiovascular tract
500	skeleton
600	nervous system
700	blood
800	other organs
900	"body as whole"

A sub-division of complications, e.g., in the respiratory tract, is given in table 6.

Table 6. Sub-division of the anatomy/respiratory tract

Code	Anatomy
300	respiratory tract, misc.
310	nose
320	paranasal sinuses
330	mouth/throat/tongue/ tonsils
334	larynx
340	bronchial system
350	lung
360	pleura

2. *The symptoms*
Here we also have endeavoured to groupe the symptoms at closely adjoining positions. Thus, for example, all signs of respiratory distress are included in one of the groups. "Oedema" comes before this group ; "asphyxia" follows.

This allows us not only to inquire about the symptom "respiratory distress" in the individuel case, but in the instance of imprecises definition to call up all respiratory symptoms from "pulmonary oedema" up to asphyxia.

At this point we should mention an ever intellectual difficulty : We endeavour to

Table 7. Coding of the symptoms (e.g., of the respiration)

Code	Anatomy
1851	oedema
1951	asthma
1952	respiratory distress/dyspnoea
1953	bronchospasm
1954	hyperventilation
1955	spasm
1956	stridor
1957	laryngospasm
2051	asphyxia

adapt the reported AR far as possible to the medical description, and to state it without diagnostic evaluation.

The medical diagnosis is irrelevant here. This of course already involves an interpretation of the AR, making a subsequent corrective amendment impossible. We have there-fore strictly separated the symptomatology from our interpretation.

3. *The interpretation of the AR*

After input of the symptoms and anatomy, we have provided its own input for our interpretation of the cases. Here an assessment of the connection is possible from a scientific point of view.

Table 8. Possible inputs for assessment, causes and sequelae

Causal relation	Causes (examp)	sequelae
Proved	Congenital	No
Not to be excluded	rimary disease	Yes*
	Allergic	Not yet
To be excluded	perceptible	
	Contra-indication	
Iatrogenic		No entry
	Preparation or	
inexplicable	vaccine	
Vaccination-Breakthrough/ Lack of effect	Summation Effect/ interaction	

*This statement is usually explained in clear text.

The following are coded for this purpose :
a. the assessment
b. the possible causes
c. the sequelae.

In addition to the coded data it is possibl to add at the end a short input in clear text for each case.

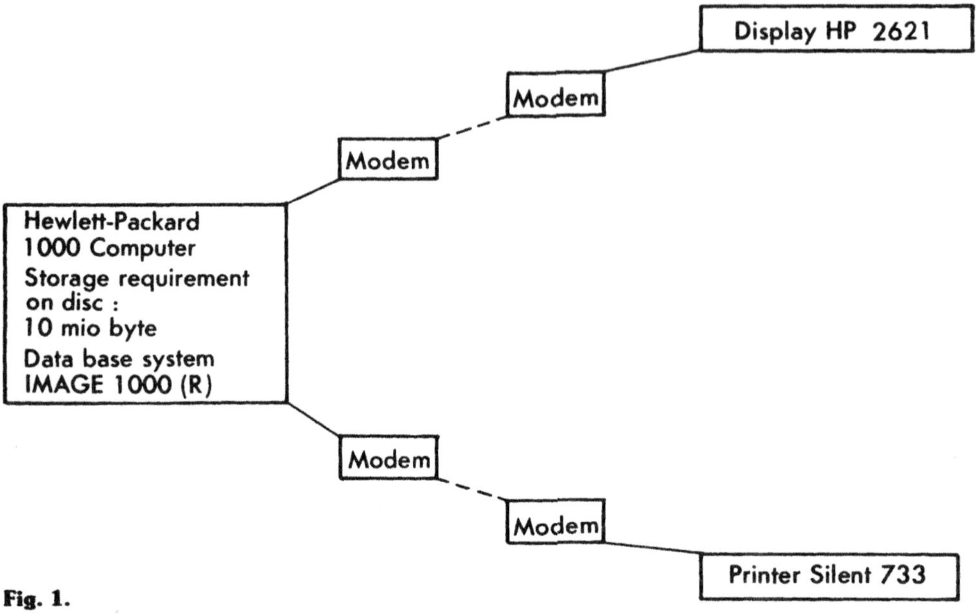

Fig. 1.

The program system is based on the following hardware.

The Medical Department has available a display terminal Type HP 2621(R) for the dialog, and a Silent 733 for print-outs which is also used for other pruposes.
The computer serves primarily as laboratory computer for other applications (on-line acquisition and processing of measurement data).
The required data management was effected with the data base system IMAGE 1000(R) from Hewlett-Packard and the described self-written programs. The capacity is such that all reports arising until the year 2000 can be stored.

The amount of medical information stored per case reported could be increased five-fold in comparison with the former technique with margin-punched cards. Moreover, a very much greater accuracy in classification of a case reported is possible. Thus, for example, 80 different side-effects could be classified on the punched cards, whereas in the computer about 3000 varying side-effects can be described.

The program system is designed for use by medical scientists and secretaries in the Medical Department. Knowledge of computer-handling is not necessary. Various measures were taken for data security and data protection, and all the conditions of German legislation on data protection have been fulfilled.

The structure of the data base is the following :

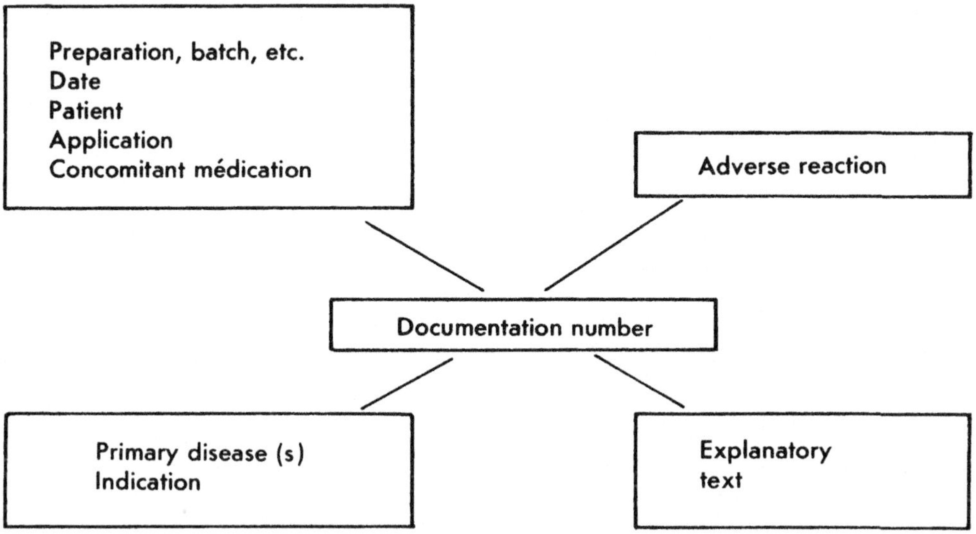
Preparation, batch, etc.
Date
Patient
Application
Concomitant médication
Adverse reaction
Documentation number
Primary disease (s)
Indication
Explanatory
text

Fig. 2.

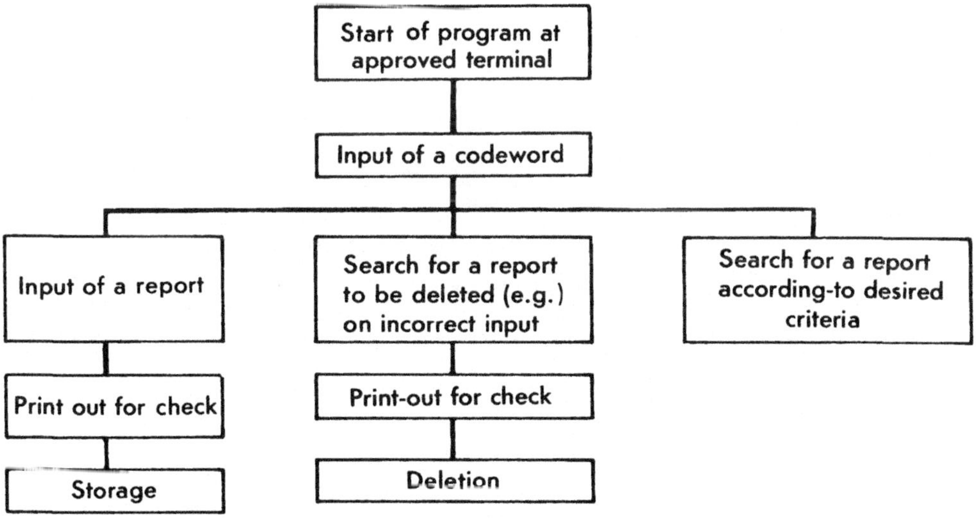
Start of program at approved terminal
Input of a codeword
Input of a report
Search for a report to be deleted (e.g.) on incorrect input
Search for a report according-to desired criteria
Print out for check
Print-out for check
Storage
Deletion

Fig. 3.

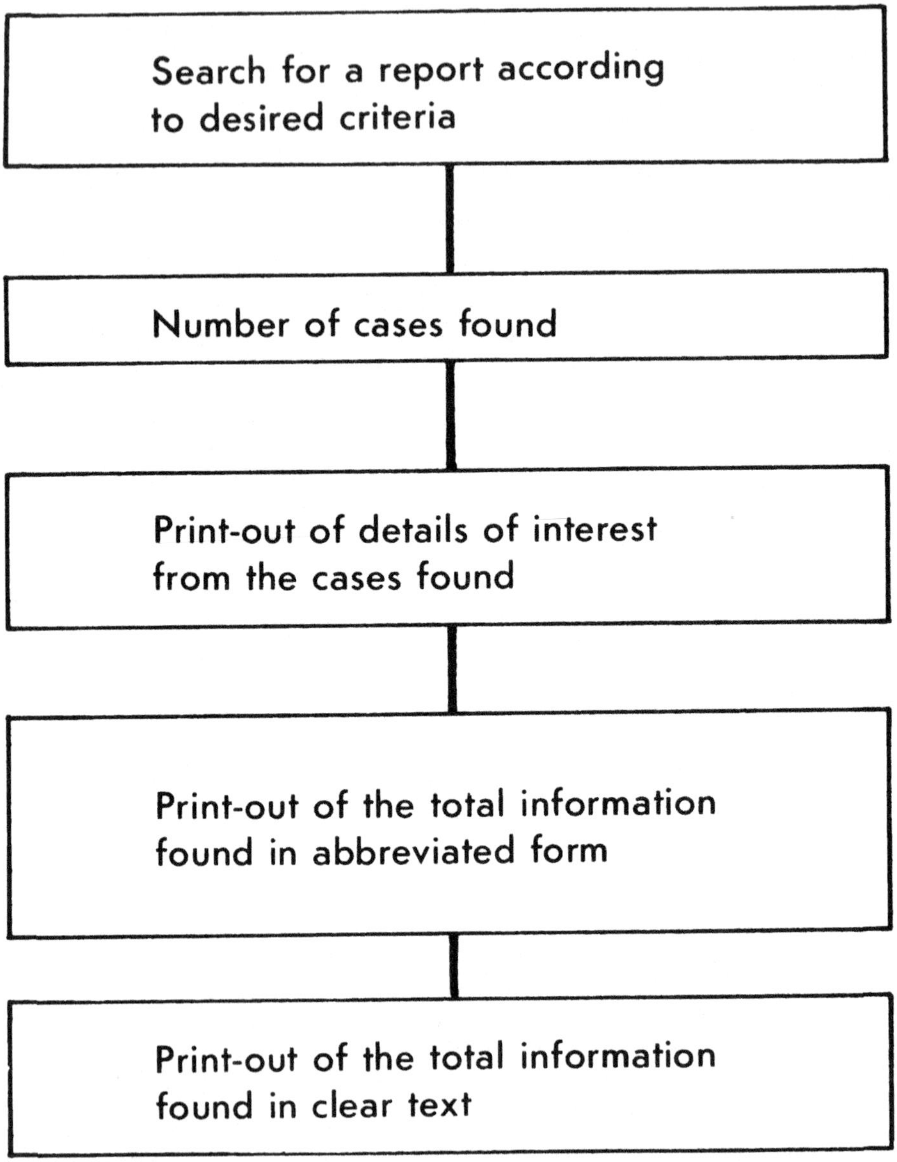

Fig. 4.

Four files are combined by the documentation number. A number of sub-files is grouped around these four files. It is not important for the user to know the structure of the data base. Operation takes place via a dialog with hierarchic graduation and menu selection.

```
************************************************************ 4228  5933*** *
MELDUNG EINER NEBENWIRKUNG
                                          MELDUNG AN BGA / PEI AM ..........
                                          MED.ABT. / DR.QUAST / TH.

                                          KOPIE AN ARZNEIMITTELKOMMISSION

    PRAEPARAT :                     DIPHTERIE-ADSORBAT-IMPFSTOFF
    CHARGENNR. :                    0000
    L - NR. :                        438
    MELDUNG EINGANG :               3/ 1981
    KONTOR :                        MUENCHEN

            PATIENT

    INITIALEN        NN
    ALTER            15-19 JAHRE
    GESCHLECHT       M
    WOHNORT (PLZ)    1000

    ALLERGIKER :          JA
    GRUNDKRANKHEIT(EN) :
     581  NEPHROTISCHES SYNDROM
     250  DIABETES MELLITUS

    INDIKATION ZUR ANWENDUNG :
                          IMPFUNG (PROPH.)
                          IMMUNSTIMULATION
                          KLINISCHE PRUEFUNG

            NEBENREAKTION
            =============

     1. HAUT, PARTIELL
         PETECHIEN
              ZUSAMMENHANG : NICHT AUSZUSCHLIESSEN
   >>         URSACHEN :     ALLERGISCH
   >>         URSACHEN :     PRAEPARAT BZW. IMPFSTOFF
              FOLGEN :       NOCH NICHT ABZUSEHEN

     2. THROMBOZYTEN
         ..PENIE
              ZUSAMMENHANG : NICHT AUSZUSCHLIESSEN
   >>         URSACHEN :     INFEKTIONSKRANKHEIT
              FOLGEN :       KEIN EINTRAG

     3. GELENKE, MEHRERE
         BLUTUNG

     4. GELENKE, MEHRERE
         SCHWELLUNG

     5. LOKALREAKT. SONST.  IMPFORT
         BLUTUNG

    VERABREICHUNGSDATUM :                    2/ 1981
    INTERVALL BIS ZUM AUFTRETEN DER NR :     >12STD - 2TAGE
    APPLIKATIONSART :                        I.M. (PISTOLENIMPFUNG)
    VORBEHANDLUNG MIT PRAEP. :               3 MAL
    BEGLEITMEDIKATION (ANZAHL) :             2
    ARZNEIMITTEL :
    11  ANTIDIABETIKA
    30  CORTICOIDE

    ARZT (NAME) :          SCHM
    ARZT (PLZ) :           1000
    ERLEDIGUNGSDATUM :     4/ 1981

         SIMULATED CASE (SIMULIERTER FALL )
         SHOULD BE EXTINGUISHED AFTER INPUT !
         (MUSS NACH DER EINGABE GELOESCHT WERDEN !)

***********************************************************************
```

After the start of the program a basic function is chosen, i. e., after the computer-question — N E X T ? —
It is keyed in : "input" or
"delete" or
"search" etc.

Incorrect inputs are immediately recognized by the computer and rejected.

Since 1978 the computer has been in routine operation for management of the data on adverse reactions. At the beginning (for approx. one year) mainly inputs were carried out in order to acquire all reports retrospectively, so that we overlook now more than 11 years. Now the data base is used very intensively for inquiries.

The coding and input of one case takes usually 5 minutes. A normal inquiry usually needs the same time and can be done by one intelligent secretary.

Knowledge of all reported ARs makes a scientific treatment of each individual case possible.
We give the enquiring physician information of a possible connection to the AR reported, since with the computer it is easy for us to find similar cases and compare them with the case reported.

For the reports desired in the Federal Republic of Germany to the superior federal authorities — Federal Public Health Authority or Paul-Ehrlich-Institut — we similarly use the easily comprehensible computer print-out, also reporting here all cases which have become known to us, regardless of their degree of severity or of the interpretation of the causal connection with our preparation.
At the moment the management of clinical trials of Behring-werke is being taken onto the same computer according to the same concept.

REFERENCES

1. 2. Arzneimittelgesetz, Gesetz zur Neurodnung des Arzneimittelrechts, vom 1.9.1976.
2. Bock H.E., Die Arzneimittelprüfung am Menschen, *Med. Pharma. Studienges* (1976).
3. Bock K.D., *Diagnostik* **10** (1977), 586.
4. Handbuch der Internationalen Klassifikation der Krankheiten, Verletzungen und Todesursachen (ICD), Kohlhammer-Verlag 8. Rev. (1968).
5. Karch F.-D. *et al*, *JAMA* **234** (1965), 1236.
6. Rote Liste 1980, Verzeichnis von Fertigarzneimitteln, Bundesverband der Pharmazeutischen Industrie e. V. Ffm.
7. Venulet J., *Int. J. Clin. Pharmacol.* **7** (1973), 253.
8. Walter E., *Med. Welt* **30** (1979), 437.
9. W.H.O.-World Health Organization, Adverse Reaction Terminology, doc. DEM/RDM 73 11.

Sécurité et médicaments (1982), p. 301

CNS Safety Evaluations of New Drugs Based on Computerized Bio-electrical Potentials

T. M. ITIL, D. M. SHAPIRO, G. N. MENON and K. Z. ITIL*

*150 White Plains Road Tarrytown NY 10591 USA

Abstract — It is required that all new compounds undergo "Safety" evaluations in healthy subjects before being administered in patient populations. During these so-called phase I safety trials, the "toxic" effects of compounds on peripherical organs is the primary area of concern. Cardio-toxicity, liver toxicity, renal toxicity and hematopoietic toxicity, after single and multiple dosages, are studies extensively based on objective data. Central nervous system (CNS) safety, however, is usually not established by objective means.

In order to determine the "abnormal" CNS effects of compounds, we have developed a system using computer-power spectrum analysis of the bio-electrical potentials of the brain (computer-analyzed EEG, or CEEG). The occipital and central CEEG leads are analyzed before and after drug administration. At these times, for each lead, power spectral values of individual subjects are compared with those for normal subjects of comparable age from the computer data base. If any doses of the drug induce CEEG alterations outside normal ranges, the significant effects of the drug are established. If the compound is predicted by animal pharmacology to be therapeutically useful for illnesses of the peripheral organs, these CNS effects are detrimental for peripheral use and may be considered as "toxic". Further development as a peripheral agent is contraindicated.

ALLOCUTION DE CLOTURE

Messieurs, Mesdames, mes Chers Confrères,

Je serai très bref car vous avez hâte de profiter du soleil parisien, mais je ne veux pas que ce congrès se termine sans que vous soyez remerciés de l'intérêt que vous avez témoigné pour les diverses sessions de cette réunion et de votre assiduité. Je remercie collectivement tous ceux et celles qui nous ont déjà fait part de leur satisfaction tant sur le contenu du congrès que sur son déroulement matériel.

Votre satisfaction est pour le Comité d'Organisation la plus belle des récompenses.

Je souhaitais dans mon introduction que vos débats contribuent à faire évoluer un certain nombre de questions.

Avons-nous réussi ? Je suis pour ma part persuadé que des prises de conscience de certaines vérités, que des évolutions de pensées se sont faites au cours de ces trois jours, tant au cours des sessions elles-mêmes que grâce aux contacts personnels que ce congrès a permis.

C'est cela qui est important.

La répétition est l'âme de l'enseignement, et c'est à force d'appuyer toujours dans le même sens avec patience et persévérance que l'on réussit à faire évoluer les situations apparemment les plus figées.

Je vais vous donner la primeur d'une information qui vous intéresse certainement tous :

Nos collègues et amis allemands dont l'association est une des plus actives ont accepté d'organiser le 5e Congrès International des M.I.P. Celui-ci aura donc lieu en 1984 en République Fédérale Allemande.

Je suis sûr d'être votre interprète à tous en les en remerciant et en les félicitant. Je leur souhaite aussi beaucoup de courage.

Je ne veux pas terminer sans remercier les traductrices qui ont assumé de façon remarquable un travail difficile.

Merci encore aux orateurs et aux participants.

Bon séjour à Paris pour ceux qui restent encore un peu !

Bon retour pour les autres !

Et à dans trois ans en Allemagne !

Avril 1981

Michel AURICHE
Président du Congrès

TABLE OF SPEAKERS

Alder S. Institut Für Toxikologie Schorenstrasse 16 CH 8603 Schwerzenbach bei Zürich Switzerland	**Alexandre J.M.** Hôpital Broussais Service de Pharmacologie Clinique 96, rue Didot 75674 Paris Cedex 14 France	**Amos J.C.** Smith Kline & French Laboratories Ltd Mundells, Welwyn Garden City, Herts AL 7 1 EY United Kingdom	**Auriche M.** Rhône Poulenc Santé 22, Cours Albert 1er 75008 Paris France
Bass R. Bundesgesundheitsamt (B.G.A) Postfach 1000 Berlin 33 West Germany	**Bax R.P.** Roussel Lab. Ltd. Roussel House Wembley Park Middlessex HA 9 ONF United Kingdom	**Beckwith L.D.** 40 Grevillea Way Blackwood South Australia 5051 Australia	**Berneker G.C.** Medical Department Clinical Drug Safety Ciba Geigy Ltd 4002 Basle Switzerland
Blanc Ph. Laboratoires M.S.D. Chibret 3, avenue Hoche 75008 Paris France	**Bossi L.** L.E.R.S. 58, rue de la Glacière 75013 Paris France	**Burke J.T.** Merrell 168, rue de Rivoli 75044 Paris Cedex 01 France	**Burley D.M.** Ciba Geigy Pharmaceuticals Division Horsham, West Sussex, RH 12 4 AB United Kingdom
Carpentier P. Unicet (Schering USA) 92, rue Baudin 92300 Levallois-Perret France	**Champey Y.** Théraplix 46-52, rue Albert 75640 Paris Cedex 13 France	**Ciampini M.** c/o Medical Department Pfizer Italiana Via del Fornetto 85 00149 Rome Italy	**Ciucci A.G.** Medical Department Clinical Drug Safety Ciba Geigy Ltd 4002 Basle Switzerland

Cohen B.M. 546 Irvington Avenue Elizabeth New Jersey 07 208 USA	**Crooks J.** University Department of Pharmacology and Therapeutics Ninewells Hospital & Medical School, Dundee, DD 1 9 SY Scotland, United Kingdom	**Crowder D.** Sandoz Products Ltd Feltham United Kingdom	**Culley Mc.** Roussel Lab. Ltd Roussel House Wembley Park Middlesex HA 9 ONF United Kingdom
Duchêne-Marullaz P. Pharmacologie Médicale Faculté de Médecine 28, place Henri Dunant 63001 Clermont-Ferrand cedex France	**Duchier J.** Thérapharm 49, rue St-André des Arts 75006 Paris France	**Ducrot H.** Groupe Hospitalier Necker Enfants Malades Consultation de Médecine 149, rue de Sèvres 75730 Paris Cedex 15 France	**Dukes M.N.G.** c/o Netherlands Committee for the Evaluation of Medicines P.O. Box 5811 2280 HV Rijswijk The Netherlands
Dunne J.F. Senior Medical Officer Pharmaceuticals W.H.O. 1211 Geneve 27 Switzerland	**Emanueli A.** Funzione Medica Divisione Farmaceutica Italia Farmitalia Carlo Erba Via Imbonati, 24 Milano Italy	**Espie J.R.** Laboratoires MSD - Chibret 3, avenue Hoche 75008 Paris France	**Faccini J.M.** Centre de Recherches Laboratoires Pfizer 37400 Amboise France
Farina J.C. Sandoz Ltd 4002 Basle Switzerland	**Flind A.C.** Smith Kline & French Laboratories Ltd Mundells, Welwyn Garden City, Herts AL 7 1 EY United Kingdom	**Forte V.** c/o Medical Department Pfizer Italiana Via del Fornetto 85 00149 Rome Italy	**Frederick G.L.** Senior Toxicologist Drugs Directorate Santé et Bien-être Social Place Vanier, Tower B 355 River Road Vanier Ontario K 1 A - 1 B 8 Canada
Glocklin V. Food and Drug Administration Bureau of Drugs Rockville Maryland 20857 USA	**Griffin J.P.** Dept. of Health and Social Security Medicines Division Market Tower 1 Nine Elms Lane London SW 8 5 NQ United Kingdom	**Grimbert J.H.** Riker 92, boulevard du Montparnasse 75014 Paris France	**Grimm R.** Wander Ltd Berne Switzerland
Grohmann R. Psychiatrische Klinik der Universität München Nußbaumstr. 7, 8000 München 2 West Germany	**Gross F.H.** Pharmakologisches Institut der Universitat in Neuenheimer Feld 366 D. 6900 Heidelberg West Germany	**Guillet P.** 21, rue Cujas 75005 Paris France	**Hamilton M.P.** Canon Washington Cathedral Mt St Alban Washington DC 20016 USA
Hasford J. Institut für Medizinische Informationsverarbeitung, Statistik und Biomathematik der Universität München, Marchioninistr. 15 D. 8000 München 70 West Germany	**Henry J.F.** L.E.R.S. 58, rue de la Glacière 75013 Paris France	**Herxheimer A.** Department of Pharmacology Charing Cross Hospital Medical School, Fulham Palace Road, Hammersmith, London W 6 8 RF United Kingdom	**Horsnell S.T.** 40 Grevillea Way Blackwood South Australia 5051 Australia
Idänpään-Heikkilä J.E. National Board of Health Siltasaarenkatu 18 00530 Helsinki 53 Finland	**Inman W.H.W.** Drug Surveillance Research Unit, the University of Southampton, 34 Bassett Crescent East, Southampton, England SO2 3 FL United Kingdom	**Itil K.Z.** 150 White Plains Road Tarrytown NY 10591 USA	**Itil T.M.** 150 White Plains Road Tarrytown NY 10591 USA

Janton C. 33, avenue Maréchal Lyautey 75016 Paris France Rhône Poulenc Santé 22, cours Albert 1er 75008 Paris France	**Jick H.** Boston Collaborative Drug Surveillance Program 400 Totten Pond Road Waltham, Massachusetts 02154 USA	**Kerr L.** c/o Medical Department Pfizer Italiana Via del Fornetto 85 00149 Rome Italy	**Krupp P.** Sandoz Ltd. Pharmaceutical Division Clinical Research, Drug Monitoring Centre 4002 Basle Switzerland
Lawson P.H. Dept. of Clinical Pharmacology Wards 4/5. Royal Infirmary, Glasgow G 4 OSF Scotland United Kingdom	**Lucchelli P.E.** Direttore Medico Smith Kline & French S.p.A. Viale Ortles, 12 20139 Milano Italy	**Lunde I.** Statens Legenmidde Kontroll National Center for medical product control Norway Sven Oftedals Vei 6 Oslo 9 Norway	**Luscombe D.K.** Leo Laboratories Ltd., Longwick Road, Princes Risborough, Aylesbury, Bucks England and Division of Applied Pharmacology, University of Wales Institute of Science & Technology, Cardiff-Wales-United Kingdom
De Maar E.W.J. W.H.O. avenue Appia 1211 Geneve Switzerland	**Maclay W.P.** Sandoz Products Ltd. Feltham United Kingdom	**Marsh B.T.** Leo Laboratories Ltd., Longwick Road, Princes Risborough, Aylesbury, Bucks England and Division of Applied Pharmacology, University of Wales Institute of Science & Technology, Cardiff-Wales-United Kingdom	**Martel F.** Rhône Poulenc Secrétariat Général 22, avenue Montaigne 75008 Paris France
Melmon K.L. Stanford University Medical Center Department of Medicine S102 D Stanford, California 94305 USA	**Menon G.N.** 150 White Plains Road Tarrytown NY 10591 USA	**Micheletti E.** Department of Pharmacy Policlinico Umberto I Roma Italy	**Millstein L.G.** Food & Drug Administration (HFD-107) 5600 Fishers Lane Rockville, Maryland 20857 USA
Olive G. Chargé de Mission auprès de la Direction Générale de l'INSERM "Pharmacologie Toxicologie" 101, rue de Tolbiac 75654 Paris Cedex 13 France	**Phillips J.S.** Division of Clinical Services Department of Health P O BOX 5013 Wellington New Zealand	**Prella P.G.** Pharmaceutical Division Pfizer Italiana S.p.A. Roma Italy	**Quast U.** Behringwerke AG. Postfach 11 40 D- 3550 Marburg/L. West Germany
Rondel R. K. Bristol Myers Int. Corp. 185 chaussée de la Hulpe 1170 Bruxelles Belgique	**Rowley-Jones D.** Smith Kline & French Laboratories Ltd. Mundells, Welwyn Garden City, Herts AL 7 1 EY United Kingdom	**Rumeau-Rouquette C.** Unité 149 de l'INSERM 44, chemin de Ronde 78110 Le Vésinet France	**Sacchetti G.** Funzione Medica Divisione Farmaceutica Italia Farmitalia Carlo Erba Via Imbonati, 24 Milano Italy
Salako L.A. Department of Pharmacology & Therapeutics, University of Ibadan Ibadan Nigeria	**Sanderson R.** Smith Kline & French Laboratories Ltd. Mundells, Welwyn Garden City, Herts AL 7 1 EY United Kingdom	**Scherer J.** Psychiatric Clinic of the University of Munich Nussbaumstrasse 7 8000 München 2 West Germany	**Schlumberger J.F.** Pharmuka 35, quai du Moulin de Cage 92231 Gennevilliers Cedex France
Semler-Collery J. F.N.C.C. 27-33, quai A. Le Gallo 92517 Boulogne France	**Shapiro D.M.** 150 White Plains Road Tarrytown NY 10591 USA	**Simon P.** Département de Pharmacologie Clinique Groupe Hospitalier Pitié - Salpétrière 47, Bd. de l'Hôpital 75651 Paris Cedex 13 France	**Spriet-Pourra C.** Hoechst 3, avenue du Général de Gaulle 92800 Puteaux France

Stevens E.A. Pfizer limited Sandwich Kent CT 13 9 NJ United Kingdom	**Strauss A.** Psychiatric Clinic of the University of Munich Nussbaumstrasse 7, 8000 München 2 West Germany	**Talbot P.S.** 40 Grevillea Way Blackwood South Australia 5051 Australia	**Tuck G.C.** Miles Laboratories Ltd., Stoke court - Stoke Poges Slough Bershire United Kingdom
Vadrot M. L.E.R.S. 58, rue de la Glacière 75013 Paris France	**Van Landeghem V.H.** L.E.R.S. 58, rue de la Glacière 75013 Paris France	**Venulet J.** Ciba Geigy Medical Department 4002 Basle Switzerland	**Vessey M.P.** University Department of Community Medicine and General Practice 8 Keble Road, Oxford, OX1 Oxford, OX1 3 QN United Kingdom
Wardell W.M. University of Rochester Medical School Rochester NY 14642 USA	**Weber E.** Abteilung Klinische Pharmakologie der Medizinis- chen Universitätsklinik Heidelberg, Bergheimer Straße 58, D-6900 Heidelberg West Germany	**Werb. M.** Behringwerke AG. Postfach 1140 D- 3550 Marburg / L. West Germany	**Westerholm B.** General Director National Board of Health and Welfare Linnégatan 87 S-106 30 Stockholm Sweden
Wheeley M. St. G. Servier Lab. Ltd. Horsenden Lane South Greenford Middlessex UB 6 7 PN United Kingdom	**Wiholm B.E.** National Board of Health and Welfare Linnégatan 87 S-106 30 Stockholm Sweden	**Wolff F.W.** Institute for Drug Development 800 Notley Road Silver Spring, Maryland 20904 USA	**Wuest J.R.** College of Pharmacy Cincinnati OH 45267 USA
Zbinden G. Institut Für Toxikologie Schorenstrasse 16 CH. 8603 Schwerzenbach bei Zürich Switzerland			